114.8

Perspectives on Disaster Recovery

Perspectives on Disaster Recovery

Jerri Laube, R.N., Ph.D., F.A.A.N.
Dean and Professor of Nursing
University of Southern Mississippi
Hattiesburg, Mississippi

Shirley A. Murphy, R.N., Ph.D.
Professor
Department of Mental Health Nursing
Oregon Health Sciences University
Portland, Oregon

Foreword by
Roy Popkin
Deputy Director, Disaster Services
American Red Cross
Washington, D.C.

WARNER MEMORIAL LIBRARY
EASTERN COLLEGE
ST. DAVIDS, PA. 19087

 APPLETON-CENTURY-CROFTS/Norwalk, Connecticut

0-8385-7835-7

Copyright © 1985 by Appleton-Century-Crofts
A Publishing Division of Prentice-Hall, Inc.

85 86 87 88 89 90 / 10 9 8 7 6 5 4 3 2 1

Prentice-Hall International, Inc., London
Prentice-Hall of Australia, Pty. Ltd., Sydney
Prentice-Hall Canada, Inc.
Prentice-Hall of India Private Limited, New Delhi
Prentice-Hall of Japan, Inc., Tokyo
Prentice-Hall of Southeast Asia (Pte.) Ltd., Singapore
Whitehall Books Ltd., Wellington, New Zealand
Editora Prentice-Hall do Brasil Ltda., Rio de Janeiro

Library of Congress Cataloging in Publication Data

Laube, Jerri.
  Perspectives on disaster recovery.

  Includes index.
  1. Disaster relief. 2. Disasters—Psychological
aspects. I. Murphy, Shirley A. II. Title.
HV553.L38 1984   363.3'4   84-12405
ISBN 0-8385-7835-7

Design: Lynn M. Luchetti

Contributors

Frederick L. Ahearn, Jr., D.S.W.
Chair and Associate Professor
Community Organization and Social Planning
Graduate School of Social Work
Boston College
Chestnut Hill, Massachusetts

Connie J. Boatright, R.N., M.S.N., C.S.
Clinical Specialist in Psychiatric Nursing
Roudebush Veterans Administration Medical Center
Clinical Assistant Professor of Nursing
Indiana University
Indianapolis, Indiana

Mary E. Cowan, R.N., M.N.
Instructor and Research Assistant
Department of Mental Health Nursing
The Oregon Health Sciences University
Portland, Oregon

Thomas Eisentrout, D. Min.
Diplomat, American Association of Pastoral Counseling
Private Practice, Pastoral Psychotherapy
Fort Thomas, Kentucky

Calvin J. Frederick, Ph.D.
Professor
Department of Psychiatry and Biobehavioral Sciences
University of California at Los Angeles
Chief, Psychology Service
Veterans Administration Medical Center
West Los Angeles, California
Formerly Chief of Disaster Assistance and Emergency
    Mental Health
National Institutes of Mental Health

JoAnn Glittenberg, R.N., Ph.D., F.A.A.N.
Professor of Nursing and Anthropology
University of Colorado Health Sciences Center
Denver, Colorado

Don M. Hartsough, Ph.D.
Associate Professor
Department of Psychological Sciences
Purdue University
West Lafayette, Indiana

Jerri Laube, R.N., Ph.D., F.A.A.N.
Dean and Professor of Nursing
University of Southern Mississippi
Hattiesburg, Mississippi

Jacob D. Lindy, M.D.
Associate Professor of Clinical Psychiatry
Co-Director, Traumatic Stress Study Center
University of Cincinnati
Cincinnati, Ohio

Joanne G. Lindy, Ph.D.
Associate Professor
Department of Psychiatry
University of Cincinnati
Director of Consultation and Education
Central Psychiatric Clinic
Cincinnati, Ohio

Mary Evans Melick, R.N., Ph.D.
Principal Research Scientist
Special Projects Research Unit
Office of Mental Health
State of New York
Albany, New York

Dennis S. Mileti, Ph.D.
Associate Professor of Sociology
Colorado State University
Fort Collins, Colorado

Shirley A. Murphy, R.N., Ph.D.
Professor
Department of Mental Health Nursing
Oregon Health Sciences University
Portland, Oregon

Martin E. Silverstein, M.D.
Associate Professor of Surgery
University of Arizona
Tucson, Arizona
Senior Fellow in Science and Technology
Georgetown University Center for Strategic and
    International Studies
Washington, D.C.

Contents

Foreword

Twenty-two years ago, *Man and Society in Disaster* presented practitioners in the field of disaster preparedness and relief with a variety of perspectives on what they were doing and how the condition of human beings and social organizations was affected by catastrophic events.

Since the publication of that volume, the working world of the disaster responder and the people in trouble has changed. New kinds of disasters have been added to the lexicon of planners and managers. New agencies and programs have come into the field. The role of the Federal government has expanded and has been institutionalized, largely within the Federal Emergency Management Agency. State and local agencies are now involved in comprehensive emergency planning. Hazard mitigation—prevention, loss reduction through preparedness planning, building codes, land use controls, and other components—has been given tremendous new emphasis primarily through the National Flood Insurance Program and the Earthquake Hazards Reduction Act. We have experienced Three Mile Island and critical hazardous material spills like Love Canal and Times Beach. Sociopolitical expectations of what will be done for disaster victims have broadened.

During this same period, there have been no new comprehensive multidisciplinary publications on disasters and their impacts. There have been many fine studies of one kind or another, but the present volume, *Perspectives on Disaster Recovery* is the first to follow *Man and Society in Disaster* with a look at disaster from a variety of social science viewpoints.

The present work also introduces new elements, such as mental health perspectives ranging from Frederick L. Ahearn's experience with the 1977 Blizzard in Boston, Don Hartsough's experiences with floods and tornadoes, Connie Boatright's study of what happened to children after a tornado, Jerri Laube's experiences during Hurricane Celia and other disasters, and the work that Jacob Lindy and Thomas Eisentrout did following the Beverly Hills Supper Club fire and a plane crash near the Cincinnati airport.

For practitioners in the disaster field, such perspectives are extremely important, for until 1972 little attention was given to the mental health aspects of disaster because the single authoritative study in the field had said there were no problems. Now we know there are problems and human needs. We need advice and guidance as to how to deal with such problems. As nonclinicians, disaster workers need guidance as to what the state of the art may be.

Also, the role of the mass media in disaster by the Lindys, Hartsough, and Mileti instructs practitioners, as well as the news media themselves that they play much more than a mere reporter's role. They disseminate warnings, and inform victims as to what has happened to their community and what is or isn't being done to help. When the media oversensationalize or emphasize the negative, they become part of the recovery problem. Like it or not, the mass media are part of disaster preparedness and recovery. This book provides important perspectives on this subject.

Underpinning these very specific perspectives are others, on theoretical and methodological issues and clinical applications presented by Shirley Murphy, Don Hartsough, Mary E. Cowan, Martin E. Silverstein, and Mary Evans Melick. While *Perspectives on Disaster Recovery* may focus largely on medical and mental health aspects of disaster, the background and experience of the authors tends to give the present work a broader scope and thus it becomes a potentially important adjunct to the practitioner's library of things to know and do about planning for and implementing disaster recovery.

At a time when a court of law rules that victims can sue for "psychic damage," when Three Mile Island, Love Canal, and Times Beach added new dimensions to human concerns about disaster recovery, and when psychological reactions have become part of "environmental impact studies," all of us who are in the field of emergency management realize we can no longer rely solely on the old way of doing things. It is hoped that by reading *Perspectives on Disaster Recovery,* emergency managers will be able to transfuse into that realization new insights which can be applied to the job of picking up the pieces or bandaging the hurts that disasters create. The authors of this book, Jerri Laube and Shirley Murphy, and their fellow contributors to this volume, have given us much to think about and to act upon. For this alone, they are to be commended . . . and thanked.

Roy Popkin
Deputy Director, Disaster Services
American Red Cross
Washington D.C.
March 1984

Preface

This book was developed in response to the need of disaster researchers, educators, and practitioners. The objective was to present a perspective on disaster research, clinical and community issues, without sacrifice of depth. The topics were chosen in consideration of this intention and in accord with the contributors' current interest and expertise. Pictures, courtesy of the American National Red Cross, which vividly record scenes from actual disasters, have been included.

Part One deals with theoretical and methodological issues. While the study of disasters has escalated dramatically during the past decade, research has focused on the traumatic effects of victims and communities, evaluation of disaster recovery programs, and policy implications. Theory generation and instrument standardization have not been major research objectives.

In Chapter 1, Murphy identifies concepts and theories that would be appropriate to test and thus expand the currently limited theory base of disaster inquiry. A comprehensive framework for research and interventions is proposed.

Hartsough identifies and discusses major methodological issues in disaster research in Chapter 2. He also describes a number of instruments that are appropriate to assess psychological effects of disasters.

In Chapter 3, Murphy and Cowan present the process of designing and implementing a disaster study based on information presented in the first two chapters.

Part Two focuses on clinical applications for disaster populations. Despite the fact that about 75,000 disaster injuries were treated in the United States between 1971 and 1980, there is no disaster literature that reports the influence of physical injury on the overall disaster recovery process. Silverstein's chapter fills this void. In addition, he describes the impact of disaster injury on the emerging medical care system, which has not been included in past disaster literature.

Frederick's chapter provides important material on the newly classified phenomenon of Posttraumatic Stress Disorders. Diagnostic and treatment issues are presented along with case examples. Of major importance in this chapter is the measurement instrument he developed.

Boatright's chapter describing a study of absenteeism among elementary school children following a tornado is a unique contribution to the literature. The study raises many interesting questions which have not been examined in depth.

The unique stresses of disaster and the emotional responses which may be expected from victims of disasters are discussed by Laube in Chapter 7. She uses a case example to illustrate the time phases of disaster.

A comprehensive current review and critique of physical and mental health status of postdisaster victims is presented by Melick. Tropical Storm Agnes (1972) serves as a case study to report life changes and illness among working class male disaster victims and comparison subjects.

Chapter 9, the final chapter in Part Two, also by Laube, reports the results of a study she conducted among health professionals following a disaster. Helpers conceptualized as victims is not a common approach. Laube has made a unique contribution to the disaster literature through this creatively designed and carefully conducted study.

In Part Three, the focus is on the interface between victims, health professionals, and community systems. Since disasters are largely unpreventable and uncontrollable, efforts of helping organizations can be best directed toward alleviating the effects of loss. Recovery is dependent upon the exchange or fit between the kind of aid needed as it is perceived by disaster victims and the availability and value choices of aid as perceived by organizations that control resources. Thus a common theme for the final four chapters is person/environment "fit."

Ahearn addresses the issues and problems associated with designing and implementing mental health programs that must be responsive to individual and collective trauma following a disaster. In addition to the analytical skills required to carry out successful interventions, Ahearn stresses the sociopolitical skills required to interact with community and relief organizations.

Chapter 11, by Lindy and Eisentrout is best described as a "sensitive critique" of the collaborative efforts in crisis of mental health professionals and the clergy. Their account of joint efforts to aid victims following the Beverly Hills Supper Club (Kentucky) fire serves as a model from which other communities may derive benefit.

Glittenberg uses findings from a longitudinal 5-year study following the 1976 Guatemalan earthquake to demonstrate the effects of disaster relief at both the individual and aggregate levels. The exchange between external aid and internal settlement decision-making profoundly affected health and well-being of the victims.

Hartsough and Mileti discuss the role of yet another major environmental influence on disaster loss and recovery, the mass media.

Their chapter represents the first comprehensive paper to be published on this topic.

Lindy and Lindy conclude Part Three by exemplifying several disasters in order to assess both positive and negative impacts of the mass media on disaster victims. The Powell and Rayner conceptual model is used to demonstrate the quality of information exchange between the victims, the general public, health, and community professionals during each time phase of disastrous events.

A personal account of Laube's experience in the Blizzard of 1978, Indianapolis, has been included as an epilogue. A researcher, educator, and worker in the field of disaster, she suddenly found herself in a role reversal. This material deals with the feelings she experienced as the victim.

A summary table of behavior symptoms and treatment options for children who have experienced a disaster is included in the Appendix. The table was developed by the Institute for the Studies of Destructive Behaviors and the Los Angeles Suicide Prevention Center under contract with the National Institutes of Mental Health.

In conclusion, this book is written for the student and professional in nursing, medicine, social work, pyschology, the ministry and related disciplines. The research findings and methodological issues plus the multifaceted approach to the problems of disaster provide new knowledge in the field and should serve as a valuable text and reference.

J.L.
S.M.

Acknowledgments

We wish to acknowledge all those who have extended their assistance, encouragement, and support throughout the preparation of this book. Important among them are our respective family members who loved and supported us throughout our writing pains and growths; the victims of disaster who have taught us much of what we know; Hazel Newsom, formerly with the Dallas Chapter of the American Red Cross; Jeanne Durr formerly with the American Red Cross, Washington, D.C.; and all those dedicated individuals who gave of their talent, time, and energy in disaster work, without whom this book could never have been written.

Our appreciation also goes to our contributors, esteemed researchers and scholars, who prepared the chapters; to Roy Popkin of the American Red Cross for writing the foreword; at Appleton-Century-Crofts, Leslie Boyer, former Assistant Editor, who was responsible for the initiation of this work; and Charles Bollinger, Senior Editor, and Susan Neitlich, Production Editor, for their trust, patience, and invaluable assistance.

Jerri Laube
Shirley Murphy

Perspectives on Disaster Recovery

Theoretical and Methodological Issues

The Conceptual Bases for Disaster Research and Intervention

Shirley A. Murphy

The study of disasters has escalated dramatically during the past decade, but as Perry and Lindell (1978) point out, research has been conducted with limited conceptualization. That is, concepts and theories thought to be pertinent are described, but linkages between them and the research proposed are frequently left unexplained. Several publications address this void. Conceptual models have been put forth regarding individual, community, family, and organizational responses (Bolin, 1982; Kreps, 1978). Similarly, stress, crisis, loss, grieving, coping, and support have been suggested as pertinent concepts regarding individual responses to recovery (Cohen and Ahearn, 1980). The degree of personal impact, type of disaster, potential for recurrence, control over future impact, and duration of the event have been proposed as an intervention typology by Berren et al. (1982). Finally, Green (1982) critiqued 16 disaster studies whose findings are virtually noncomparable because of conceptual and methodological variability.

While the studies identified in the previous paragraph have delineated issues and suggested directions to guide disaster research, a number of problems are yet to be addressed: (1) lists of concepts identified and described for disaster research are incomplete; (2) no comprehensive models for individual recovery have been published; (3) published conceptual frameworks have not specified testable linkages between concepts; (4) no studies have been published that have identified theory testing as a specific research objective; and (5) the process of conceptualization has been primarily deductive. Chapter 1 has three purposes: (1) to discuss briefly the interrelationship between conceptual development, research, and intervention; (2) to describe pertinent con-

cepts and theories; and (3) to exemplify some conceptual frameworks
which specify linkages between concepts.

THE INTERDEPENDENT RELATIONSHIP OF THEORY, RESEARCH, AND INTERVENTION

Theory generates knowledge which can be used to guide intervention;
research builds and tests theory; and clinical intervention provides an
opportunity to apply theory and to generate researchable questions.
The process of theory building is deductive, inductive, and retroduc-
tive. For example, disaster workers find concepts from a crisis intervention framework very useful for counseling victims in the immediate postdisaster period. Likewise, disaster researchers may use a crisis
intervention model to generate hypotheses. In both cases, a written
theoretical framework was selected a priori to guide interventions or
research. These are examples of the deductive method. Alternatively,
Lindemann (1944) used the inductive method when he counseled victims following the Coconut Grove fire and subsequently developed concepts of loss and grief, based on his clinical observations. Over the past
40 years, the concepts of loss and grief have been refined by their use
both inductively and deductively. This process is often referred to as
retroduction (Willer and Webster, 1970).

Since the terms theory, concept, construct, conceptual framework,
theoretical framework, conceptual model, and theoretical model appear
frequently in the literature, but without consensual definitions, the
terms are defined here to avoid ambiguity in the remainder of the chapter. A theory is "a set of interrelated constructs (concepts), definitions,
and propositions that present a systematic view of phenomena by spec-
ifying relations among variables, with the purpose of explaining and
predicting the phenomena" (Kerlinger, 1973, p. 9). A concept is "a complex mental formulation of an object, property, or event that is derived
from individual perception and experience" (Chinn and Jacobs, 1983,
p. 200). For example, "recovery" is an important disaster concept. A
construct is "a highly abstract and complex concept whose reality base
can only be inferred" (Chinn and Jacobs, 1983, p. 200). "Vulnerability"
of disaster victims is a construct.

The terms conceptual framework, conceptual model, theoretical
framework, and theoretical model can be used synonymously and generally refer to global ideas about individuals, groups, and events of interest to a discipline. The terms are interchanged in this chapter,
although "conceptual framework" appears most frequently.

Conceptual frameworks are made up of concepts and propositions.

Therefore, a conceptual framework is defined as a set of concepts and statements that organize phenomena of interest. Put simply, they serve as frames of reference. Moreover, they are not universal. That is, they vary among investigators studying the same phenomena. For example, several investigators studied the Buffalo Creek disaster. Erikson (1976) assessed the loss of communality, while Titchener and Kapp (1976) identified long-term psychological trauma. Thus, it becomes apparent that differing conceptualizations would be appropriate.

Conceptual frameworks are not directly testable because the concepts and propositions that make up a framework are too abstract. In other words, more specificity is required if they are to be testable hypotheses. For example, the disaster conceptual framework of Powell and Rayner (1952) is composed of concepts that describe disasters over time: warning, threat, impact, inventory, rescue, remedy, and recovery. Even though each concept is described briefly by the authors, to become testable, concepts must specify an individual or group, identify relationships with other concepts, and be developed into testable hypotheses. Laube has made a beginning step in Chapter 7. She takes the reader through each time period by using examples from recent disasters and begins the initial task of linking one time phase with the next. Developing testable hypotheses is the next step. As Hartsough points out in Chapter 2, some researchers have attempted to separate stresses directly associated with an event from stresses associated with the response to the same event (agent-produced versus response-produced). See Chapters 3 and 14 for additional applications. However, many investigators have used the Powell and Rayner model since its inception in its highly abstract form.

This chapter incorporates disaster concepts from other published typologies into the time sequence of Powell and Rayner. Since this volume focuses on recovery, concepts associated with the recovery process are emphasized. The model is diagramed in Figure 1.1. While the concepts are presented in a time sequence, it is important to note that the process of disaster recovery is not completely linear; that is, events occur simultaneously and sometimes out of the order of discussion.

PERTINENT CONCEPTS

Causal Agents

Natural Disasters. The Disaster Relief Act of 1974 defined a major disaster as "any hurricane, tornado, storm, flood, high-water, wind-driven water, tidal wave, tsunami, earthquake, volcanic eruption, landslide,

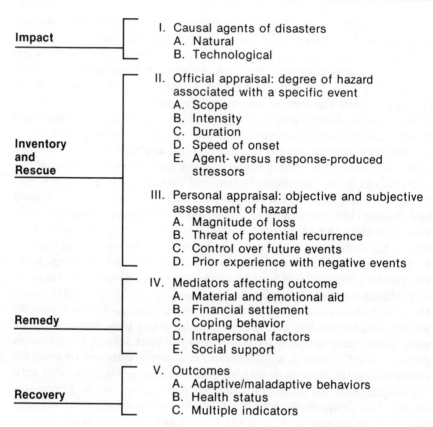

Figure 1.1. Classification System for Disaster Research.

snow storm, drought, fire, explosion, or other catastrophe in any part of the continental United States, or its territories, which causes damage of sufficient severity and magnitude to warrant major disaster assistance" (U.S. Public Health Service, 1976). From January 1, 1971 to June 30, 1980, 326 events were declared major disasters by U.S. Presidents. During this $9\frac{1}{2}$-year period, over 2100 disaster-related deaths and 72,000 injuries were reported. Another major category of disasters, technological or man-made, is not included in the above definition.

Technological/Human Influence. The media have brought to our attention an increasing number of mass emergencies that have arisen from technological failure and/or human errors, either of judgment or direct action. Examples are hotel fires, airplane crashes, nuclear reactor accidents, and the dumping of toxic wastes. There is no official consensual definition of these traumatic events; however, they have some salient characteristics which may or may not differentiate them from natural disasters. First, the extent to which one believes an incident could have been prevented may have a direct relationship to the amount of anger and blame generated. Next, the extent to which hostile feelings are expressed may affect mental health outcomes. It may be that if blame can be attributed to a specific person or organization, more energy is devoted to seeking retribution rather than integration of the event into the life experience. Finally, errors in human judgment that ultimately harm others evoke responses contrary to human values. Examples of recent technological disasters are Love Canal (New York), Three Mile Island (Pennsylvania), and Times Beach (Missouri). Alternatively, if one believes events such as hurricanes and tornadoes are caused by an agent over which one has no control (i.e., the weather), it may be that one will formulate the attribution, "nothing could be done." Recovery may be different in the latter circumstances; however, the human factors associated with adequate warning and rescue operations are indeed present, and hence may be sources of error which also result in beliefs that the consequences could have been less damaging. Thus, both natural and technological events involve potential human error, which points up an important similarity between the two kinds of disasters. At the present time, little comparative analysis between events caused by different causative agents has been done.

Official Appraisal: The Degree of Hazard Associated with a Specific Event

Scope of Impact. "Scope" refers primarily to the geographical impact of an event. Assessment of scope includes loss of life, the extent of property damage, and whether losses are confined to a specific area or are widespread.

Event Intensity. "Intensity" refers to the magnitude of an event. Assessment includes disruption of essential services such as water, electricity, and transportation.

Event Duration. The longer the duration of an event, the greater the anxiety is likely to be. Some individuals, after a brief period of disorientation, will adapt; others will not.

Speed of Onset. Theoretically, the more warning or preparation one has, the less serious the effect. For example, a flash flood allows little warning, whereas continuous rainfall leading to gradually rising water and then flooding should provoke different responses. This will be true only insofar as those potentially affected can accept and make use of warnings. Harry Truman, a colorful character who lived in the shadow of Mount St. Helens, reportedly had several opportunities to leave his property but refused to do so. At present, research regarding responses to warning has not yielded conclusive evidence.

Agent- Versus Response-Produced Stressors. "Agent-produced" refers to those stresses directly associated with the event, such as property devastation following a hurricane. "Response-produced" refers to those stresses indirectly associated with the event, such as dissatisfaction with temporary housing provided by government agencies following the loss of property.

Arguments have been advanced favoring the separation of these stresses for purposes of analysis. Such information is essential in evaluating victim response to services offered, adequacy of services, and stresses experienced by service providers who can appropriately be considered victims.

Taken together, these five factors constitute the hazard, or potential degree of harm that may arise. Assessment of hazard is primarily carried out by authorities in official capacity, such as the Federal Emergency Management Agency (FEMA), the Red Cross, and local emergency preparedness agencies. Next, we examine disaster response at the individual level. Even though the appraisal of the degree of hazard has been presented first, official and personal appraisals are most likely to occur simultaneously.

Personal Appraisal: Objective and Subjective Impact

Magnitude of Loss. In general, the greater the scope, intensity, and suddenness of onset of an event, the greater the loss. Personal survival, deaths of significant others, and property loss are seldom mutually exclusive. Research findings are limited regarding differential magnitude of loss. It is reasonable to assume that deaths of loved ones represent a greater magnitude of loss than loss of personal property; however, it may be that these two magnitudes of loss differ in qualities other than magnitude and thus defy direct comparison.

Bereavement Loss. The death of a significant other is reportedly the most stressful event experienced (Bugen, 1977; Schulz, 1978; Shneidman, 1976; Weisman, 1973). While there is little empirical evidence, it could be argued that the mode of death, the cause of death one assigns, the importance of the deceased person, and whether the deceased is confirmed or presumed dead are additional factors that may differentiate the bereavement experience and ultimate recovery of the bereaved. Weisman (1973) differentiates timely (expected and accepted) from untimely (premature, unexpected, and violent) death. Bugen (1977) focuses on the relationship between the deceased and bereaved. He states that the bereaved's belief that the death was preventable is the most important factor in predicting the recovery outcome. Shneidman (1976), discussing the availability of death certificates in the case of confirmed but not presumed death, states, "The impact of the death certificate is considerable. It can affect the fact and fortune of a family, touching both its affluence and mental health" (p. 241). Death certificates are required for claims for life insurance, property rights, and social security benefits for dependent children. Moreover, war experiences suggest that confirmed death, however brutal, contributes to the reality and finality of death (McCubbin, 1976). Alternatively, when a person is missing and therefore presumed dead, relatives and friends continue to hope that the person escaped, will be found alive, or was not in the area at the time, until sufficient contrary evidence surfaces. In addition, there are no generally accepted norms for grieving, nor any legal avenues to financial resolution of presumptive death. Thus, many factors in the conceptualization of disaster bereavement need to be considered.

Property Loss. While the loss of one's home is thought to be much less traumatic than the death of a loved one, property loss presents its own unique set of problems that require appraisal, coping, and adaptation. Frequently, entire neighborhoods are destroyed; thus shelter, treasured items, clothing, supportive others, and familiar surroundings are gone. Relocation may bring about lowered socioeconomic status, change in schools for children, interruption of employment, social, and leisure activities, financial ruin to homeowners, and countless hassles such as filling out forms and having to accept government-supplied furniture and cooking utensils. Disaster researchers have reported long-term stresses associated with property loss (Bolin, 1982; Kilijanek and Drabek, 1979). Lawsuits are common, sometimes families must relocate more than once, and some victims perceive their lives never returning to predisaster quality of living (Bolin, 1982; Murphy, 1981; Titchener and Kapp, 1976).

Threat of Potential Recurrence. Unfortunately, natural disasters pose threats of repeated attack, particularly in some geographical areas. Thus, disasters with a high probability for recurrence call for prevention and intervention strategies of extended proportions, particularly program awareness on community-wide levels. However, encouraging homeowners to "take out flood plan insurance next time" does not guarantee that prior losses will not be incurred again, which produces feelings of grief, anger, and helplessness.

Control over Future Events. Social psychologists have studied the concepts of control and predictability extensively over the past decade (Abramson et al., 1978; Hanusa and Schulz, 1977; Wortman and Dintzer, 1978). In general, the more predictable one's environment and the more ability one has to control his or her environment, the more likely coping with negative life events will be adaptive. Conversely, the less predictability and control one has, the more likely one gives up, or copes maladaptively. Since many disasters are neither preventable nor their impacts controllable, those responsible for helping can concentrate only on reducing consequences, such as improving warning and evacuation systems and maintaining ample temporary shelter.

Prior Experience with Negative Events. The more opportunity to have experienced crisis situations, and the more similar to the current event, the more resources the individual has to draw upon, the more likely the coping behavior adopted will be successful. Therefore, if an individual has lived through a hurricane, or loss through death, he or she will have similar experiences to draw upon and thus the probability of successful coping is increased. The key to this concept is previous success. If the prior experiences have not been successful, the probability of adaptive coping in the situation decreases. However, data from disaster situations are limited. In support of the notion that prior successful coping leads to current adaptation, Kilijanek and Drabek (1979) report that the elderly are less likely than younger disaster subjects to perceive significant long-term negative consequences regarding either their physical or mental health. Similar findings for elderly disaster victims are reported by Bell (1978). These findings indicate that older persons' experience with negative life events aids in coping with present events. By contrast, when victims of the volcanic eruption of Mount St. Helens, whose mean age was 39, were asked the question, "What past loss experience helped you get through the current crisis?" 35 percent of those responding replied "nothing." Other responses in order of importance were "prior death of a significant other" 29 percent, and "personal belief system" 23 percent. Many of the victims had experienced divorce, but did not report that this loss experience helped them cope with their disaster losses (Murphy, 1981).

In summary, both official and personal appraisals occur during the early post-disaster periods, namely the inventory and rescue phases. Having briefly described the factors that influence the appraisal of hazard that follows a disaster, the discussion shifts to concepts and/or theories that serve as part of an overall conceptual framework for research or intervention, or that may have the potential to be study hypotheses. The following concepts and/or theories are included: crisis intervention, untimely death including predictors of grief response, stressful life events and illness, learned helplessness, and high risk and vulnerability.

CONCEPTUALIZATION OF THE EARLY POSTDISASTER PERIOD

Crisis Intervention Theory

Burgess and Baldwin (1981), in a recent typology of crises, discuss specific emotional outcomes resulting from traumatic stress: "such crises are precipitated by strong, externally imposed stresses or traumatic situations that are unexpected and uncontrolled and that are emotionally overwhelming to individuals" (p. 183). Mass emergencies such as disasters would constitute crises as described by Burgess and Baldwin, and others.

Crisis frameworks have been used frequently by disaster workers and researchers because the use of a crisis framework accounts for a precipitating event or hazard, recognizes the extreme state of disequilibrium of the individual, assumes that circumstances surrounding the crisis are time-limited, and proposes that appropriate intervention has the potential for growth and positive influence. Application of crisis concepts in disasters have been illustrated by numerous authors (Cohen and Ahearn, 1980; Hoff, 1978) and need not be elaborated on here. It is important to note that the "theory" is a descriptive theory at the present time and has not been subjected to empirical tests. However, clear descriptions by numerous authorities make it a very attractive framework for professionals and paraprofessionals alike, who must work under emotionally draining circumstances and time pressures. It was not until 1972 that the National Institute of Mental Health provided funds for crisis services for disaster victims. Only limited efforts have been made to evaluate the effectiveness of these services. Two relevant studies regarding the use of crisis services are reported by Baisden and Quarantelli (1978) and Lindy et al. (1981). Both studies indicate the reluctance of "normal" populations to use available services.

Untimely Death

As Weisman (1973) so aptly states, most individuals can accept the universality of death as a concept, but, with few exceptions, tend to believe every death is unnecessary and preventable, and therefore untimely. "When someone we care about dies, it is almost always untimely and the only timely death happens to someone who, in our opinion, richly deserves it" (p. 368).

Weisman conceptualizes untimely death as three distinguishable mode of death characteristics: premature, unexpected, and calamitous. Untimely death can occur in combinations of the above conditions and have pertinent application to disaster death. Premature death is the demise of an individual prior to one's expected old age. Unexpected death is sudden and unpredicted and can produce grave emotional impact because it violates one's inner timetable of expectation. Calamitous death occurs under violent circumstances such as murder, car accidents, fires, and so forth. At the present time, the theory is descriptive and thus not amenable to empirical testing in its present form.

The Concept of Grief. The most common conceptualization of grief used by health practitioners is the five-stage model developed by Kubler-Ross (1969): denial, anger, bargaining, depression, and acceptance. Similar stage models have been advanced by others. In general, two important assumptions have emerged from these models: (1) individuals go through a series of stages; (2) almost without exception, stage models postulate that recovery is the final outcome. However, empirical evidence gathered over the past two decades does not support these assumptions. Rather, the data suggest that levels of adaptation, particularly following the death of a significant other, are dependent on a complex set of variables which include the mode of death, predictability, belief of preventability, the ages of both the deceased and bereaved, the relationship between the deceased and bereaved, required role changes, and cultural and financial factors.

Bugen's model of bereavement grief, first published in 1977, asserts that grief is a dynamic concept whose outcomes are best predicted by a combination of two factors: whether the relationship between the deceased and bereaved is central or peripheral and whether the bereaved believes the death was preventable or unpreventable. The model is a 2 × 2 matrix in which the vertical axis represents the closeness of the relationship while the horizontal axis represents the extent to which the bereaved believes the death was preventable. These two factors interact to create four grief states predicting both intensity and duration. Thus, if the relationship between the deceased and bereaved prior to death was central, and if the bereaved believed the death was preventable, the grieving process is predicted to be intense and prolonged. Whereas, if the relationship was peripheral and death was believed unpreventable, grieving is predicted to be mild and brief. The Bugen model is included here because the concept can be empirically tested without additional development. Concepts of loss and grief described elsewhere are still in the descriptive theory stage and hence are not testable.

Concurrent Stressful Life Events

The impact of a disaster is influenced by both the intensity and additivity of the events experienced. Many investigators have attempted to establish a causal relationship between stressful life events and the onset of illness as well as the extent to which the stress-illness process can be mediated by supportive mechanisms (Dean and Lin, 1977; Dohrenwend and Dohrenwend, 1974; Lin et al., 1979). By contrast, Lazarus and Cohen (1977) suggest that less-intense stressors that are frequent and persistent may be better overall measures of life stress than major events. Hence, both major life events and daily "hassles" might be incorporated in disaster research. The reader is referred to Chapter 3 for additional conceptual development, and to Chapter 2 for measurement issues. The opportunities for including the concept of stress in disaster research are many and varied.

The Theory of Learned Helplessness

According to learned helplessness theory (Abramson et al., 1978), when individuals are exposed to uncontrollable outcomes and develop inappropriate expectations that future outcomes will also be uncontrollable, they will experience helplessness. In other words, two *necessary* conditions must be present in order for helplessness to occur: (1) one must be exposed to an uncontrollable event, and (2) one must believe that nothing can be done to change the outcome.

The theory has had widespread empirical testing with a number of uncontrollable life events, and would appear to be useful in preventing helpless behavior in disaster victims, particularly in areas where disasters are known to recur. Despite the apparent relevance of the theory to disasters, there are no published accounts of its application in disaster research or intervention. Space limitations prevent discussion of the dimensions of the theory that are testable. Rather, the reader is referred to the initial work (Abramson et al., 1978) and subsequent development and application (Murphy, 1982).

Concepts of Risk and Vulnerability

Populations at risk can be defined as those individuals, groups, and families who are particularly susceptible to mental distress and physical illness by virture of selected characteristics and exposure to unpredictable and uncontrollable factors in the environment, and who have inadequate resources with which to respond to environmental stressors. The terms "risk" and "vulnerability" have frequently been interchanged; however, recently Clarke and Driever (1983) have defined "at-risk" as an objective indicator, whereas "vulnerability" refers to a subjective orientation. Both are pertinent assessment concepts regarding the ability of health professionals to predict outcomes and intervene with disaster victims. "At-risk" disaster populations have received very limited attention, both theoretically and practically.

Factors that may differentiate those disaster victims most likely to have a traumatic and delayed recovery are: demographic variables such as age of the victims and the deceased in cases of disaster death (generally the younger, the more traumatic), numbers and ages of dependent children, and income; central relationship between the deceased and bereaved prior to death; belief that death was preventable even though the event may not have been; the number of deaths of significant persons; concurrent negative life events, including recent events unrelated to the disaster as well as response-produced stresses; limited coping repertoire; and limited supportive network of significant others. Readers are referred to Chapter 3 for measurement issues regarding high-risk variables, and to Chapters 4, 5, and 6 for application of risk variables with disaster victims.

In summary, all of the concepts and theories are appropriate for inclusion in conceptual frameworks to guide research and interventions. However, all require explicit operational definitions and linkages between concepts prior to becoming testable hypotheses.

MEDIATING FACTORS IN DISASTER LOSS

Since disasters are primarily unpreventable and uncontrollable, efforts of health professionals can best be directed toward alleviating the effects of loss. The majority of disaster victims are offered material and financial aid during the early postdisaster period. For example, FEMA provides temporary housing and grants to facilitate repair and early return to damaged residences. The SBA (Small Business Administration) provides low-interest loans to victims. Volunteer agencies such as the Red Cross also provide material aid. However, it has been reported that disaster victims' need for mental health services may persist over time. Thus, the questions can be raised: if postdisaster stress persists over time, how do disaster victims cope, adapt, and/or recover? The conceptual basis for the questions can be found in the coping literature. A synthesis of this literature is briefly summarized next.

The Coping Process
The coping literature is a vast one, and like many other constructs studied by health and social scientists, is fraught with conceptual and measurement problems. Coping has been conceptualized as an ego process (Vaillant, 1977), a personality trait (Lazarus et al., 1974), and a person/environment transaction (Moos, 1977; Pearlin and Schooler.

1978). In the latter, special situational demands requiring the individual to tolerate, master, or reduce demands, is pertinent to disaster response. What an individual thinks and does in a particular situation, or how coping mediates in stressful situations, has been conceptualized by Folkman and Lazarus (1980) as being both problem-focused and emotion-focused. The Ways of Coping Scale developed by Folkman and Lazarus is comprised of both cognitive and affective components and provides an opportunity for individuals to self-report how they feel and behave in response to specific stressors. Two additional theoretical perspectives of the person/environment interaction conceptualization to coping are self-expectancy, the extent to which one believes he or she should be able to master a problem alone, and social support, the extent to which others help to mediate stressors.

Self-Efficacy Theory. A major intrapersonal resource may be one's ability to effect outcomes. Self-efficacy theory (Bandura, 1977) is based on the premise that "expectations have a profound effect on behavior. An outcome expectancy is defined as a person's estimate that a given behavior will lead to certain outcomes. An efficacy expectation is the conviction that one can successfully initiate and execute the behavior required to produce the desired outcome" (p. 193). Thus, whether a person initiates coping and how long that person will persist in coping depends on the belief or expectation one has at the outset. Bandura notes that role models and past successes or failures in coping are factors that affect the development of self-efficacy or self-reliant behavior.

Other important personal resources may be a positive view of the world based on positive life experiences and strong, stable social ties (Antonovsky, 1979). Perceptions of stress as challenge, commitment, and control have also been found to maintain health (Kobasa et al., 1979).

Interpersonal Supports. The construct of social support as an antecedent in preventing illness and as an intervenor in ameliorating the effects of stress on illness has received widespread attention over the past decade. The intervening or buffering hypothesis is the more frequently reported role, and the most controversial regarding how it works. At the present time, there is no consensual definition of social support, little agreement on its function, and widespread debate over its measurement (Heller, 1979; Norbeck, 1981; Thoits, 1982). Like stress, it is a multidimensional concept, generally consisting of both material and emotional aid. Widely quoted definitions are those of Caplan (1974) and Cobb (1976). Social support as defined by Caplan (1974) is "that continuing set of social aggregates that provide individuals with opportunities for feedback about themselves and for validations of their expectations about others, which may offset deficiencies in these communications within the larger community context" (p. 4). Cobb (1976) defined social support as information leading a person to believe that he or she is: (1) cared for and loved, (2) esteemed and valued, and (3) belonging to a network of communication and mutual obligation. More recently, House (1981) defined social support as "an interpersonal transaction involving one or more of the following: (1) emotional concern (liking, love, empathy); (2) instrumental aid (goods and services); (3) information (about the environment); and (4) appraisal (information relevant to self-evaluation)" (p. 39).

Numerous investigators report that the importance of a relationship with a confidant acts as either an antecedent that reduces the likelihood of illness or buffers the impact following the occurrence of negative life events (Brown et al., 1975; Burke and Weir, 1977; Miller et al., 1976). A number of other investigators have reported support for the buffering hypothesis (Cobb, 1976; Gore, 1978; MacElveen-Hoehn and Smith-DiJulio, 1978; Pearlin et al., 1981).

Lin et al. (1979) point out that the mediating or buffering role of social supports is becoming widely accepted, yet there is no theoretical explanation as to *why* the mediating effect occurs. Lin et al. (1979) offers two explanations: (1) Social groups may exert pressure to conform to norms regarding involvement in preventive health behaviors. This is a plausible explanation if one accepts the notion that persons maintain familial and confidant ties and interactions even in times of stress. (2) Interaction patterns provide practical information, such as where to look for work, or how to locate a counselor. Authors of two critical reviews of the social support literature (Heller, 1979; Thoits, 1982) advise caution in the interpretation of study results, citing both complex conceptual and methodological problems with the majority of published studies claiming support of the buffering hypothesis. In general, there is no consistency across studies regarding the amount, types, or sources of support that should be measured (Thoits, 1982). Moreover, life events and social support may be confounded since many life events scales used in measurement include events that can be interpreted as losses or gains in social supportive relationships (death of spouse, divorce, marriage, change in leisure activities) (Gore, 1981; Heller, 1979; Thoits, 1982). Both Heller (1979) and Lin et al. (1979) assert that social support instruments may also measure social competence, or one's ability to seek help. Based on current literature, the following suggestions are offered by the author when attempting to conceptualize and measure the buffering or moderating effects of social support: (1) longitudinal data are necessary to rule out confounding of independent and dependent variables; (2) social competence, self-esteem, and self-efficacy may be enhanced by supportive inputs and should be measured separately; and (3) supportive relationships have functional, structural, reciprocal, and negative properties which need to be taken into account.

The assessment of the role of supportive relationships following a disaster has received limited attention. Bolin (1982) gathered information from tornado victims regarding numbers and types of material aid obtained, sources of social support, and perceptions regarding its usefulness toward recovery. Fleming et al. (1982) examined the mediating influences of social support on stress resulting from the nuclear reactor accident at Three Mile Island. The author is currently studying the effects of self-efficacy and social support as mediators between stress and illness in a longitudinal study following the volcanic eruption of Mount St. Helens.

In summary, actions taken to ameliorate the loss effects following disasters have had little conceptual basis beyond the attempts to separate agent-produced and response-produced effects. As pointed out here, it is important to select the conceptualization of a given concept that best explains what one is attempting to define and measure.

Conceptualizing Recovery Outcomes

Conceptualization of variables incorporated in disaster research is evolving. The limited conceptual bases for disaster interventions and research are understandable due to unique aspects of disasters. Moreover, the need to save lives and minimize injuries places priorities on immediate activities, and only recently have review and funding protocols been established for quick-response research proposals. At the present time, it appears that human responses to aversive events in general can be predicted only in very general terms. Silver and Wortman (1980) conducted an exhaustive review of the literature on coping with uncontrollable aversive events. They concluded that, to date, there is no universal coping response. These data suggest that "phase" analyses (heroic, honeymoon, disillusionment, reconstruction) have very limited value in conceptualization.

A second pertinent point is that there is no clear definition of adaptive and maladaptive behavior. Wortman and Dintzer (1978) assert that depression and helplessness, for example, are maladaptive *only* when an outcome can be changed by an individual. Thus, the concept of recovery demands our attention.

Health Status. Health is a frequent and important indicator of disaster outcomes because of the relationship between environmental stressors over which one has little control and onset of illness. Both mental and physical health status following disasters have been reported. However, as Melick points out in Chapter 8, there is little consistency in conceptualization across studies. For example, "emotional effects," "psychological effects," and "mental impairment" may measure similar variables. Similarly, measurement of these constructs varies widely from study to study. Examples are given by Hartsough in Chapter 2. While health status has been found to be an important recovery indicator, some recent well-conducted studies would suggest that recovery is a multivariate phenomenon.

Multiple Indicators of Recovery. To assess family recovery following the effects of tornadoes at two sites, Bolin (1982) conceptualized recovery along four dimensions: emotional, economic, housing, and perceived quality of life. Similarly, Berren et al. (1982) use the combined measures of causal agent, duration, magnitude of personal impact, potential for recurrence, and perceptions of control to predict services necessary for adaptive outcomes. Logue et al. (1981) applied a complex stress model. Finally, the use of the legal system in loss resolution is on the increase and should be examined as a recovery variable (Rabin, 1978).

CONCLUSION

This chapter has argued for increased theory-based disaster research and intervention. Some basic terms were defined to eliminate the fear and mystery that surrounds theory-building. An expanded list of appropriate concepts and theories has been identified and described to offer concrete suggestions for researchers and practitioners.

REFERENCES

Abramson, L., Seligman, M., Teasdale, J. Learned helplessness in humans: Critique and reformulation. Journal of Abnormal Psychology, 1978, *87*, 49–74.

Antonovsky, A. Health, Stress and Coping. San Francisco: Jossey-Bass, 1979.

Baisden, B., Quarantelli, E. The delivery of mental health services in community disasters: An outline of research findings. Journal of Community Psychology, 1981, *9*, 195–203.

Bandura, A. Self-efficacy: Toward a unifying theory of behavioral change. Psychological Review, 1977, *84*, 191–215.

Bell, W. Disaster impact and response, overcoming the thousand natural shocks. Gerontologist, 1978, *18*, 531–540.

Berren, M., Beigel, A., Barker, G. A typology for the classification of disasters: Implications for intervention. Community Mental Health Journal, 1982, *18*, 120–134.

Bolin, R. C. Long-term Recovery from Disasters. Boulder: University of Colorado Press, 1982.

Brown, G., Bhrolchain, M., Harris, T. Social class and psychiatric disturbances among women in an urban population. Sociology, 1975, 9, 225.

Bugen, L. Human grief: A model for prediction and intervention. American Journal of Orthopsychiatry, 1977, 47, 196–206.

Burgess, A., Baldwin, B. Crisis Intervention Theory and Practice. Englewood Cliffs, N.J.: Prentice-Hall, 1981.

Burke, R., Weir, T. Marital helping relationships: Moderators between stress and well-being. The Journal of Psychology, 1977, 95, 121–130.

Caplan, G. Support Systems and Community Mental Health. New York: Behavioral Publications, 1974.

Chinn, P., Jacobs, M. Theory and Nursing. St. Louis: C.V. Mosby, 1983.

Clarke, H., Driever, M. Vulnerability: The Development of a Construct for Nursing. In P. Chinn (Ed.), Advances in Nursing Theory Development. Rockville, Md.: Aspen Systems, 1983.

Cobb, S. Social support as a moderator of life stress. Psychosomatic Medicine, 1976, 38, 300–314.

Cohen, R. E., Ahearn, F.L., Jr. Handbook for Mental Health Care of Disaster Victims. Baltimore: Johns Hopkins University Press, 1980.

Dean, A., Lin, N. The stress-buffering role of social support: Problems and prospects for systematic investigation. Journal of Nervous and Mental Disease, 1977, 165, 403–417.

Dohrenwend, B., Dohrenwend, B. Stressful Life Events: Their Nature and Effects. New York: Wiley, 1974.

Erikson, K. Everything in Its Path. Destruction of Community in the Buffalo Creek Flood. New York: Simon & Schuster, 1976.

Fleming, R., Baum, A., Gisriel, M., Gatchel, R. Mediating influences of social support on stress at Three Mile Island. Journal of Human Stress, 1982, 8, 14–22.

Folkman, S., Lazarus, R. An analysis of coping in a middle-aged community sample. Journal of Health and Social Behavior, 1980, 21, 219–239.

Gore, S. The effect of social support in moderating the health consequences of unemployment. Journal of Health and Social Behavior, 1978, 19, 157–165.

Gore, S. Stress-buffering functions of social supports: An appraisal and clarification of research models. In B. Dohrenwend, B. Dohrenwend (Eds.), Stressful Life Events and Their Contexts. New York: Neale Watson Academic Publications, 1981.

Green, B. Assessing levels of psychological impairment following disaster. Journal of Nervous and Mental Disease, 1982, 170, 544–552.

Hanusa, B., Schulz, R. Attributional mediators of learned helplessness. Journal of Personality and Social Psychology, 1977, 35, 602–611.

Heller, K. The effects of social support: Prevention and treatment applications. In A. Goldstein, R. Kanfer (Eds.), Maximizing Treatment Gains. New York: Academic Press, 1979.

Hoff, L. People in Crisis. Menlo Park, Calif.: Addison-Wesley, 1978.

House, J. Work Stress and Social Support. Reading, Mass.: Addison-Wesley, 1981.

Kerlinger, F. Foundations of Behavioral Research. New York: Holt, Rinehart, & Winston, 1973.

Kilijanek, T., Drabek, T. Assessing long-term impacts of a natural disaster: A focus on the elderly. Gerontologist, 1979, 19, 555-556.

Kobasa, S., Hilker, R., Maddi, S. Who stays healthy under stress? Journal of Occupational Medicine, 1979, 21, 595-598.

Kreps, G. The organization of disaster response: Some fundamental theoretical issues. In E. Quarantelli (Ed.), Disasters: Theory and Research. Beverly Hills, Calif.: Sage Publications, 1978.

Kubler-Ross, E. On Death and Dying. New York: Macmillan, 1969.

Lazarus, R., Averill, J., Opton, E. The psychology of coping: Issues of research and assessment. In G. Coelho, D. Hamburg, J. Adams (Eds.), Coping and Adaptation. New York: Basic Books, 1974.

Lazarus, R., Cohen, J. Environmental Stress. In I. Altman, J. Wohlwill (Eds.), Human Behavior and the Environment: Current Theory and Research. New York: Plenum, 1977.

Lin, N., Simeone, R., Ensel, W., Kuo, W. Social support, stressful life events and illness: A model and an empirical test. Journal of Health and Social Behavior, 1979, 20, 108-119.

Lindemann, E. Symptomatology and management of acute grief. American Journal of Psychiatry, 1944, 101, 141-148.

Lindy, J., Grace, M., Green, G. Survivors: Outreach to a reluctant population. American Journal of Orthopsychiatry, 1981, 51, 468-478.

Logue, J.N., Melick, M.E., Struening, E. A study of health and mental health status following a major natural disaster. In R. Simmons, (Ed.), Research in Community and Mental Health: An Annual Compilation of Research. 2, 217-274. Greenwich, Conn.: JAI Press, 1981.

MacElveen-Hoehn, R., Smith-DiJulio, K. Social network behavior in long-term illness: Preliminary analysis. Paper presented at Social Networks Conference, Portland State University, 1978.

McCubbin, H. Coping repertoires of families adapting to prolonged war-induced separations. Journal of Marriage and the Family, 1976, 38, 461-471.

Miller, P., Ingram, J., Davidson, S. Life events, symptoms and social support. Journal of Psychosomatic Research, 1976, 20, 515-522.

Moos, R. Coping with Physical Illness. New York: Plenum, 1977.

Murphy, S. Coping with stress following a natural disaster: The volcanic eruption of Mount St. Helens (Doctoral dissertation, Portland State University, 1981). Dissertation Abstracts International (University Microfilms, No. 82-07, 42 10B, 4014).

Murphy, S. Learned helplessness: From concept to comprehension. Perspectives in Psychiatric Care, 1982, 20, 27-32.

Murphy, S. Stress levels and health status of victims of a natural disaster. Research in Nursing and Health, 1984, 7, 205-215.

Norbeck, J. Social support: A model for clinical research and application. Advances in Nursing Science, 1981, 3, 43-60.

Pearlin, L., Lieberman, M., Managham, E., Mullon, J. The stress process. Journal of Health and Social Behavior, 1981, 22, 333-356.

Pearlin, L., Schooler, C. The structure of coping. Journal of Health and Social Behavior, 1978, *19*, 2–21.

Perry, R., Lindell, M. The psychological consequences of natural disaster: A review of research on American communities. Mass Emergencies, 1978, *3*, 105–115.

Powell, J., Rayner, J. Progress Notes: Disaster Investigation, July 1, 1951–June 30, 1952. Englewood, Md.: Army Chemical Corps Medical Laboratories, 1952.

Rabin, R. Dealing with disasters: Some thoughts on the adequacy of the legal system. Stanford Law Review, 1978, *30*, 281–298.

Schulz, R. The Psychology of Death, Dying, and Bereavement. Menlo Park, Calif.: Addison-Wesley, 1978.

Shneidman, E. Death: Current Perspectives. Palo Alto, Calif.: Mayfield, 1976.

Silver, R., Wortman, C. Coping with undesirable life events. In J. Garber, M. Seligman (Eds.), Human Helplessness: Theory and Applications. New York: Academic Press, 1980.

Thoits, P. Conceptual, methodological and theoretical problems in studying social support as a buffer against life stress. Journal of Health and Social Behavior, 1982, *23*, 145–159.

Titchener, J., Kapp, F.T. Family and character change at Buffalo Creek. American Journal of Psychiatry, 1976, *133*, 295–299.

U.S. Public Health Service. Disaster assistance and emergency mental health. DHEW Pub. No. (ADM) 76–327. Washington, D.C.: Department of Health, Education and Welfare, 1976.

Vaillant, G. Adaptation to Life. Boston: Little, Brown, 1977.

Weisman, A. Coping with untimely death. Psychiatry, 1973, *36*, 366–379.

Willer, D., Webster, M. Theoretical concepts and observables. American Sociological Review, 1970, *35*, 748–757.

Wortman, C., Dintzer, L. Is an attributional analysis of learned helplessness phenomenon viable? A critique. Journal of Abnormal Psychology, 1978, *87*, 75–90.

2

Measurement of the Psychological Effects of Disaster

Don M. Hartsough

The focus of this chapter is on the measurement of individual psychological effects following a community disaster. The concepts and measurement instruments discussed are also relevant to assessment in other stress situations, including individual trauma (rape, accidents) but these are beyond the scope of the present discussion. The chapter has two purposes: (1) to show that assessing the aftereffects of a disaster should be based upon an understanding of disaster phenomena; and (2) to assist the individual investigator in selecting appropriate measurement instruments or in developing new ones. It is not unusual to find a prospective disaster researcher sandwiched between the need to gather data quickly (presumably before the effects disappear) and the desire to create a clean, well-designed study. It is hoped that the material herein will make the latter task easier. The chapter will have achieved its purposes if it promotes attention to critical issues in the planning of disaster research, a thoughtful and deliberate selection of instruments, and a better understanding of the complexity of the psychological effects of disasters.

We will first examine briefly what is meant by psychological effects and why it is important to measure them. Some of the unique challenges that face the disaster researcher and some issues in measurement are then described. A transactional model for psychological disaster research is presented and discussed. It was not the author's intention to clutter the literature with yet another model, and in fact I have borrowed freely from two conceptualizations which may be well known to the reader. The model provides a framework for discussing assessment alternatives open to the investigator, such as checklists and scales, structured interviews, clinical assessment, questionnaires, psychophysiological measures, and psychosocial indicators. A list of specific measurement instruments that have been employed with disaster populations is also included and discussed. In spite of the barriers and pitfalls along the path, disaster research and mitigation are significant, stimulating areas of professional endeavor, and promise to benefit both victim populations and workers who have come to their aid.

SUBJECT DOMAIN OF THE CHAPTER

Psychological effects refer to a wide range of negative feelings, somatic symptoms, upsetting thoughts, and dysfunctional behaviors that are precipitated by an unusual and compelling experience. Psychological effects include both those that are considered normal in light of the upsetting experience and those that indicate a functional disorder, including diagnosable anxiety and depression. The psychological effects of disasters are now considered to be normal reactions to abnormal circumstances; that is, such effects are not considered to be psychopathologic in the conventional sense, and a high rate of recovery is usually expected. This does not mean that postdisaster effects should be taken lightly by mental health professionals, as disaster victims are truly traumatized and highly vulnerable, and consequences in the long run may be quite negative if the curative process does not take place. Thus, psychological effects can also refer to rates of psychiatric disorder that are linked to disasters. Effects are not found uniformly in a disaster population. Discovering which groups are at-risk following a disaster defines one of the purposes for measurement.

Perhaps it would be useful at the outset of this report to spell out some of the author's positions with regard to the measurement of psychological effects of disaster. It has already been mentioned that the aftereffects of disasters are interpreted as *normal responses to unusually upsetting circumstances,* and that they are part of a healing process that has the ultimate goal of restoring or at least approximating a prior state of psychological health. A second position concerns the *interaction of psychological effects with the personality of the victim.* Psychological effects are considered to be primarily situationally determined (Gleser et al., 1981; Melick et al., 1982). It is possible that there is a U-shaped interaction between severity of the disaster event and the influence of personality, such that both very minor events (e.g., temporary evacuation from home) and extremely severe events (e.g., concentration camp or extended torture) have very little interaction with the personality of the participant or victim, because the stimulus characteristics of the situation are prepotent. On the other hand, incidents that have a moderate to severe stimulus characteristic may increase the interaction with personality in terms of the measurement of psychological effects. This hypothesis is highly speculative. A third position of the author states that psychological effects are influenced by two major sources in the disaster situation. The first source is the agent of disaster, such as a tornado, earthquake, nuclear plant accident, or terrorist attack. The second source is the response of society, in particular, rescuers, disaster workers, and the victim's support group to the disaster. Following Quarantelli (1979) these sources of influence are labeled *agent-produced effects* and *response-produced effects*, respectively.

While measurement in this report is meant to convey the understanding and assessment of psychological effects in the broadest sense, I must admit to a certain bias in terms of disaster affects research. The use of standardized measurement instruments is strongly recommended because of their potential for generating knowledge about disaster effects across different situations. The use of homemade questionnaires and inventories may be the path of least resistance at the time a study is planned, but after the data are in what can they tell us about a disaster population in comparison with others? Another recommendation is for the use of multiple procedures or techniques for measuring the same set of psychological effects. Psychological measurement is not an exact science and one way to correct for the inevitable slippage in measurement is the use of a multimethod approach. Also, the use of a comparison group is to be strongly recommended for most disaster studies. While this recommendation may seem elementary for experienced research workers, who must meet the requirements of granting agencies, it has been too often ignored by the occasional disaster researcher. The definition of a proper comparison group is a design and measurement issue discussed later in the chapter. Finally, one must observe that research on psychological effects that is grounded in a theoretical framework usually has been more effective than atheoretical research. As indicated in the next section, disaster research has been primarily descriptive until the recent past. Fortunately we seem to be entering into an era where greater concern for theory is in evidence.

OVERVIEW OF DISASTER EFFECTS MEASUREMENT

The measurement of psychological effects has evolved considerably over the last half century as a result of changes in the purposes of the measurement and the professional and scientific orientations of the investigators. There appear to be at least three basic goals for the measurement of psychological effects following disasters: (1) to understand the phenomena in human terms, including their complexity and their meaning for the people whose lives have been touched, and sometimes profoundly altered; (2) for the documentation of scientific evidence about both psychological effects in general and about their manifestation for any individual victim or group of victims; and (3) to provide a basis for public policy regarding the response to disasters, including planned interventions for the mitigation of psychological effects in victims and in disaster workers. There has been a progression from the early descriptive studies which focused on the objective of understanding to the more recent investigations of a more analytic nature. The flurry of research activity that took place following the nuclear reactor accident at Three Mile Island (TMI) in 1979 would appear to be a bench mark in the recent history of research on psychological effects.

DESCRIPTIVE STUDIES

The majority of studies on the psychological effects of disaster through the mid-1970s used either naturalistic observation or clinical interviews to study victims, or were sociological investigations employing unstandardized questionnaires (Kinston and Rosser, 1974; Melick et al., 1982; Perry and Lindell, 1978). A fascinating exception was the clinical study by Beach and Lucas (1960) which employed standard clinical measurement techniques and a control group of peers to determine the effects of being trapped in a coal mine for many days. A major effort was launched during the 1950s by the National Research Council to study interpersonal and social behavior following natural disasters. These studies collectively have provided an important empirical basis for an understanding of the social context for individual behavior in disasters. They have exploded a number of myths about disaster behavior (Quarantelli and Dynes, 1973) and have provided a basis for more refined measurement of psychological effects. These investigators represent a more global approach to disaster research, in contrast to the more specific and analytic approach favored by recent investigators. Moos (1974) describes the legitimacy of both research orientations:

> The goals of understanding and prediction often lead to the choice of quite different assessment methods. Investigators interested primarily in understanding have tended to utilize more complex, intuitive, clinical, and global assessment methods; investigators interested primarily in accurate prediction have tended to utilize simple, objective, specific, and

actuarial methods. Whether this is necessary, because different ends require different means, or whether the development of methods of intermediate complexity can effectively combine these goals is still unclear. For the present at least, understanding and prediction must be dealt with as somewhat separate goals, even though in the deepest and most relevant sense all of us fervently wish we could do both (pp. 335–336).

The goal of prediction as described by Moos is a subset of the broader goals of scientific documentation. To meet these goals the investigator typically must employ a more refined approach to measurement of psychological effects than is found in most descriptive studies, although in the process much of the richness of understanding generated by descriptive methods is lost.

Analytic Studies

Analytic studies are those that frame a question about the psychological effects of disaster so that it may be tested by use of the scientific method. Analytic studies are likely to answer more refined questions than simply "Are there any psychological effects?" or "Do disaster victims describe themselves as emotionally upset?" Investigators with an analytic bent are likely to formulate hypotheses about specific at-risk populations or to make predictions about what their measures will produce. As indicated earlier, the use of hypothesis testing was the exception rather than the rule until the mid-1970s. It is instructive, for example, to read an assessment of the disaster literature as it pertains to an important subset of victims (psychiatric patients), written by a research group with expertise in epidemologic methods:

> It revealed a surprising dearth of knowledge about the reactions of psychiatric patients to any type of disaster. Furthermore, the few studies reported during the past two decades are conceptually and methodologically deficient. They failed to specify independent and mediating variables relating to the effects of disaster; outcome usually was assessed in a narrow if not simplistic manner; data were gathered through observation rather than standardized instruments; comparison groups were not included to control for confounding variables; and longitudinal follow-ups were not conducted despite the report of profound long-term effects of exposure to disaster. (Bromet et al., 1982, pp. 725 to 726.)

One may empathize with the frustration experienced by these authors on finding previous research so unhelpful. An investigator may "know" in a personal way that there are profound postdisaster psychological effects; yet if these effects cannot be demonstrated scientifically, the investigator's efforts may be for naught.

Three Mile Island—A Bench Mark in Disaster Effects Research

The nuclear reactor accident at TMI in 1979 has been described as the most studied accident in America (Report to Congress, 1980) and with respect to psychological effects, this characterization is particularly apt. Because the accident was ominously threatening and drew worldwide attention, but did not cause injury or death, or result in community destruction, the effects on the mental health of the surrounding population became identified as the major impact of the accident. Psychological stress became the major variable of study and debate with regard to the restart of an undamaged reactor at TMI (Hartsough and Savitsky, in press). Thus, emotional, attitudinal, and behavioral responses to a major incident, on both individual and collective levels, had ceased to become a by-product of research interest, and instead occupied center stage. The TMI-2 accident attracted several major research efforts (Baum et al., 1981; Bromet et al., 1980; Dohrenwend et al., 1979; Flynn and Chalmers, 1980; Houts et al., 1980, 1981; Mileti et al., 1982). Thus, it became possible for the first time to have consensual validation for the psychological effects of a particular incident, based upon scientific evidence from several sources. Three Mile Island research also sampled a broad range of methods including standard symptoms checklists and interview schedules (Bromet et al., 1980) and psychosocial indicator data (Mileti et al., 1982). A multimethod design was successfully employed within one study (Collins et al., 1983), which employed self-report, behavioral, and psychophysiologic measures on the same sample of subjects. Also, all of the TMI investigators attempted to use control or comparison groups, with varying success. In addition to the higher quality and greater quantity of research produced by the TMI incident, findings became an important body of evidence for public policy and regulatory decisions at the highest level of government (Hartsough and Savitsky, in press).

THE SIGNIFICANCE OF MEASURING PSYCHOLOGICAL EFFECTS

Theoretical Questions

There are a number of questions that remain to be answered by future research on disaster effects. A comprehensive review of the theoretical aspects of disaster psychology falls outside the scope of this chapter, but a few instances of theoretical issues will be mentioned to highlight the significance of measurement. I previously stated a position on the normality versus the pathology of psychological effects following disasters. The fact is that the precise linkage between disaster experience and subsequent psychiatric disorders is largely unknown, especially the mediating variables that are middle links in the network from independent to dependent variables. Mediating variables are socially significant because most disaster events are practically impossible to influence, while mediating variables (such as social support, crisis counseling intervention, and financial assistance) can be manipulated.

A second major theoretical question pertains to the event-effects relationship. Reviews of the literature (see Chapter 8) point toward a major situational influence for psychological effects. Authors have hypothesized a number of variables as situational determinants (Berren et al., 1980), and these hypotheses should be subjected to research. A third issue pertains to the dynamics of a disaster experience. Do psychological effects of disasters and other traumatic experiences progress from initial shock through a series of predictable phases that end with acceptance or assimilation of the disquieting experience? This theoretical issue is critical to an understanding of the basic coping process and also for planning interventions for disaster victims. Horowitz (1976) posits the existence of a stress response syndrome with alternating intrusion and denial phases, but Silver and Wortman (1980) cite a number of studies that cast doubt on the whole notion of a phasic process. The longitudinal measurement of psychological effects following different types of events and for different at-risk groups would assist in answering these questions.

Legal, Policy, and Accountability Needs

Over 600 individuals in 178 families who survived the Buffalo Creek disaster in 1972 became litigants in a legal action against the Pittston Company, which they considered responsible for the disaster. Each of the victims was examined clinically by both sides, and in an out-of-court settlement they were awarded 13.5 million dollars, including 8 million dollars for psychic impairment stemming from the disaster. Gleser et al., (1981) provide a fascinating account of the comprehensive clinical and scientific investigation conducted on behalf of the victims. Although lacking a comparison group, their study presents compelling evidence for both short-term distress and long-term impairment among many citizens of the Buffalo Creek region. The work of these authors and their colleagues is an excellent example of the use of measurement for humanitarian purposes, that is, the proper assessment of damages so that legal redress to victims is possible.

Mention has already been made of the role of measurement in the assessment of psychological aftermath of TMI. The Supreme Court in 1983 ruled that psychological stress should not be considered as an environmental impact under the National Environmental Policy Act, unless there is a physical impact on victims (Hartsough and Savitsky, in press). To the extent that future regulatory or civil court proceedings allow for the consideration of psychological effects of disasters, a precise measurement of these effects will be important not only to the policy makers and litigants, but to investigators who are charged with proper management of evidence.

Following a Presidentially declared disaster it is possible for mental health centers and other service providers to apply for federal funds through Public Law 93-288, Section 413 for the provision of crisis counseling to disaster victims. Part of the application process is a requirement for a needs assessment for crisis counseling in the affected area. At the present time such assessments are by necessity quite crude, usually depending upon the observations of key informants, and demographic characteristics of the population. With an increased knowledge of the effects of disasters on particular populations a high level of accountability to the funding agencies will be possible, as will be more effective predisaster planning (Hartsough, 1982).

Evaluative Research on Interventions

There has been little research on the effectiveness of postdisaster interventions that are designed to mitigate psychological effects. The primary reasons appear to be the relative recency of such services, the lack of requirements for evaluative studies, and the lack of precision in measuring psychological effects. This state of affairs may not continue, however, because those who contend that more services for disaster victims are needed also bear the responsibility to demonstrate that the requested services are effective. A careful assessment of planned interventions would seem to be critical, especially in light of the common perception that psychological effects are part of a normal healing process that will occur even in the absence of mitigation. To pose the evaluation question in a cumbersome sentence: It would seem incumbent upon researchers to demonstrate what *events* produce what sorts of *reactions* in what *types of populations* over what *length of time;* and to show that such reactions are susceptible to what kinds of *interventions* performed by what kinds of *personnel.* Measurement is obviously a critical component of this effort.

CHALLENGES TO MEASURING PSYCHOLOGICAL EFFECTS

Defining and Gaining Access to a Subject Population

Subject populations should be defined with specific criteria. The term "victim" is ambiguous if it is not further qualified. There is no standard definition or set of criteria for defining a disaster victim, thus, the individual research investigator must provide an operational definition. Victims often refer to individuals or families who have been subjected to property loss, injury, or death of a close family member. However, victim status may also be applied to evacuees or to anyone who lives within a prescribed geographical area surrounding a disaster site. The term "secondary victim" has been applied to disaster workers and others with close, extended contact with either the disaster site or with primary victims. Some authors prefer the term "survivor" because they feel it has fewer negative connotations. The definition of the population under study is largely a matter of matching the realities of the disaster situation to the research needs of the investigator and should not be of great concern except to make clear what the criteria for selection are.

Gaining access to a subject population is not always so easily accomplished as defining it. Immediately following natural disasters or large-scale evacuations, the affected populations scatter to both private residences (friends, relatives) and commercial accommodations. Only a small fraction will be found in evacuation shelters provided by the American Red Cross or the National Guard, and it is commonly observed that this group is highly selected in terms of financial resources and ties (or lack of them) to the community. The disaster populations that are geographically located provide much easier access than those whose home residence has no relation to the disaster, for example, transportation accidents. Lindy et al. (1981) documented the difficulty of maintaining contact with a disaster population from the Beverly Hills Supper Club fire. They noted that the victims were scattered over a wide geographical area and were reluctant to maintain contact with an intervention program during the months following the disaster.

Defining a Valid Comparison Group

Analytic studies (discussed in a following section) often require the use of a comparison group in order to test a set of hypotheses of interest to the investigator. Generally speaking the more specific or refined the research question, the greater the need for carefully drawn experimental and comparison groups. For example, Bromet et al. (1980) tested the effects of the TMI nuclear reactor accident on mothers of preschool children who lived within a defined distance of the accident site. Their comparison group was a similar group of mothers from a comparable locality in Pennsylvania that also had a nuclear generating plant, but one that had experienced no accident. The investigators considered that a complete design would call for a second comparison group of mothers who lived near a generating plant that was not nuclear-fired; however this group had to be dropped for financial and administrative considerations (Bromet E., personal communication, 1979). Another research group at TMI (Houts et al. 1980, 1981) employed a much looser definition of a comparison group by taking subjects who were over 40 miles from TMI in comparison with the experimental group who lived close to TMI. The more careful definition of the comparison group in the Bromet et al. (1980) study allowed for greater confidence in its findings in contrast with the Houts et al. (1980, 1981) research.

Murphy and Stewart (1982) employed linked pairs and comparison group technique to control for age, occupation and related variables in a study of the effects of bereavement following the Mount St. Helen's eruption. Such designs are especially effective where the research focus is exclusively on individual variables rather than community or organizational variables.

Selecting Measurement Instruments

The proper selection of measurement instruments is a critical step for obtaining an accurate assessment of psychological effects following a disaster. It is unfortunate that selections are too often made hurriedly and without full consideration of the choices available. Apparently there has been a strong temptation to develop questionnaires anew for each incident. Until the recent past the unfortunate result was an unrelated assortment of measures, employing rather casual designs, and producing unintelligible results across a nonrepeated set of incidents! Consequently, the research on psychological effects has not produced a consistent pattern of results. It is hoped that the transactional model of psychological effects presented later will offer some structure for the process of considering which measurement instruments to use.

Timing

It is quite likely that the nature and intensity of psychological effects varies with the time at which they are measured. Theoretical notions of the effects of traumatic experiences generally include a phasic perspective (Melick et al., 1982) although, as previously mentioned, a phase interpretation of response to trauma has been criticized.

Assessing Causality

An accurate assessment of the sources of psychological effects is an important task for the researcher, especially where findings may be utilized by policy makers or in civil courts. Yet it is often impossible to separate effects attributable to the event itself from effects that are linked to society's response to the incident (Quarantelli, 1979). The mismanagement of housing assignments following the Buffalo Creek flood (Erikson, 1976) is a classic example of effects from the latter source. The role of the media in disaster as discussed in Chapter 13, (Hartsough and Mileti, 1982) is another source of secondary influence.

An in-depth discussion of this problem is beyond the scope of this chapter, but longitudinal designs with identical or highly correlated measures offer one solution, while path analysis with several different measures is another variation of the same idea. It is sufficient to note here that it may be possible with careful planning and instrument selection to develop a study which makes meaningful assignments of causality to mediating variables in addition to exposure to the precipitating agent.

A TRANSACTIONAL MODEL

A model of some of the important transactions between the individual and the environment regarding psychological effects from a traumatic event is portrayed in Figure 2.1. The model displays a series of critical steps between the occurrence of an event in the environment and outcomes linked to that event that occur both at the individual level and to aggregates of individuals at the community level. The model is based primarily on the concepts of stress and coping described by Lazarus (1966) and his colleagues (Aldwin et al., 1980; Folkman and Lazarus, 1980). It also contains the contribution of Quarantelli (1979), who pointed out that mental health effects from a disaster may be response-produced as well as event-produced, that is, society's response to disaster is often a significant source of distress at the individual level. The task of the model in the present context is to suggest appropriate measures for the various steps that link the occurrence of an event to its outcomes. The facets of the model and measures appropriate for each are described below.

Hazard

The intensity and nature of hazards sustained by disaster victims vary across individuals within one event (some lose more than others) and also vary from one type of event to another. Riverine floods are gener-

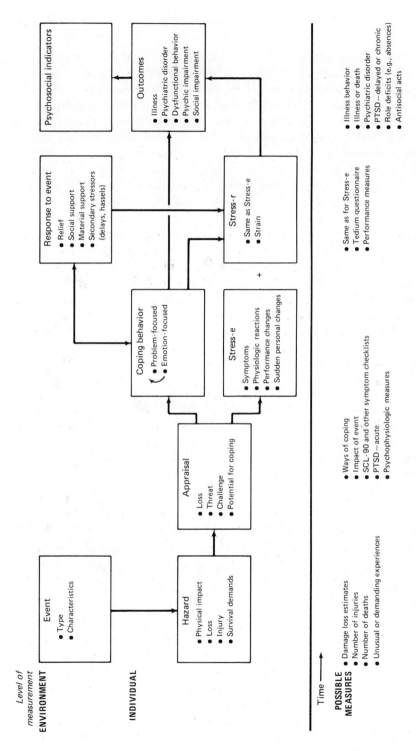

Figure 2.1. A Transactional Model of Psychological Effects and Associated Measures.

Level of
measurement
ENVIRONMENT

INDIVIDUAL

Event
• Type
• Characteristics

Hazard
• Physical impact
• Loss
• Injury
• Survival demands

Appraisal
• Loss
• Threat
• Challenge
• Potential for coping

Coping behavior
• Problem-focused
• Emotion-focused

Stress-e
• Symptoms
• Physiologic reactions
• Performance changes
• Sudden personal changes

Response to event
• Relief
• Social support
• Material support
• Secondary stressors (delays, hassels)

Stress-r
• Same as Stress-e
• Strain

Psychosocial indicators

Outcomes
• Illness
• Psychiatric disorder
• Dysfunctional behavior
• Psychic impairment
• Social impairment

Time ⟶

POSSIBLE
MEASURES
• Damage loss estimates
• Number of injuries
• Number of deaths
• Unusual or demanding experiences

• Ways of coping
• Impact of event
• SCL-90 and other symptom checklists
• PTSD—acute
• Psychophysiologic measures

• Same as for Stress-e
• Tedium questionnaire
• Performance measures

• Illness behavior
• Illness or death
• Psychiatric disorder
• PTSD—delayed or chronic
• Role deficits (e.g., absences)
• Antisocial acts

ally conceded to produce hazards of a less-severe nature than tornados or jetliner air crashes. Hazards refer to the "objective" evidence of harm precipitated by an event on an individual. Factors such as the physical impact of the agent on the individual and injuries suffered are included here, as well as loss of property, loss of a significant relationship through death, and the extra demands placed on the individual in order to survive. Measurements of hazards include damage loss estimates, loss of a job, loss of a family member through death, the frequency and severity of injury to the individual victim or significant others, loss of housing, and whether the individual had to endure unusual or demanding experiences, such as extended exposure to the elements. Hazard measurements should be objective and verifiable; the significance of the hazard to the individual should not be included. Hazard data may be available shortly following a disaster from property loss estimates, verified deaths, medically diagnosed injuries, and event-oriented interviews of victims in temporary shelters. The use of such data for predicting subsequent negative effects has been explored by Papperman (1981).

Appraisal

Appraisal has been hypothesized as a two-part perceptual process by which the individual ascribes meaning to environmental events and their hazards. Primary appraisal results in the interpretation of environmental events as loss, threat, or challenge (Folkman and Lazarus, 1980) and secondary appraisal relates to the individual's perceptions of the potential for coping (Lazarus, 1966). There appear to be no measures that are related exclusively to this particular facet of the model.

Coping Behavior

According to Folkman and Lazarus (1980) coping is typically a combination of two underlying strategies, one of which focuses on the environment and attempts to solve the problem by making changes in the external world, and the other which is directed toward making internal changes in order to adjust to the new circumstances. The two strategies are labeled *problem-focused coping* and *emotion-focused coping*, respectively. The Ways of Coping Inventory has been designed by the Lazarus research group to measure an individual's employment of these strategies.

Stress Produced by the Event

The first major source of stress from disaster stems directly from an appraisal of the hazards produced by the agent of disaster. In Figure 2.1 these stresses are labeled "Stress-e" to identify them as agent-produced. Included here are the symptoms and physiologic reactions that typically occur following a traumatic experience, such as surviving a tornado, evacuating through flood waters, escaping from a burning building, and so on. Posttraumatic symptoms include sleep disturbances, unwanted thoughts, and other intrusions into the cognitive life of the survivor, plus feelings of anxiety, fear, and greatly elevated tension. Periods of hypervigilance, hyperactivity, and affectivity seem to fluctuate with other periods of emotional numbness, avoidance of anything associated with the incident, and defensive denial. Aspects of this pattern have been studied clinically by Horowitz and his colleagues, and expressed in the Impact of Event Scale (Horowitz et al., 1979). A psychiatric diagnosis of Posttraumatic Stress Disorder—acute type (PTSD) provides another means of labeling the Stress-e phenomena, but has been rarely used following disasters. Symptom checklists and inventories of various types have been employed to measure a range of subclinical emotional, behavioral, and psychophysiological reactions, and are reviewed in a later section of the chapter.

Society's Response to the Event

This model makes the point that the response of a community to disaster victims has a potential for both increasing and decreasing the stress experienced by the survivor population. Rescue or evacuation may be quite stressful, even though the actions may be necessary to protect the lives of those involved. Relief activities like those performed by the Red Cross or the Church of the Brethren Disaster Services are presumed to enhance coping and reduce stress, but even these may be stressful if accompanied by unexpected delays and frustrations. An individual's social support network has the potential for both positive and negative effects although the positive ones are commonly observed to predominate following disasters. Secondary stressors following disasters may range from the inconveniences caused by new living arrangements to serious barriers or delays in obtaining recovery resources. According to the transactional model, each of the foregoing variables interacts with both the individual's coping (especially problem-focused coping) and his or her stress responses. In the ideal situation coping behaviors are enhanced and stresses are reduced by the net effect of society's response to a disaster.

Response-Produced Stress

It is unclear whether the stresses created from the response to disaster are different in nature than those generated by the agent itself. It seems reasonable to hypothesize less of a traumatic character in the response-produced precipitants, and therefore a diminished likelihood of stresses associated with anxiety and with fear. Likewise, one would expect to find greater evidence of stress from frustration, unfulfilled expectations, and negative reactions to novel living situations. Stress-r may also be a by-product of coping, as for example, when problem-focused coping leads to overwork during cleanup and thus to physical and emotional exhaustion. Measures of Stress-r overlap considerably with measures for Stress-e. Kanner et al. (1978) have developed an experimental Tedium Questionnaire which may tap some of the negative feelings survivors may have about the postdisaster environment. On the other hand such environments are also characterized as altruistic (Barton, 1970) and many social barriers are temporarily removed, with the net effect of enhancing the social environment. Only two research efforts have linked physiologic measurement with a disaster population (Collins et al., 1983; Hurst, 1980) but this form of assessment seems to offer great possibilities for cross-validating findings based on scales and questionnaires. The same may be said for performance tasks which were also utilized independently by Hurst (1980) and the research group at the Uniform Services University. Both types of measures are reviewed briefly in a later section of this chapter.

Outcomes

Outcomes are separated from stresses in the transactional model even though both of them represent forms of psychological effects. This bifurcation permits a differential emphasis on process and outcome, according to the needs of the investigator; the stresses previously discussed can be easily conceptualized as transitory states that will result in some form of outcome with the passage of time. Outcomes represent the "bottom line" in terms of the permanent, individual, and collective damages precipitated by disaster. Outcomes at the individual level include psychiatric disorders, and specifically the chronic form of the PTSD. Other forms of negative outcomes are illness, social impairment (e.g., role deficits, inability to maintain employment) and other dysfunctional behavior. In the context of the model, outcomes have the connotation of relative stability, for example, behaviors still in evidence 6 months postdisaster and beyond. Measurement of outcomes at the individual level include illness behavior (Mechanic, 1974), and episodes of illness or psychiatric disorder. The measurement of role deficits and dysfunctional social behavior has usually been accomplished by sociological questionnaires and has not been subjected to standardized psychometric measurement.

Psychosocial Indicators

Outcomes at the individual level can be summed to provide data on population aggregates and permit comparison of a disaster community with a nondisaster counterpart. Psychosocial indicators are the best means of gathering data unobtrusively on disaster victims—an advantage over measures that may be reactive (Campbell and Stanley, 1963) to the phenomena under study. Such indicators include the frequency of illnesses hypothesized to be related to the disaster agent (e.g., cardiac problems), the frequency of PTSD episodes, psychiatric disorders, and other mental health indicators such as hospitalization and suicide rates. As indicators of psychological effects, measurement of psychosocial outcomes at the community level have been underutilized in disaster research. Mileti et al. (1982) report the successful use of six indicators to assess the psychological impact of TMI: (1) sales of alcoholic beverages, (2) cardiovascular deaths, (3) criminal arrests, (4) admissions to psychiatric facilities, (5) suicides, and (6) automobile accidents. The use of psychosocial indicators has the advantage of access to epidemiologic techniques and perspectives, and should be considered a priority type of research where questions of social policy are involved. Screening inventories and mental health status measures used for survey research are also good candidates for measurement of outcomes. Measures with a previous disaster use, such as the Schedule of Affective Disorders and Schizophrenia (SADS) and the Gurin Checklist, are reviewed in a later section. Such measures have the advantage of providing information at the individual level (that is, could be used in case-finding surveys) and also data for population estimates.

The transactional model provides only one means of conceptualizing the psychological impact of exposure to a disaster and its aftermath. It is a linear model, whereas the actual processes, such as appraisal and coping, continue to operate throughout recovery. The advantage of using such a model, however, is the perspective it may yield for deciding when and how to assess psychological effects, and how the findings from one measurement procedure may relate to other results. The model separates outcome from process, although both facets of the model may be considered as disaster-produced effects. Finally, the model attempts to portray some of the richness of the psychological processes that are interposed between the occurrence of an event in the environment and the individual or collective outcomes that may be evidenced weeks or months later.

ISSUES IN MEASUREMENT

The way in which an investigator resolves measurement issues that arise naturally from the assessment task will give shape and character to the research project. A few of these issues are proposed here to highlight typical concerns in disaster research.

UNITS OF ANALYSIS

The investigator should frame the research question in the most specific language possible. This step should indicate the appropriate level of units of analysis to be used in this study. The question, "Has there been an increase in emotional ill health in Santa Royale since the earthquake that cannot be detected for the non-earthquake city of Doe-ville?" implies an epidemiologic approach, whereas the question, "What is the nature and frequency of psychological stress experienced by Santa Royale residents who lost their homes in the earthquake, as compared with Santa Royale residents whose homes were spared?" suggests a house-to-house survey approach with individual interviews or a symptom checklist.

Short-Term Versus Long-Term Assessment
Is the event of short duration like a tornado, or of extended duration as may be found in riverine floods and some technological disasters? Will the measurements be taken during the event, shortly following its occurrence or many months into its recovery period, when the event has long since come and gone? Typically disaster investigators strive to get into the field as soon as possible and are usually limited to data gathering during one period of time, with the result that disaster literature related to psychological effects is weak in terms of long-term assessments. Repeated measures with the same instruments in the same population considerably enhances the interpretation of findings. If the same individuals are used for repeated measures, care should be taken that the practice effect is not confounded with the followup data. If the same measures are repeated with different individuals from the same population, care should be taken that the two samples do not differ significantly on variables related to the phenomena under study.

Descriptive Versus Analytic Studies
In descriptive studies the purpose of the investigator is to obtain a sample of responses from a defined disaster population that are believed related to the disaster experience. If several measures are used, the intercorrelations among measures may yield some insight into effects for the population studied. In operational terms, descriptive studies answer the question, "What results will be obtained if we administer this measure to this population at this point in time?" Descriptive studies may seem intuitively reasonable to the beginning investigator, and in fact, descriptive studies are useful in the exploratory phases of research in a new area, but they are weak in terms of giving convincing proof

that psychological effects exist. An example of the relative impotence of the descriptive approach is provided by Dohrenwend et al. (1979) in studying the psychological aftermath of TMI. In the rush of complying with urgent requests from the President's Commission on the Accident at Three Mile Island, control groups were omitted for several groups sampled, including the general population living adjacent to TMI. The authors' conclusions regarding distress in the general population, based upon data from the Demoralization Scale and an experimental scale of upsettingness can not be substantiated by their findings. Demoralization Scale scores of TMI residents could only be compared with those for clients of community mental health centers (the former were substantially lower) and the upsettingness scores could only be described by resorting to anchor points on the scale, a very risky basis for data interpretation.

The purpose of analytic studies is to test a hypothesis about a disaster population or subgroup that is based upon an understanding of the current state of knowledge about disaster psychological effects. Analytic studies earn their power by using designs that control for rival hypotheses concerning the predicted outcome. Investigators who seek both theoretical and practical guidance regarding design of analytic studies are referred to Campbell and Stanley (1963) and Cook and Campbell (1979).

Idiographic Versus Nomothetic Approach

Allport (1937) argues for the legitimacy of studying the individual personality as a lawful, integrated system—the idiographic approach—in contrast to the search for general laws of personality—the nomothetic approach. It may prove highly useful for certain purposes to study the life of one individual or one family to appraise the influence of exposure to a disaster and its aftermath. An idiographic philosophy was the basis for Lifton's (1967) famous studies of Hiroshima survivors. The advantage of an idiographic approach is the preservation of the complex, anfractuous nature of psychological effects on the individual. Its limitation lies in the ability to make legitimate generalizations beyond the individual case. The conclusions advanced by Lifton, for example, about "survival guilt" and the existance of a "death imprint" among Hiroshima survivors were not reached through the scientific method, but instead came from a sensitive clinician who immersed himself in a post-disaster community. Investigators who use an idiographic approach become experts on the effect of a particular incident on a particular life; they should be wary of generalizing to the population from which the individual comes.

Legal, Medical, and Sociological Definitions of Impact

The term "psychological effects" as used in this chapter conveys the notion of using scientific and/or professional methods to reach a set of conclusions about states of feeling, thoughts, and behaviors linked to exposure to an unusual incident. The investigator should be forewarned that stepping into the arena of a different discipline frequently requires the use of a different set of assumptions and the translation of psychological concepts into a different language. Legal definitions of impact may include the necessity for a physical contact between the disaster agent and the victim (Hartsough and Savitsky, in press). Impact from an incident which merely frightens a survivor without a physical confrontation is usually less credible in the eyes of the law. Psychological effects from a disaster are translated into damages in legal terms, and in order to prove damages one usually has to present behavioral evidence of negative changes in the individual's life. It has usually been insufficient to plead negative feelings and upsetting memories. (This may change with increasing sophistication in the measurement of psychological effects.)

There is a considerable overlap between medicine and psychology on definitions of disaster impact, for example, the use of symptoms as indicators of impact, and the concepts of defense, healing, and homeostasis. The major difference between the two approaches is medicine's reliance on a practitioner's diagnosis without resort to standardized psychological assessment devices.

In terms of sociological research, impact is usually assessed by means of questionnaire items rather than clinical evaluation or standardized instruments. Also, impact may be used as an independent variable, whereas in most psychological research it is a dependent variable (Bolin and Trainer, 1978). Bolin (1982) assessed impact by a series of questions in a structured interview. Items concerning psychological effects included "comparing your situation to others"; and items on injury, death and hospitalization of family and neighbors; geographic displacement; workloss of primary breadwinners; and extent of disruption from living in a trailer court. One interest of these investigators is the role of impact on family recovery.

UNIFYING CONCEPTS IN PSYCHOLOGICAL DISASTER RESEARCH

Reviewers of the disaster literature (Cohen and Ahearn, 1980; Melick et al., 1982; Perry and Lindell, 1978) have pointed out the lack of a unifying theoretical framework for disaster psychology. This deficit is most pronounced when comparisons are made between studies employing dissimilar methods, conducted by investigators with different backgrounds and objectives, and gathering data on a wide range of types of incidents. Research in the last decade has reflected more consistency in the use of both measurement devices and concepts. Several concepts are presented here in terms of their relation to the transactional model presented earlier. It is perhaps too early to determine whether further use of these concepts will culminate in the cohesive theoretical framework that is now lacking, but at least in the interim research investigators have succeeded in obtaining a kind of construct reliability. Six of the most prominent unifying concepts are *stress, coping, psychic impairment*, the stress response syndrome based upon symptoms of *intrusion* and *avoidance*, the *Posttraumatic Stress Disorder*, and *psychosocial indicators*.

In terms of the transactional model, stress and coping are process concepts. Stress became the concept which unified major research projects following TMI (Baum et al., 1981; Bromet et al., 1980; Collins et al., 1983; Dohrenwend et al., 1979; Hartsough and Savitsky, in press; Houts et al., 1980, 1981; Mileti et al., 1982). While stress was sometimes treated as an outcome measure, especially with regard to the legal conflict over the restart issue, some investigators (Bromet et al., 1980; Mileti et al., 1982) also focused on the outcomes of stress such as behavioral or clinical dysfunction. Access to measurements of coping has been lacking, but the existence of measurement instruments is expected to increase the use of the concept.

The concept of psychic impairment was employed to serve both clinical and legal purposes for victims of the Buffalo Creek Flood (Church, 1974; Gleser et al., 1981; Stern, 1976; Titchener and Kapp, 1976). The connotation of impairment places this term in an outcome category in the transactional model. Perhaps it is significant that the Buffalo Creek investigators, with a foreknowledge that findings would have to meet legal tests of impact, bypassed the use of stress as a unifying concept in favor of one that more clearly implies a behavioral outcome.

Horowitz (1976) has contributed the process concepts of intrusiveness and denial or avoidance, the former appearing as a symptom pattern and the latter as a major coping strategy. The significance of these two process concepts is their apparent universality following exposure to trauma. Various manifestations of intrusiveness and avoidance (or denial) are prominent in the PTSD, which was first offered as a medical diagnosis in the Diagnostic and Statistical Manual for Mental Disorders (DSM-III) (1980). The PTSD is clearly an outcome concept and although it has been rarely used following major disaster, a study by

McDonald (1981) indicates that diagnosticians familiar with the criteria for its use, would use it appropriately. Finally, another source of outcomes is provided by the concept of psychosocial indicators of psychological effects due to disasters. Psychosocial indicators are archival and behavioral measures that apply more appropriately to the effects of disasters on population aggregates rather than individuals, but the use of this source of information about psychological effects provides a context for the evaluation of the individual survivor.

MEASUREMENT ALTERNATIVES

The selection of measurement instruments for disaster research is often based upon an investigator's familiarity with specific measures, his or her professional background, or a preference toward one class of measurement procedures. Unfortunately, there is also a temptation for the uncritical use of what is "hot" at the moment. It is suggested here that measures be selected after a review of the alternatives, including successful performance in previous disaster research, and a decision that the specific measures chosen fit the needs of the project. The following discussion is for the reader who may be relatively unfamiliar with measurement alternatives or one who wishes to review these alternatives. The following eight types of procedures probably do not exhaust all possibilities, but do reflect the kinds of measures that have been used in disaster research: standardized scales, inventories and checklists; experimental scales, inventories and checklists; clinical assessment; structured interviews; questionnaires; performance measures; psychophysiologic measures; and psychosocial indicators.

Standardized Scales, Inventories, and Checklists
These devices offer a straightforward measurement procedure—they require the respondent (or a rater) to indicate whether or not an item applies, or to rate the strength or intensity of its application. These procedures may be self-administered (self-report) or used by someone who is familiar with the respondent. Such procedures have the advantage of being objective, easily scored, and applicable to a wide range of situations. The information gained from standardized scales, inventories, and checklists has the definite research advantage of allowing comparison across incidents. The major disadvantage is in the limitation of item content.

Helmstadter (1964) provides an excellent basic discussion of qualities that should be met by good measurement instruments. The author lists: (1) appropriateness to the group to be tested, (2) feasibility of use, (3) ease of administering and scoring, and (4) its qualities as a measurement instrument. The qualities of concern for all measures, but especially for research instruments where generalization to other work is a prime concern, include (1) standardization and the availability of normative data on a group of interest; (2) reliability; (3) objectivity—the specificity of response and reference to observable behaviors, and (4) validity, including content, criterion, and construct validities. For a more advanced discussion of these concepts, plus discussion of a wide range of specific psychological measurements, the reader is referred to Cronbach (1970) and Aiken (1976).

Experimental Scales, Inventories, and Checklists

These procedures have the same test characteristics as those previously discussed with the exception that no standardization data exist, and the investigator will not be able to compare his or her data with that from a common reference group. Most of these devices were employed one or two times by the investigators who made them up. The lack of standardization data need not be a deterrent to their use, especially if they are currently under development and information about their reliability and validity is available from the author of the test. Experimental scales, inventories, and checklists without accompanying data as to their psychometric properties offer little advantage to the researcher over fresh instruments. It behooves the author reporting use of experimental procedures to make available information about their psychometric properties to overcome this deficit.

Clinical Assessment

Clinical assessment may be performed in conjunction with clinical intervention or for documenting damages for legal purposes (Gleser et al., 1981) although it may be a rather cumbersome procedure in that latter instance. A fascinating example of the use of standard clinical instruments is provided by Beach and Lucas (1960). The DSM-III (1980) includes a diagnostic category specifically designed to document an assessment of discernible behavior changes following unusual environmental events. The PTSD may be applied to acute or delayed patterns, and in addition to disasters, it is appropriate for use following individual trauma such as rape or an automobile accident. The PTSD shows promise for providing a baseline measurement in medical settings for psychological effects following disasters. Whether the criterion behaviors of the PTSD are to be considered pathologic (as are other disorders in the DSM-III) or a normal reaction remains to be determined by future use.

Structured Interviews

Structured interviews and questionnaires were the procedures most frequently chosen by sociological investigators in the decades of the innovative research begun in the 1950s and sponsored by the National Research Council (cf. Barton, 1970). These methods are still used frequently to assess family and community responses (e.g., Bolin and Bolton, 1980), and their utility has been increased by more sophisticated designs and the repeated use across different incidents by the same investigators. As used in sociological research, structured interviews are usually not subjected to an analysis of their psychometric properties. Interpretation of the results, therefore, requires faith on the part of the reader that the interviews have been reliable and valid. Put another way, the use of structured interviews demands technical skills on the part of those who use them that are more demanding than the skills required by the users of checklists and other standardized instruments.

A variation on the structured interview has been used successfully to make clinical-type assessments of mental health status in survivor populations. These include the SADS, the Gurin Checklist, and the Health Opinion Survey, all of which are discussed in the following list of specific measures. Many of these measures have been assessed for their reliability and validity, and usually will yield either a yes–no decision on the presence of psychopathology or a total score that can be used for quantitative comparison.

QUESTIONNAIRES

A questionnaire provides the most straightforward method of self-report. The replies of respondents are accepted as a literal and honest depiction of their response to an event, and the questions are framed so that the intent of the investigator is quite obvious ("How upset were you about TMI?"). Questionnaires have been used in sociological studies to obtain information on social and interpersonal behaviors of disaster victims. These include communication patterns, affiliation, disaster-related behaviors (cleanup, rescue), giving and receiving aid, and so on (Barton, 1970). The questionnaire method has been extended into the more subjective areas of attitudes about disaster situations and symptom descriptions (e.g., see Bromet et al., 1980; Dohrenwend et al., 1979; Houts et al., 1980, 1981). It may be speculated with some logic that such findings, based on questionnaires, about subjective topics are less reliable than those with reference to interpersonal and social behaviors. The difficulty with questionnaires for assessment of psychological effects is that they require honest self-description (Cronbach, 1970), with a minimum response set toward social desirability. If there are strong feelings in the disaster population about organizations perceived as causing the disaster, as is often the case in man-made and technological incidents (Erikson, 1976; Melick et al., 1982) then the responses to questionnaires may be highly reactive to the phenomena under study. Reactivity is a source of error in measurement related to bias, and is caused when the measurement process itself slants a respondent's answers one way or another (Campbell and Stanley, 1963).

Performance Measures
Performance measures refer to standardized performance tests which are highly sensitive to a subject's ability to perform certain tasks, often ones related to concentration, rigidity, and ability to stay on track in spite of minor stress. The first use of such tests appears to have been made by Hurst (1980), and different tests were later employed by the Uniformed Services University Research group (Baum et al., 1981; Baum et al., 1982; Collins et al., 1983).

Psychophysiologic Measures
The same two sets of investigators using performance measures also employed psychophysiological measures of stress with disaster populations. Hurst (1980) used the palmar sweat technique and Baum et al. (1981, 1982) and Collins et al. (1982) made use of the extensive research on catecholamine levels in urine as a measure of stress. As interpreted by the transactional model in Figure 2.1, such measures are process measures of response to stress, that is, they have little clinical significance for outcomes per se but are valuable for testing for the existence of stress at a different level (somatic) of measurement.

Psychosocial Indicators
Psychosocial indicators are measures that reflect outcomes of the psychological effects of disasters at the population level of measurement. Data routinely collected on illness, admissions, accidents, crime, absences from school or work, purchases of medication or alcohol, rates of suicide, divorce and homocide, and the like have the potential for reflecting altered patterns of stress in a disaster population. There are clear advantages to this method of assessment. First, data on these behaviors are routinely collected and thus enable periodic comparisons. Second, psychosocial indicators may be obtained from a carefully defined comparison group. Third, these measures are unobtrusive; that is, they can be gathered without people knowing that the observations are being taken. Fourth, results from a psychosocial measure are not

contaminated by bias or reactivity in the measurement process (as might be true of questionnaires or structured interviews). There are shortcomings, as well, to this approach. Archival data varies in its accuracy and availability. There are also normal, seasonal, or yearly data fluctuations, which must be controlled statistically for accuracy in interpretation.

MEASURES USED WITH DISASTER POPULATIONS

The preponderance of research on the psychological aftermath of disasters has employed a survey method (sometimes by telephone) and a questionnaire or self-report technique. Hurst (1980) appears to have been the only investigator to experimentally manipulate variables in research with a disaster population. The following list of instruments that have previously been employed in disaster research is offered to expedite the investigator's search for an appropriate measuring tool. It is not possible to provide more than a cursory examination of these measures, and most of the single-purpose questionnaires designed for one-time use have been omitted. It is hoped that the awareness of previous utilization of specific measures will lead to replication studies and an accumulation of knowledge so that base-rate information will become available for comparison of specific events.

Clinically Oriented Scales, Checklists, and Interviews

The *Symptom Checklist-90 (SCL-90)* is a 90-item self-report symptom inventory designed to reflect the psychological symptom patterns of psychiatric and medical patients, and is a measure of current, point-in-time psychological symptom status (Derogatis, 1977; Derogatis et al., 1976). It is not a measure of personality or of past psychiatric history. A 56-item short form is also available. Nine scales can be calculated for both versions (e.g., somatization, obsessive-compulsive, depression, anxiety) as well as three global indexes, including a Global Severity Index. Items appear as brief phrases which are rated for intensity on a five-point scale. Administration time is typically 15 to 20 minutes, and although the SCL-90 has been used with a number of groups, the primary standardization groups are psychiatric and medical patients. Test-retest reliabilities for individual symptom dimensions (scales) range from 0.78 to 0.90. The manual reports no significant practice effect with repeated administrations. The standardized frame of reference for the respondent is "the last 7 days including today," but the measure may be used without distortion for upward to 2 weeks. Gleser et al. (1981) used an early form of the SCL-90 in the Buffalo Creek studies. Murphy (1981, 1984, and Chapter 3) used the Depression and Somatization Scales of the Symptom Checklist-90-R. The SCL-90 proved to be sensitive to differences between samples from the TMI population and comparison groups (Bromet et al., 1980; Collins et al., 1983). Hartsough and Papperman (in preparation) used the short form to test for flood–non-flood differences following the severe flooding of Fort Wayne, Indiana.

The *Langner Index of Psychological Distress* is a 22-item screening score developed during the Midtown Manhattan study. Unlike the SCL-90, which appears to be sensitive to subclinical levels of psychopathology, the Langner appears most suitable for detecting more severe psychopathology. It is a screening instrument, meant for "mass surveys of large populations" (Langner, 1962, p. 270). Its items were drawn principally from the Minnesota Multiphasic Personality Inventory (MMPI); nearly half of them relate to physical or somatic symptoms. The scale was validated through comparisons of patients with known psychiatric diagnoses from persons known to be well. The scale was used by Houts et al. (1980, 1981) in TMI research.

The *Gurin Symptom Checklist* is an anxiety and psychosomatic checklist with items drawn from community-wide surveys, and it serves the purpose of eliciting symptom patterns from normal populations (Gurin et al., 1960). Items selected for the Gurin Symptom Checklist were those that discriminated previous survey respondents diagnosed as having psychological problems from those diagnosed as having no problems. In its development research, the Gurin produced four factors: psychological anxiety, physical health, immobilization, and physical anxiety. (The physical health factor had only two items.) This scale was used by Melick (1978) to test for differences in emotional health between flood and nonflood subgroups.

The *Health Opinion Survey* appears to have been a forerunner of the Gurin Symptom Checklist (Christensen, 1981), and is described by MacMillan (1957) as a short inventory of psychoneurotic indicators, developed as a population screening test. It uses a three-point rating scale and is not a tool for individual diagnostic assessment. It was validated by MacMillan against the results of clinical interviews but may also reflect the presence of poor physical health (Tousignant et al., 1970). The Health Opinion Survey was utilized by Murphy (1977) in a study of war stresses on Vietnamese civilians.

The *General Health Questionnaire* (Goldberg, 1972) was developed as a 140-item measure to test for current and emotional reactions related to psychiatric disturbance. Shorter versions of 12 to 60 items exclude physical illness content. A 30-item questionnaire was used by Parker (1977) to test for psychiatric disturbance after evacuation from

Cyclone Tracy and at two follow-ups. A score of 5 or more on this version was taken as strongly suggestive of psychiatric disturbance. Originally standardized in Great Britian, the measure has also been used in Australia (Andrews et al., 1978; Andrews et al., 1975). The measure is a screening instrument for community surveys and case identification, but not a diagnostic tool. Item content is related to non-psychcotic psychiatric illness.

The *Schedule of Affective Disorders and Schizophrenia* (Endicott and Spitzer, 1978) was "designed to elicit information necessary for making diagnosis using the Research Diagnostic Criteria as well as to describe the subjects' symptoms and levels of functioning" (p. 837). The Research Diagnostic Criteria were developed by Spitzer et al. (1978) to provide consistency in the criteria that research investigators used for the description or selection of subjects with functional psychiatric illnesses. The SADS uses an interview format and takes $1\frac{1}{2}$ to 2 hours for completion. Interviewers should be experienced in making diagnoses of psychopathology. There are several versions of the SADS, including one which assesses current functioning in the week prior to the interview, with emphasis on a current illness episode; and a more general version which evaluates functioning over one's lifetime. Bromet et al. (1980) used a modified lifetime version of the Schedule of Affective Disorders and Schizophrenia-Lifetime (SADS-L) for an assessment of a respondent's mental health history. The SADS appears to be a valuable but time-consuming procedure for providing a clinical assessment of victims of disaster research. Its advantage over a conventional, nonstandardized, clinical assessment interview is that it reduces error variance for the information gathered through a structured interview format. It also reduces criterion variance with the use of a common standard for all assessments.

The *Psychiatric Evaluation Form (PEF)* appears to have been an earlier form of the SADS and is described by Endicott and Spitzer (1972) and Spitzer et al. (1968) as a comprehensive instrument, with 20 scales, including one on Overall Severity. Gleser et al. (1981) found an advantage in its flexibility and used the PEF for quantifying clinical interview data for Buffalo Creek flood victims. They used five scales: alcohol abuse, overall severity, anxiety, depression, and belligerence.

Impact of Event Measures

The *Schedule of Recent Experience (SRE)* (Hawkins et al., 1957), the *Social Readjustment Rating Scale (SRRS)* (Holmes and Rahe, 1967), and many later models and variations are the primary means of measuring stressors as independent of their effects. In most versions of life events questionnaires the respondent indicates the presence or intensity of an event within a specified period in the immediate past. A typical time window is 12 or 18 months. The events to be rated having previously been graded for their change-causing value, a total score for life change units (LCU) is calculated for each respondent. Life change and illness susceptibility (Holmes and Masuda, 1974) has been the focus of most of the life events research; for a comprehensive review see Christensen (1981). Critics have pointed out the confounding of life event items with illness outcomes and other methodological problems of the earlier questionnaires (Christensen, 1981). None of the questionnaires has item content directly related to disasters, but Melick (1978) used the SRE to study flood victims. She found LCU scores higher for a flood group shortly following the flood and returning to normal later; the scores were also positively related to the number of illnesses reported. The measures have been used with a wide range of patient and normal populations.

The *Life Experience Survey (LES)* was designed by Sarason et al. (1978) to compensate for some of the measurement deficiencies of the SRE and the SRRS. The LES is a 47-item self-report measure of stressful life events. Unlike its predecessors, it permits a rating of intensity of impact and the positive or negative quality of events rated. It is reported to have stable test-retest scores over 6 weeks and no significant correlations between positive and negative scores. The LES has been used by Murphy (1981, 1984, and Chapter 3) and Hartsough and Papperman (in preparation) in psychological effects research.

The *Impact Event Scale* is a self-report instrument "that measures the current degree of subjective impact experienced as a result of a specific event" (Horowitz et al., 1979). Unlike the impact measures discussed above, it *does* measure stress by its effects and is clinically oriented due to the intrapersonal set of item content. Items were derived from clinic work and research around concepts related to the stress response syndrome of Horowitz (1976), although details regarding item selection are not available. The revised scale of 15 items reflects a focus on symptom clusters essential to the Horowitz stress response syndrome and labeled intrusion (7 items) and avoidance (8 items). Respondents rate reactions such as, "I had dreams about it," and "I tried to remove it from memory," on a four-point frequency scale and a three-point intensity scale. Respondents rate themselves with reference to a specific event happening anytime in their past; the typical *effects* time-window is within the last week. The test-retest reliabilities of the total scale (0.87) and the subscales (intrusion, 0.89; avoidance, 0.79) indicate high stability of response. Some standardization data are presented by Horowitz et al. (1979) and Zilberg et al. (1982). There appear to be some psychometric problems; for example, an extremely high response frequency suggests a positive response bias to be operating with this scale. This scale has been used mostly in a clinical setting and there is no evidence of use for a disaster population, although this would be a natural extension in its development (Horowitz et al., 1980; Zilberg et al., 1982).

The *Disaster Impact Scale* was developed by Western and Milne (1976) with the apparent purpose of assessing effects directly related to a disaster agent, Cyclone Tracy. The measure was one of five questionnaires used by Milne (1977), and four variables—psychological stress, physical injury, loss of possessions, and damage to dwellings—were summed to create the Disaster Impact Scale. No psychometric properties of the questionnaire were reported. The scale should be considered experimental.

The *Disaster Stress Reaction Assessment* is another experimental device, reported by Demi and Miles (1983). This inventory reflects directly the wording of the PTSD, and is intended to be an efficient means of analyzing criteria for this diagnosis. Three questions qualify the event and further questions relate to symptoms indicative of reactions to disasters. No data or theoretical foundations are provided by the authors, nor has its use with a disaster population been reported.

The *Hassles Scale* was developed by Lazarus and Cohen (1977) to focus on stressors and psychological effects of apparently less intensity than typical items for the LES, SRE, and SRRS. The Hassles Scale is experimental, an 117-item inventory that ranges from minor item content (filling out forms) to moderately intense personal problems (sexual problems without a physical basis). Three-point persistence and irritability rating scales are provided for the respondent. The scale was used by Murphy in her work following the disaster at Mount St. Helens.

Special Purpose Measures

The categorization of the above measures is only approximate; the measures in this category seemed to reflect more specialized interest, but they may have characteristics related to those already described.

The *Demoralization Scale* (Link and Dohrenwend, 1980) is a 26-item inventory which describes the psychological symptoms and reactions likely to be developed when a person cannot meet environmental demands but also cannot extricate himself or herself from the predicament. Items are rated on a 5-point scale for content such as helplessness, trouble in concentrating, frightening dreams, poor appetite, and so on. Internal consistency is reported to be above 0.90 and the scale has been used with patients from mental health centers. According to the authors, scores can reflect psychiatric disorder, but also a pattern of attitudes and symptoms that may be separate from psychiatric illness. The scale was altered by Dohrenwend et al. (1979) for use with the population surrounding TMI, and reflected sharp increases in demoralization following the accident.

The *Ways of Coping Inventory* (Aldwin et al., 1980) is "a checklist of 68 items describing a broad range of behavioral and cognitive coping strategies that an individual might use in a specific stressful episode" (Folkman and Lazarus, 1980, p. 224). Items are drawn from the domains of defensive coping, information seeking, problem solving, palliation, inhibition of action, direct action, and magical thinking. The scale is based upon theoretical formulations of Lazarus and his colleagues that coping refers to both overt and intrapsychic behavior that has the goal of preventing, avoiding, or controlling a source of stress (Lazarus, 1966). The bidirectional view of coping is reflected in the revised ways of coping inventory, which contains a 24-item problem-focused subscale and a 40-item emotion-focused subscale. This measure was utilized by Collins et al. (1983) in association with both physiologic and performance measures of stress on a TMI population. The investigators created two new "highly exploratory" scales of denial (four items) and reappraisal (five items).

The *Sleep Disruption Questionnaire* is a research-oriented tool described by Karacan, et al. (1973) which inquires about the recurrence of problems in the area of sleep, including nightmares, early awakening, insomnia, and medication taking. This instrument was used by Gleser et al., (1981) at Buffalo Creek.

The *Self-Anchoring Scale (SAS)* does not describe psychological effects directly but is used as a measure of the respondent's perception of his or her life situation, and can be used to compare current with former living conditions, and those expected in the future. This measure was developed by a social psychologist (Cantril, 1965) and has been widely used in international research. It is taken to indicate individuals' attitudes and opinions about the best possible circumstances that could characterize their lives at various specified times. Self-defined anchor points are used in conjunction with a 10-point rating scale. The SAS is a brief survey instrument that was used by Murphy (1977) on studies of civilian Vietnamese refugees.

The *Tedium Questionnaire* is an experimental measure of 21 items created by Kanner et al. (1978). The authors see as one source of stress the absence of positive conditions, and propose the concept of tedium as reflecting physical, emotional and attitudinal exhaustion. The Tedium Questionnaire was designed to reflect an individual's appraisal of these three aspects of tedium. Test-retest reliability is reported as 0.89 and research by the authors indicates that the negative features and lack of positive features are unrelated to each other in studies of students and professionals. This measure has not been employed by the investigators of disaster effects, but shows promise for detecting some of the strain effects produced by extended disaster work (see Fig. 2.1).

The *Subjective Stress Scale* is an experimental measure designed to reflect the degree of felt stress (Kerle and Bialek, 1958). The scale was used by Anderson (1976) to study 93 randomly selected business-men from a sample of 432 who had sustained business losses following a flood. Apparently used as an interview questionnaire, Kendall's co-efficient was 0.58 for six of the eight questions used.

The *Affect Rating Scale* (Sipprelle et al., 1981) employs 30 adjec-tives in a Likert-scale format for respondents to indicate how they feel at that moment in time. A seven-point scale is employed, and four uni-polar dimensions have been found—potent positive, potent negative, weak positive, weak negative, and a fifth general factor, relaxation. This scale has the potential for assessment of transitory changes in affec-tive experience. It was used by Hurst (1980) to assess the impact of viewing tornado stimulus material on tornado victims and their non-victim counterparts in a disaster community.

Psychophysiologic Measures

Physiological measures of stress have been applied to populations of normals in stress (Baum et al., 1982; Rose et al., 1979), but have been underutilized in disaster research.

The *Palmar Sweat Sampling Procedure* (Strahan et al. 1974) is an experimental technique that was developed with an eye toward use in naturalistic settings. Samples of palmar sweat may be collected with the use of small sterile bottles filled with laboratory quality distilled water. The samples may be later evaluated in the laboratory by use of a Beckman Instruments model RC-16C conductivity bridge. Test-retest reliability indicates stability—for a 1-day interval, 0.84; for a 4-day interval, 0.73; and for alternate hands the range is 0.73 to 0.93. Hurst (1980) employed the palmar sweat technique in a study of tor-nado victims, and by using the measure at the same site on the same hand (before and after experimental manipulation), overcame two ma-jor criticisms of the technique (Venables and Christie, 1973). The pro-cedure would still be considered experimental for disaster populations (Fowles and Venables, 1970).

The assessment of *catecholamine levels in urine* (Frankenhaeuser et al., 1968) is another technique for measuring stress that allows for collection of samples in a naturalistic setting. Samples are collected for carefully controlled time periods in order to offset diurnal fluctuations in catecholamine levels. The purpose of this technique is to estimate sympathetic arousal by means of estimating adrenal medulary activity. This is done by measuring epinephrine and norepinephrine levels; since the proportion of epinephrine and norepinephrine in secreted catecholamines is relatively constant and since catecholamine excretion is a good index of adrenal activity, a measure of these secretions is an estimate of stress. Collins et al. (1983) used this technique with success on a TMI population, finding that norepinephrine measures were more sensitive than epinephrine measures. Like the palmar sweat technique, measurement and health consequences for different levels of catecholamine excretion have not been clearly established.

Performance Measures

A *proofreading task* (Glass and Singer, 1972) was used by Collins et al. (1983) for the TMI research. This task requires proofreading for errors of various sorts from seven typed pages taken from a book on American cities. Because of the unique and specific nature of the skill required in this task, the user should be alert for variables other than the concentration abilities presumably related to stress levels.

An *Embedded Figures Task* (Witkin, et al., 1979) was used by Collins et al. (1983) to assess concentration and motivation deficits related to stress. Subjects were asked to locate the hidden target figure embedded in a more complex geometric figure. The authors did not provide a rationale for the use of this performance test. Presumably the stress to be detected was situational, yet Witkin and his colleagues implied that the ability to separate part of an organized field from the field as a whole relates to consistent individual differences between an articulated versus a global field cognitive approach.

The *Flanagan Aptitude Classification Test* is a standard instrument in industrial settings (Buros, 1978). Hurst (1980) used 75 items from the Coding subtest and the Memory subtest in his work with the Monticello tornado victims. The measure is a standard test of concentration and short-term memory.

Psychosocial Measures

Mileti et al. (1982) used archival data on alcohol sales, cardiovascular deaths, criminal arrests, psychiatric admissions, suicides, and automobile accidents to compare TMI residents with those in comparison communities for evidence of illness and role dysfunction that would indicate stress in the TMI population. Taylor (1976) reported the use of data on arrests and alcohol sales in the community of Xenia, Ohio, following the 1974 tornado.

CONCLUSIONS

Study of the psychological effects of disasters appears to be part of a much larger effort to understand the nature of personal crises and their mitigation. Other groups targeted for study and help include those in bereavement, and victims of rape or assault. This larger movement is significant for several reasons. It is cross-disciplinary, with the potential for cross-fertilization from findings and perspectives originating in different theoretical frameworks, but also providing a challenge to professional and scientific communication. Second, it underscores the assumption that disorganized behavior and negative affective states can be precipitated in a healthy, well-functioning personality. The pendulum has swung away from the search for predisposing personality influences on traumatic effects. While a situational perspective is highly desirable as a basis for short-term therapeutic interventions, such as crisis intervention, the theoretical issue remains. How do traumatic experiences and personality interact, both in terms of effects and coping? Third, the study of trauma and disaster for its psychological effects has generated a keen interest in mitigative factors, such as social support networks. It is this area of study that offers the most hope for ways of altering psychological effects. The stress that stems directly from experiencing a large-scale community disaster is, for all practical purposes, unpreventable. On the other hand, stresses from postevent sources may be decreased through a variety of social and professional interventions.

Measurement of disaster effects appears finally to have attracted the interest of psychologists and others with commitments to a more refined measurement strategy. The design and methods of disaster effects research employed since 1975 have generally been more efficient and effective than those used previously. Many possibilities exist, however, for new instruments to be used in the future (cf. Derogatis, 1982; Reichelt, 1983). The use of multiple approaches for measuring the same construct (e.g., stress), the careful selection of victim and comparison groups, and the use of measures with a behavioral referent are the means suggested by this report for enhancing measurement of psychological effects.

REFERENCES

Aiken, L.R. Psychological Testing and Assessment (2nd ed.). Boston: Allyn and
    Bacon, 1976.
Aldwin, C., Folkman, S., Coyne, J.C., et al. The Ways of Coping: A Process

Measure. Paper presented at the American Psychological Association, Montreal, September, 1980.

Allport, G.W. Personality: A Psychological Interpretation. New York: Holt, Rinehart, & Winston, 1937.

Anderson, C. Coping behaviors as intervening mechanisms in the inverted-U stress-performance relationship. Journal of Applied Psychology, 1976, *61*, 30–34.

Andrews, G., Tennant, C., Hewson, D.M., Vaillant, G.E. Life event stress, social support, coping style, and risk of psychological impairment. Journal of Nervous and Mental Disease, 1978, *166*, 307–316.

Andrews, G., Tennant, C., Schonell, M., et al. An Approach to Measuring the Health of an Urban Population. Human Communications Laboratory, University of New South Wales, 1975.

Barton, A.H. Communities in Disaster. New York: Doubleday, 1970.

Baum, A., Gatchel, R.J., Fleming, R., Lake, C.R. Chronic and Acute Stress Associated with the Three Mile Island Accident and Decontamination: Preliminary Findings of a Longitudinal Study. Technical report submitted to the U.S. Nuclear Regulatory Commission, 1981.

Baum, A., Grunberg, N.E., Singer, J.E. The use of psychological and neuroendocrinological measurements in the study of stress. Health Psychology, 1982, *3*, 217–236.

Beach, H.D., Lucas, R.A. Individual and group behavior in a coal mine disaster. National Research Council, Disaster Research Group, (13, Publication No. 834), 1960.

Berren, M.R., Biegel, A., Ghertner, S. A typology for the classification of disaster. Community Mental Journal, 1980, *3*, 454–458.

Bolin, R.C., Long-term Family Recovery From Disaster. Monograph No. 36. Boulder, Colo.: Institute of Behavioral Sciences, 1982.

Bolin, R.C., Bolton, P.A. Family Recovery from Natural Disaster: A Comparison of Nicaraguan and United States Families. Paper presented at XVIIIth International Seminar of the Committee on Family Research, Roserberg Castle, Sweden, June, 1980.

Bolin, R.C., Trainer, P. Modes of family recovery following disaster: A cross-validational study. In E.L. Quarantelli (Ed.), Disasters: Theory and Research. Beverly Hills, Calif.: Sage Publications, 1978.

Bromet, E., Parkinson, D., Schulberg, H.C., et al. Three Mile Island: Mental Health Findings. Washington, D.C.: National Institute of Mental Health, 1980.

Bromet, E., Schulberg, H.C., Dunn, L. Reactions of psychiatric patients to the Three Mile Island nuclear accident. Archives of General Psychiatry, 1982, *39*, 725–730.

Buros, O.K. (Ed.) The Eighth Mental Measurement Yearbook. Highland Park, N.J.: Gryphon Press, 1978.

Campbell, D.T., Stanley, J.C. Experimental and Quasi-Experimental Designs for research. Chicago: Rand McNally, 1963.

Cantril, H. The Pattern of Human Concerns. New Brunswick, N.J.: Rutgers University Press, 1965.

Christensen, J.F. Assessment of stress: Environmental, intrapersonal, and outcome issues. In P. McReynolds (Ed.), Advances in Psychological Assessment. San Francisco: Jossey-Bass, 1981.

Church, J.S. The Buffalo Creek disaster: Extent and range of emotional and behavioral problems. Omega: The Journal of Death and Dying, 1974, 5, 61-63.

Cohen R.E., Ahearn, F.L., Jr. Handbook for Mental Health Care of Disaster Victims. Baltimore: Johns Hopkins University Press, 1980.

Collins, D.L., Baum, A., Singer, J.E. Coping with chronic stress at Three Mile Island: Psychological and biochemical evidence. Health Psychology, 1983, 2, 149-176.

Cook, T.D., Campbell, D.T. Quasi-Experimentation: Design and Analysis Issues for Field Experimentation. Chicago: Rand McNally, 1979.

Cronbach, L.J. Essentials of Psychological Testing (3rd ed.). New York: Harper & Row Pub., 1970.

Demi, A.S., Miles, M.S. Understanding psychologic reactions to disaster. Journal of Emergency Nursing, 1983, 9, 11-16.

Derogatis, L.R. SCL-90: Administration, Scoring and Procedures Manual-I for the Revised Version and Other Instruments of the Psychopathology Rating Scale Series. Baltimore: John Hopkins University School of Medicine, Clinical Psychometrics Unit, 1977.

Derogatis, L.R. Self-report measures of stress. In L. Goldberger, S. Breznitz (Eds.), Handbook of Stress: Theoretical and Clinical Aspects. New York: Free Press, 1982.

Derogatis, L.R., Lipman, R., Rickels, K., et al. The Hopkins Symptom Checklist (HSCL): A measure of primary symptom dimensions. Modern Problems in Pharmacopsychiatry, 1978, 7, 79-110.

Derogatis, L.R., Rickels, K., Rock, A.F. The SCL-90 and the MMPI: A step in the validation of a new self-report scale. British Journal of Psychiatry, 1976, 128, 280-289.

Diagnostic and Statistical Manual for Mental Disorders (3rd Ed.). Washington, D.C.: American Psychiatric Association, 1980.

Dohrenwend, B.P., Dohrenwend, B.S., Kasl, S.V., Warheit, G.J. Technical staff analysis report on behavioral affects to President's Commission on the Accident at Three Mile Island. Washington, D.C.: President's Commission on the Accident at Three Mile Island, 1979.

Endicott, J., Spitzer, R.L. What! Another rating scale? The psychiatric evaluation form. Journal of Nervous and Mental Disease, 1972, 154, 88-104.

Endicott, J., Spitzer, R.L. A diagnostic interview: The schedule for affective disorders and schizophrenia. Archives of General Psychiatry, 1978, 35, 837-844.

Erikson, K.T. Everything in Its Path: Destruction of Community in the Buffalo Creek Flood. New York: Simon & Schuster, 1976.

Flynn, C.B., Chalmers, J.A. The Social and Economic Effects of the Accident at Three Mile Island. Washington, D.C.: Office of Nuclear Regulatory Research, U.S. Nuclear Regulatory Commission, 1980.

Folkman, S., Lazarus, R.S. An analysis of coping in a middle-aged community sample. Journal of Health and Social Behavior, 1980, *21*, 219-239.

Fowles, D.C., Venables, P.H. The effects of epidermal hydration and sodium reabsorbtion on palmar skin potential. Psychological Bulletin, 1970, *73*, 363-378.

Frankenhaeuser, M., Mellis, I., Rissler, A., et al: Catecholamine excretion as related to cognitive and emotional reaction patterns. Psychosomatic Medicine, 1968, *39*, 109-120.

Glass, C.C., Singer, J.E. Urban Stress. New York: Academic Press, 1972.

Gleser, G.C., Green, B.L., Winget, C. Prolonged Psychosocial Effects of Disaster: A Study of Buffalo Creek. New York: Academic Press, 1981.

Goldberg, D.P. The Detection of Psychiatric Illness. London: Oxford University Press, 1972.

Gurin, G., Veroff, J., Field, S. Americans View Their Mental Health. New York: Basic Books, 1960.

Hartsough, D.M. Planning for disaster: A new community outreach program for mental health centers. Journal of Community Psychology, 1982, *10*, 255-264.

Hartsough, D.M., Papperman, T.J. Psychological Effects of Exposure to Urban Floods. In preparation.

Hartsough, D.M., Savitsky, J.C. Three Mile Island: Psychology and Environmental Policy at a Cross-roads. American Psychologist. In press.

Hawkins, N.G., Davies, R., Holmes, T.H. Evidence of psychosocial factors in the development of pulmonary tuberculosis. American Review of Tuberculosis and Pulmonary Disease, 1957, *75*, 768-780.

Helmstadter, G.C. Principles of Psychological Measurement. New York: Appleton-Century-Crofts, 1964.

Holmes, T.H., Masuda, M. Life change and illness susceptibility. In B.S. Dohrenwend and B.P. Dohrenwend (Eds.), Stressful Life Events: Their Nature and Effects. New York: Wiley, 1974.

Holmes, T.H., Rahe, R.H. The Social Readjustment Rating Scale. Journal of Psychosomatic Research, 1967, *11*, 213-218.

Horowitz, M. Stress Response Syndromes. New York: Aronson, 1976.

Horowitz, M., Wilner, N., Alvarez, W. Impact of event scale: A measure of subjective stress. Psychosomatic Medicine, 1979, *41*, 209-218.

Horowitz, M.J., Wilner, N., Kaltreider, N. Signs and symptoms of post-traumatic stress disorder. Archives of General Psychiatry, 1980, *37*, 85-92.

Houts, P.S., Miller, R.W., Tokuhata, G.K., Hamm, K.S. Health-related behavioral impact of the Three Mile Island Nuclear Accident: Part I (April, 1980) Part II (November, 1980), and Part III (May, 1981). Report to the TMI Advisory Panel of Health Research Studies, Pennsylvania Department of Health. Hershey, Penn.: Pennsylvania State University College of Medicine, 1970, 1981.

Hurst, J.L. Psychological effects of exposure to natural disaster. Unpublished dissertation. West Lafayette, Ind.: Purdue University, 1980.

Kanner, A.D., Kafry, D., Pines, A. Conspicuous in its absence: The lack of positive conditions as a source of stress. Journal of Human Stress, 1978, *4*, 33-39.

Karacan, I., Warheit, G.J., Thornby, J.I., et al. Prevalence of sleep disturbance in the general population. In M.H. Chase et al. (Eds.), Sleep Research (Vol. 2). Los Angeles: University of California, Brain Information Service, 1973.

Kerle, H.H., Bialek, H.M. Construction, Validation and Application of a Subjective Stress Scale (staff memorandum). Monterey, Calif.: Presidio of Monterey, U.S. Army Leadership Unit, 1958.

Kinston, W., Rosser, R. Disaster: Effects on mental and physical state. Journal of Psychosomatic Research, 1974, 18, 437–456.

Langner, T.S. A 22-item screening score of psychiatric symptoms indicating impairment. Journal of Health and Human Behavior, 1962, 3, 269–276.

Lazarus, R.S. Psychological Stress and the Coping Process. New York: McGraw-Hill, 1966.

Lazarus, R.S., Cohen, J. The Hassles Scale. Stress and coping project. Berkeley, Calif.: University of California, 1977.

Lifton, R.J. Survivors of Hiroshima: Death in Life. New York: Random House, 1967.

Lindy, J.D., Grace, M.C., Green, B.L. Survivors: Outreach to a reluctant population. American Journal of Orthopsychiatry, 1981, 51, 468–478.

Link, B., Dohrenwend, B.P. Formulation of hypotheses about the true prevalence of demoralization in the United States. In B.P. Dohrenwend, M.S. Gould, B. Link, R. Neugubauer, R. Wunsch-Hitzig, (Eds.), Mental Illness in the United States: Epidemiological Estimates. New York: Praeger, 1980.

MacMillan, A.M. The health opinion survey: Techniques for estimating prevalence of psychoneurotic and related types of disorder in communities. Psychological Reports, 1957, 3, 325–339.

McDonald, M.J. Post-traumatic stress disorder: A study of training materials for diagnosis. Unpublished Masters thesis. West Lafayette, Ind.: Purdue University, 1981.

Mechanic, D. Discussion of research programs on relations between stressful life events and episodes of physical illness. In B.S. Dohrenwend, B.P. Dohrenwend (Eds.), Stressful Life Events: Their Nature and Effects. New York: Wiley, 1974.

Melick, M.E. Life change and illness: Illness behavior of males in the recovery period of a natural disaster. Journal of Health and Social Behavior, 1978, 19, 335–342.

Melick, M.E., Logue, J.N., Frederick, C.J. Stress and disaster. In L. Goldberger, S. Breznitz (Eds.), Handbook of Stress: Theoretical and Clinical Aspects. New York: The Free Press, 1982.

Mileti, D.S., Hartsough, D.M., Madson, P. The Three Mile Island Incident: A Study of Behavioral Indicators of Human Stress. A report prepared for Shaw, Pittman, Potts, and Trowbridge, Washington, D.C., 1982.

Milne, G. Cyclone Tracy: I. Some consequences of the evacuation for adult victims. Australian Psychologist, 1977, 12, 39–54.

Moos, R.F. Psychological techniques in the assessment of adaptive behavior. In G.V. Coelho et al. (Eds.), Coping and Adaptation. New York: Basic Books, 1974.

Murphy, J.M. War stresses and civilian Vietnamese: A study of psychological effects. Acta Psychiatrica Scandinavica, 1977, 56, 92–108.

Murphy, S.A. Coping with stress following a natural disaster: The volcanic eruption of Mount St. Helens. Dissertation Abstracts International, 1981, 42 10B, 4014. (University Microfilms No. 82–07, 736).

Murphy, S.A. Stress levels and health status of victims of a natural disaster. Research in Nursing and Health, 1984, 7, 205–215.

Murphy, S.A., Stewart, B.J. Linked pairs of subjects: A method for increasing the sample size in a study of bereavement. Paper read at Americal Orthopsychiatry Association meeting, San Francisco, April 1982.

Papperman, T.J. Towards a psychology of disasters. Unpublished paper. West Lafayette, Ind.: Purdue University, 1981.

Parker, G. Cyclone Tracy and Darwin evacuees: On restoration of the species. British Journal of Psychiatry, 1977, 130, 548–555.

Perry, R.W., Lindell, M.K. The psychological consequences of natural disaster: A review of research on American communities. Mass Emergencies, 1978, 3, 105–115.

Quarantelli, E.L. The consequences of disasters for mental health: Conflicting views. University of Cincinnati: Taft Lecture Series, 1979.

Quarantelli, E.L., Dynes, R.R. When disaster strikes. New Society, 5–9, 1973.

Reichelt, P.A. Location and utilization of available behavioral measurement instruments. Professional Psychology: Research and Practice, 1983, 14, 341–345.

Report to Congress of the United States by the Comptroller General, "Three Mile Island: The most studied nuclear accident in history." September 1980.

Rose, R.M., Hurst, M.W., Herd, J.A. Cardiovascular and endocrine responses to work and the risk for psychiatric symptomatology among air traffic controllers. In J.E. Barrett et al. (Eds.), Stress and Mental Disorder. New York: Raven Press, 1979.

Sarason, I., Johnson, J., Siegel, J. Assessing the impact of life changes: Development of the life experiences survey. Journal of Consulting and Clinical Psychology, 1978, 46, 932–946.

Silver, R.L., Wortman, C.B. Coping with undesirable life events. In J. Garber, M.E.P. Seligman (Eds.), Human Helplessness: Theory and Applications. New York: Academic Press, 1980.

Sipprelle, R.C., Gilbert, F.S., Ascough, J.C. The Affect Rating Scale: Unipolar semantic space components of affective space. Unpublished manuscript submitted for publication. West Lafayette, Ind.: Purdue University, 1981.

Spitzer, R.L., Endicott, J., Mesnikoff, A.M., Cohen, M.S. The Psychiatric Evaluation Form. New York: Biometrics Research, 1968.

Spitzer, R.L., Endicott, J., Robins, E. Research dignostic criteria: Rationale and reliability. Archives of General Psychiatry, 1978, 35, 773–782.

Stern, G.M. The Buffalo Creek Disaster. New York: Random House, 1976.

Strahan, R.F., Todd, J.B., Inglis, G.B. A palmar sweat measure particularly suited for naturalistic research. Psychophysiology, 1974, 11, 715–720.

Taylor, V. Delivery of Mental Health Services in Disasters: The Xenia Tornado and Some Implications. Columbus, The Ohio State University Disaster Research Center Book and Monograph Series, 1976.

Titchener, J.L., Kapp, F.T. Family and character change at Buffalo Creek American Journal of Psychiatry, 1976, *133*, 295–299.

Tousignant, M., Denis, G., Lachapelle, R. Some considerations concerning the validity and use of the health opinion survey. Journal of Health and Social Behavior, 1970, *15*, 241–252.

Venables P.H., Christie, M.J. Mechanisms, instrumentation, recording techniques, and quantification of responses. In W.F. Prokasy, D.C. Raskin (Eds.), Electrodermal Activity in Psychological Research. New York: Academic Press, 1973.

Western, J.S., Milne, G.G. Some social effects of a natural hazard: Darwin residents and Cyclone Tracy. Paper read at a Symposium of Natural Hazards, Canberra, Australia, May 1976.

Witkins, H.A., Goodenough, D.R., Oltman, D.K. Psychological differentiation: Current status. Journal of Personality and Social Psychology, 1979, *37*, 1127–1145.

Zilberg, N.J., Weiss, D.S., Horowitz, M.J. Impact of events scale: A cross-validation study and some empirical evidence supporting a conceptual model of stress response syndromes. Journal of Consulting and Clinical Psychology, 1982, *50*, 407–414.

3

Designing and Implementing a Disaster Study

Shirley A. Murphy
Mary E. Cowan

Disasters are catastrophic stress events which expose normal populations to life-threatening situations, sudden and disfiguring deaths of relatives and friends, and massive personal and public environmental destruction (Lindy et al., 1981). As emphasized throughout this book, disasters can be conceptualized as a sequence of events over time: warning, threat, impact, inventory, rescue, remedy, and recovery (Powell and Rayner, 1952). It is known from earlier reports that many past disaster studies have focused on the first six events in the time period extending from immediately before the disaster and up to a few weeks following the impact. While it seems reasonable to assume that physical and mental health disturbances might occur during the recovery period well beyond a few weeks postimpact, controversy regarding both the magnitude and extent of health effects in the recovery period still exists.

The major purposes of this chapter are twofold. First is a detailed discussion regarding how a major research project was designed and implemented capturing the unique features of a specific disaster. The information contained in preceding chapters is applied in this process. Second, a description of the methods used to identify disaster victims believed to be "at-risk" will be reported.

DISASTER RECOVERY

Individual and community recovery responses to numerous disasters have been described during the past several decades. Lifton and Olson (1976) identified the "survivor syndrome" among victims of the Buffalo Creek flood 27 months following the disaster in 1972. According to Lifton and Olson and others, the survivor response is characterized by death imprint and anxiety (memories and images associated with dying), death guilt (why did I survive while others died?), psychic numbing (inability to express feelings, apathy, and withdrawal), and impaired human relationships (increased conflict, as well as increased interpersonal sensitivity). In order to recover, individuals must find meaning in the event, that is, an explanation, conviction, or at least resignation, that the event and its effects were unpreventable. Loss of communality, also described by Lifton and Olson (1976), is a breakdown of community structure following a disaster. The combination of suddenness of a disaster, immense destructive power within a limited circumscribed area, isolation, and human callousness in causation, are all factors that contribute to the destruction of a sense of community.

Specifically, the recovery period following a disaster gives rise to numerous additional stressful activities such as grieving, adjusting to temporary if not permanent relocation; cleaning and repairing of property when possible, providing information associated with insurance beneficiary status, and role change to widow and/or single parent (Kinston and Rosser, 1974). Typically, these disruptions extend far beyond the immediate crisis period affecting significant numbers of people. For example, guilt, phobias, sleep disturbances, hostility and rage, anxiety, depression, and cognitive impairment have been reported for many months following disasters (Cohen and Ahearn, 1980; Horowitz, 1976; Singh and Raphael, 1981; Titchener and Kapp, 1976; Wilson, 1972). Having identified some common disaster responses, what then are unique characteristics of a specific disaster?

UNIQUE ASPECTS OF THE MOUNT ST. HELENS DISASTER

In contrast to many past mass emergencies, the Mount St. Helens disaster was characterized by several novel features. The first unique aspect was that the warning period lasted nearly two months and did not appear to be taken seriously. By contrast, the very real threat lasted only a matter of minutes, and the impact was far more devastating than predicted, hampering rescue, remedy, and recovery.

On March 20, 1980, the youngest of the Cascade mountain volcanoes broke a 123-year stillness. A minor earthquake of 4.1 Richter magnitude was recorded; the first sign that an eruptive phase had begun. On both March 27 and 28, over 130 earthquakes were recorded of greater than 3.0 Richter magnitude. Ash and steam eruptions, commonly to elevations of 14,000 feet, could be seen. A large crater was formed, and extensive cracks could be observed in the ice and snow. Activity continued almost daily until April 23, 1980. Roadblocks were set up to limit travel to those living or employed nearby, but enforcement was difficult and met with resistance from homeowners, tourists, and shopkeepers alike. A need for stiffer measures to keep the general public away from the potentially dangerous area was recognized. On April 30, Washington Governor Ray's executive order established two danger zones. Access restrictions varied according to zone: the "red zone" was designated the most dangerous area, while the "blue zone" was defined as the next most dangerous area. Beautiful spring weather on May 17 attracted an onslaught of sightseers, campers, and photographers to the area. Much controversy would later surround the locations of persons who went to the red and blue zones and those who were reluctant to evacuate. Shortly after 8 A.M. on May 18, the "threat" period began, but was to last only a matter of minutes until the impact. At 8:30 A.M. a major earthquake measuring 5.1 on the Richter scale, rumbled through the mountain, causing 11 times the ground motion of the initial March 20th earthquake and releasing more than 30 times as much energy. Volcanic glass, rock, and huge uprooted trees moved downward into the valley at surface speeds nearing 100 miles per hour. Water and soil heated to over 500 °F. Thus rescue efforts were hampered by the lack of visibility, intense heat, and rapid movement of earth, water, buildings, bridges, and road surfaces. More than 200 persons who were working, camping, or sightseeing in the area escaped or were rescued and all but two survived. However, an additional 60 persons died or were reported missing and presumed dead. As would be expected, several hundred residences and farms were destroyed.

Another unique aspect of the disaster was the nature of the losses. Personal loss by death and property loss were mutually exclusive except for two cases known to the authors. Deaths could also be conceptually separated into confirmed dead and presumed dead. The impact of confirmed versus presumptive death on the bereaved was an important issue, not only for conceptual reasons, but also for practical reasons, since both known and presumptive conditions of death commonly occur as a result of accidents, disasters, and in the military. Moreover, the presumptive death status of some victims had serious legal implications for bereaved relatives since Washington state law required a 7-year time lapse before persons presumed dead could be considered officially dead. Permanent residences and recreational or vacation home losses were also mutually exclusive. That is, those persons who lived in the areas where massive property damage occurred, did not own vacation homes in the same area.

A third distinctive feature of the Mount St. Helens disaster was the extensive national, state, and local media coverage it received. The extent to which such coverage would aid or hinder the coping of disaster victims, especially the bereaved, was an issue previously unexplored in a systematic way.

Thus, the volcanic eruption of Mount St. Helens provided some unique research opportunities. First, four levels of what were to become the independent study variable, "loss," were mutually exclusive: confirmed death bereavement, presumptive death bereavement, destruction of permanent residences, and destruction of leisure residences. Second, standardized measures are now available to measure stress, coping, support, and health status, which would become the intervening and outcome variables for the study. Thus, a systematic documentation of the recovery period across varying types of loss could be conducted. It seemed important to take advantage of the opportunity to focus on recovery since, as Melick reports in Chapter 8, research on disaster recovery is lacking.

Next, as plans for the study got underway, it was learned that a number of the victims and/or their bereaved friends and relatives lived in 10 of the United States, and two Canadian provinces. Thus, proximity to the area, an important variable in the Three Mile Island disaster (Bromet and Dunn, 1981) could also be studied.

Finally, we became aware that many of the disaster victims were quite young. It soon was apparent that many high-risk variables were present and we began to wonder whether we could identify high-risk individuals or groups and how the recovery of these persons would vary with the other loss subjects. A secondary data analysis was undertaken by the second author to answer this question. Initially, we believed presumptive death bereavement would be a major distinguishing high-risk feature. Moreover, we thought that both presumed and confirmed death bereavement, both conditions of untimely death described in Chapter 1, would produce higher rates of stress and illness than that experienced by property loss and control subjects. It was also expected that stress and illness would be correlated and that self-efficacy (intrapersonal mastery) and social support (confidantes, friends, and helping professionals) would buffer the effects of stress on illness. The occurrence, then, of a natural event provided an opportunity to design a study in which three major research questions were addressed:

1. Is there a relationship between illness and presumed death of a close relative or friend or confirmed death of a close relative or friend?
2. Do self-efficacy and social supports act to buffer the negative effects of stress on health?

3. What are the perceived effects of the media on coping with loss following a disaster?

In addition to the three formal research questions, data were also gathered on many other variables including anger, blame, satisfaction with financial settlement, geographic proximity to the eruptive area, and perceived recovery status.

The conceptual framework for the study was based on a time trajectory and included a number of relevant concepts discussed in Chapter 1. Weisman's (1973) conceptualization of untimely death proposes three sufficient conditions: premature, unexpected, and violent death. Untimely death was an important reality for those bereaved as a result of the disaster. Bugen's (1977) theory of grief hypothesizes that the more central the relationship between the bereaved and deceased prior to death, and the greater the belief that death was preventable, then the more prolonged and intense the grief response. Again, this concept would be pertinent to disaster bereavement. Other concepts included were concurrent negative life events, daily hassles, the concept of self-efficacy, and theories of social support. The reader is referred to Chapter 1 for an in-depth discussion of theoretical perspectives useful in conceptualizing disaster research, and to Figure 3.1 for a visual perspective.

We would like to point out that the authors were not in the position of having to provide direct services to disaster victims. Neither were we under any time pressures to produce findings for policies or procedures. Conversely, we had sufficient time to review past published disaster studies, to design two studies that focused on the recovery

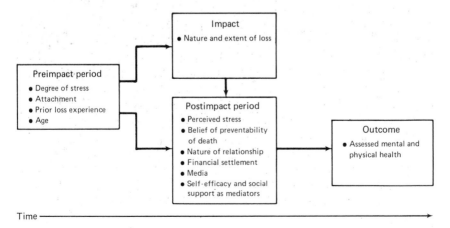

Figure 3.1. Sequence of events in coping with disaster-related loss.

process nearly a year following the disaster at which time we believed the intense grieving period would be ending, and to identify individuals considered to be "at-risk." Our intent is to provide an in-depth description of how we conducted the study and secondary data analysis over an 18-month period. Hartsough's chapter (Chapter 2) on research strategies is suggested for an in-depth discussion of disaster methodologies.

THE RESEARCH DESIGN

A five-group, posttest only, design was selected since the event leading to untimely death or property loss had already occurred.

Sampling Procedures

The Bereaved Groups. Sixty persons were officially listed as dead or missing as a result of the disaster, but only the bereaved relatives and intimate friends of adult disaster victims (N = 51) were included in the study. Persons under 18 years of age were omitted for ethical reasons. Since we knew that the potential pool of bereaved subjects for the study would be small, much effort was invested in obtaining lists of potential study subjects for the bereaved sample groups (See Table 3.1).

One method of locating potential study subjects was by obtaining death certificates for the confirmed dead disaster victims. This was a time-consuming process as some certificates were not available until 8 months after the disaster and some of the certificates could not be obtained at all. The information contained on the death certificates in-

TABLE 3.1. GROUP MEMBERSHIP, SAMPLE, AND RESPONSE RATES

	Potential No. Participants	No. Persons Contacted	No. Participants	% of Potential	% of Those Contacted
Presumed dead bereaved	62	45	39	63	87
Confirmed dead bereaved	40	36	30	75	83
Property loss (permanent residence)	—[a]	39	21	—	54
Property loss (leisure residence)	—[a]	26	15	—	58
Control subjects	—[a]	73	50	—	68
Total	—	219	155	—	71

[a]Data unavailable.

cluded names, addresses, and telephone numbers of the nearest relatives and the victims' employers.

A more difficult task was to reach bereaved relatives of persons presumed dead. Since no predisaster plan of handling deaths had been established, one county sheriff's department was assigned to establish files for confirmed dead victims, while an adjoining county sheriff's department was assigned to obtain information on the presumed dead and missing disaster victims. A list of persons who had testified at court hearings to validate presumptive death of victims of the disaster was finally obtained about 4 months postdisaster. The list included names, addresses, and telephone numbers and in some cases, the relationship to the deceased. All of these persons were not able to be contacted as many had left only local temporary phone numbers, some were no longer at the stated permanent residence, and in some cases, repeated efforts to reach the subjects by telephone were unsuccessful. In other cases, letters were intercepted by the attorneys and estate executors of the bereaved and were neither forwarded nor answered by the interceptor.

Identifying social networks was yet another means used to locate potential study subjects. Organizations, colleagues, and family members were contacted to obtain names of contact persons and possible subjects. Moreover, a local newspaper reporter who had interviewed some of the bereaved family members for a story, willingly shared several names that had not been obtained by other methods.

Since all three sampling sources yielded a small number of potential subjects, and since a number of statistical analyses requiring minimum numbers of cases was desired, two bereaved subjects for each disaster victim were sampled. In the data analysis section later in this chapter we discuss the preliminary statistical testing carried out to justify the use of each subject's scores as independent observations.

In addition to increasing sample size, the linked pairs sampling strategy also provided the opportunity to examine grieving processes based on the nature of the relationship between the deceased and bereaved. That is, the closeness of the relationship between the bereaved and deceased is said to provide useful information for predicting grief responses (Bugen, 1977). Since "close" or important relationships exist between persons who are friends as well as between relatives, one family member and one intimate friend for each disaster victim were selected as subjects. A measure of centrality of the relationship was included in the mailed questionnaire in a section pertaining to specific losses persons had experienced. Only those who ranked the importance of the deceased person at 7 or above on a nine-point scale were included in the study. The actual participants, then, included spouses, parents,

adult children, brothers, sisters, intimate friends, and colleagues of all
but eight of the 51 adult victims of the disaster (31 presumed dead and
20 confirmed dead).

The two bereaved groups consisted largely of females under 40
years of age. Thirty-three percent had completed high school and over
55 percent had some education beyond high school. Of the 55 percent,
17 percent had completed college and 14 percent had obtained advanced
degrees. The majority of bereaved persons were skilled workers (41 percent), 22 percent were self-employed, and 23 percent were professionals.
In terms of proximity to the disaster-damaged area, 9 percent of the
two bereaved groups lived in the immediate area surrounding Mount
St. Helens, 71 percent lived in Washington or the neighboring states
of Oregon and Idaho, and 20 percent lived in eight other U.S. states
and two Canadian provinces. Thus, some bereaved persons were not
directly exposed to the event itself. Rather, they learned of the magnitude of the disaster indirectly by telephone conversations with local
officials, by coming to the area, and through the media.

The Property Loss Groups. The permanent property loss group consisted
of 21 persons or 54 percent of 39 persons contacted whose residences
were in immediate proximity to Mount St. Helens; their residences were
either destroyed or damaged by flooding and massive earth slides along
the Toutle River in southwestern Washington. All 21 persons had to
leave the area at least temporarily, but most had returned to the area
by the time of data collection. Potential subjects' names were randomly selected from local telephone listings.

The recreational property loss group included 15 persons and represented 58 percent of persons randomly selected from a recreational
homeowners list. All of these vacation homes were completely destroyed, but none was occupied the morning of the volcanic eruption.
All 15 subjects owned permanent residences in either Washington or
Oregon.

The Control Group. The 50-member control group was similar to the
105 loss subjects by geographic location, occupation, age, and gender,
and primarily obtained by contacting establishments likely to employ
subjects similar to the loss subjects. For example, if a bereaved study
subject was a news photographer, another news agency of similar size
and circulation was contacted by the investigator to obtain a control
subject who met study criteria. A quota sample of control subjects was
obtained in this manner.

Seventy percent of both the bereaved and control subjects were
women whose mean age was 38.6 years. The property loss groups were

almost equally divided between men and women, and were considerably older (mean age = 48.3 years) than the bereaved and control subjects. All study participants were white. One non-English-speaking subject required an interpreter.

Designation of the Independent and Dependent Variables
Five groups of subjects were compared:

1. Thirty-nine bereaved persons of presumed dead victims known to be in the immediate disaster area, but whose bodies were not found within 7 days following the disaster
2. Thirty bereaved persons of confirmed dead victims whose bodies were found within 7 days
3. Twenty-one persons experiencing disaster-caused property loss of their permanent residences
4. Fifteen persons experiencing disaster-caused property loss of their vacation or leisure residences
5. Fifty persons experiencing no disaster-related loss.

The total number of study participants was 155. These five groups of subjects comprised four levels of the independent variable, "loss" along with the nonvictim comparator group. Dependent variables or outcomes were two measures of stress and three measures of health. Self-efficacy and social support were intervening variables.

Data-Gathering Instruments
The subjects' negative life stress, mental and physical health status, and coping patterns were assessed by the following instruments: The Life Experiences Survey (LES) (Sarason et al., 1978), The Hassles Scale (Lazarus and Cohen, 1977), The Symptom Checklist-90 (SCL-90) (Derogatis et al., 1974), The Self-Efficacy Scale (Coppel, 1980), The Coppel Index of Social Support (Coppel, 1980), and additional items written by the initial investigator (Murphy, 1981, 1982). See Table 3.2 for scoring information.

Stress Measures. The LES (Sarason et al., 1978) is a 47-item self-report measure. Respondents can select events they have experienced over two time periods in the past year and rate events according to positive or negative magnitude of the impact. Measurement of subjects' level of daily annoyances was obtained through the use of the Hassles Scale (Lazarus and Cohen, 1977). The Hassles Scale consists of 117 items which describe the ways in which a person may feel hassled (e.g., filling out forms, troublesome neighbors, worrying about one's health, ap-

TABLE 3.2. SUMMARY OF MAJOR STUDY VARIABLES AND THEIR
MEASUREMENT

Stress Variables	Measurement
Negative life events	The score on the 47-item Life Experiences Survey obtained by the impact rating of events perceived as having a negative effect at one or two designated time periods.
Daily annoyances	The score on the 117-item Hassles Scale obtained by multiplying the irritability rating of hassles by the persistence rating of hassles and summing the products of identified hassles.
	An overall measure of stress was obtained by developing a scale combining the two stress variables. This measure was used in the regression analyses in the second study question.

Outcome Variables	Measurement
Physical health	A six-item health scale was developed to measure physical health status in general.
Mental health	The Depression and Somatization subscales from the SCL-90 were analyzed in addition to the global index as measures of mental health status.
Recovery	An overall measure of perceived disaster recovery was obtained by asking participants to rate their recovery on a 1 to 9 point Likert scale.

Intervening Variables	Measurement
Self-efficacy	A total score on the Coppel Self-Efficacy Index was obtained from a 1 to 5 rating of the 22-item Self-Efficacy Index.
Social support	The quality of perceived supportive behaviors experienced was obtained by a 1 to 5 rating of 15 items on the Coppel Index of Social Support. Quantity of supports was measured size of and contact with persons in participant's social networks.
Symbolic support	An 11-item Media Scale was developed to determine whether the media was perceived as helping, hindering, or having no impact on recovery.

pearance, or employment). Respondents rate each of the 117 items on
three-point persistence and irritability scales.

Health Measures. The SCL-90 (Derogatis et al., 1974) assesses the mental health of subjects. Symptom data were collected on eight dimensions, however, only the depression and somatization scale results are reported here. Items to measure perceived physical health status were written by the investigator and used to form an index of health. Numbers of contacts with health professionals, change in status of a chronic illness, and hospitalization were some of the areas assessed (Murphy, 1981).

Support Measures. The Self-Efficacy Scale is based on Bandura's (1977) conceptualization of one's self-expectations and its relationship to one's ability to affect outcomes. Subjects rate the 22 self-descriptive statements on a five-point scale. Social support was measured by Coppel's Index of Social Support which results in three measures: perceived quality of social support, size of network, and contact with network (Coppel, 1980). Subjects' perceptions of whether the news media was supportive or invasive regarding their loss due to the volcanic eruption were assessed by an 11-item media scale written by the first author (Murphy, 1981).

Additional Items. Finally, four demographic items and 15 items pertaining to factors such as anger, blame, preventability of death, financial settlement, relationship with deceased at the time of death, coping strategies, and recovery from loss were written by the author to assess these variables.

The study instruments were either selected or designed using large numbers of items per measure, due to their generally higher sensitivity for statistical analyses when compared to measures with fewer items. *All* of the instruments were evaluated in terms of internal consistency. Coefficient alpha-reliabilities for our study sample ranged from 0.69 to 0.91. Moreover, the LES, Hassles, and SCL-90 are published instruments.

Data-Gathering Procedures

Letters mailed to potential subjects explained the nature and purpose of the study and assured confidentiality. Written informed consent was obtained from the potential subjects prior to participation. Both mail survey and interview techniques were used. Data were collected by mail primarily during the 11th month following the disaster. Follow-up personal and telephone interviews were conducted with 34 subjects in the bereaved and property loss groups. The interviews followed a standardized, semistructured format and lasted about 60 minutes. Due to the sensitive nature of the study, the lawsuits which were already emerging, and the desire to obtain a high rate of return, extreme care was taken in planning initial and replacement sampling, writing the initial letters, making follow-up phone calls, and conducting interviews to ensure optimum sample size and avoid unnecessary risks.

Data Analysis

A major task in data analyses for this study was to conduct a number
of preliminary analyses. For example, the choice of two bereaved subjects or a "linked pair" for each deceased victim improved the possibility of obtaining a representative sample for statistical analyses. This
sampling method contributed to an 80 percent participation rate. Potential methodological problems such as correlated scores on study measures between the pairs of subjects when independent observations were
desired, were ruled out prior to data analysis. The "linked pairs" sampling strategy and statistical procedures used to guard against inappropriate assumptions from the data is described elsewhere (Murphy,
1981; Murphy and Stewart, in press).

Another area of preliminary analysis consisted of building scales
in order to reduce the number of study variables. For example, an overall Stress Scale was developed by first checking the correlation between
the LES negative score and The Hassles Scale score. Their intercorre-
lation ($r = 0.77$) was high enough to warrant transforming these two
scores into Z scores and then combining them into a single measure
of stress. Likewise, 11 items regarding the media were combined to obtain a Media Scale score, 9 items were combined to form a health index, 4 items were combined to obtain a size of "social network" scale,
and 4 items were combined to obtain a "contact with social network"
scale. In order to construct scales, items were subjected to Pearson
product-moment correlations, factor analysis using the principal components method and Varimax rotation, and computation of coefficient
alpha as an index of internal consistency. Results from these analyses
demonstrate that the scales were adequate for the purposes of this research.

OUTCOMES OF DISASTER LOSS

Among the most significant study findings were that: (1) There was
an absence of statistically significant differences between the bereaved
of presumed and confirmed dead; (2) the death of a significant other
has profound negative stress and health effects on the surviving bereaved, for at least a year following death, (3) high rates of stress were
correlated with high levels of depressive symptoms among both bereaved and permanent property loss groups; (4) the high incidence of
depressive symptoms was accompanied by a low incidence of help-seeking behavior and perceived recovery; (5) there was a significant, but
lower than expected, predictive ability of social supports to buffer the
impact of stress on health; and (6) the media was perceived as a hin-

drance to recovery. Thus, the high rates of stress and illness were expected, but the similarity between the two bereaved groups was not predicted but can be attributed primarily to the time of data collection and sampling factors discussed below. The absence of predicted financial stress due to the legal definition of presumptive death, was an unexpected, positive study outcome.

The First Study Question

Since the Mount St. Helens disaster losses were mutually exclusive, a major study goal was to determine how two conditions of bereavement and two conditions of property loss affected stress, health, support. In general, the findings supported our predictions that high levels of disaster stress would lead to lowered levels of health. However, findings comparing the four magnitudes of loss did not support the entire hierarchical ordering of hypotheses that presumed death bereavement subjects would report the highest levels of stress and illness, that confirmed death bereavement subjects would report second-highest levels of stress and illness, and so forth. That is, no statistically significant differences between presumptive and confirmed death bereavement were reported on any of the five major outcome variables *11 months following the disaster.* However, in keeping with predictions, the confirmed dead bereaved group reported significantly higher scores on depression (t(49) = 2.80, p < 0.05) than permanent property loss subjects.

Data collected regarding the first study question were analyzed by a number of univariate and multivariate statistical procedures. One of the most important was the use of t tests for planned comparisons of means between groups. Results of these procedures support the hypotheses that bereaved subjects differed significantly from controls on outcome variables. That is, three of the four loss groups were significantly affected by the disaster when each group was compared to control subjects. The bereaved of presumed dead reported higher scores than controls on negative life events (t(87) = 2.70) and depression (t(87) = 2.82), both significant at the p < 0.05 level. The bereaved of confirmed dead reported higher scores than controls on negative life events (t(78) = 4.78), hassles (t(78) = 3.85), depression (t(78) = 4.57), and somatization (t(78) = 3.75), all significant at the p < 0.01 level. The permanent property loss group differed from controls on negative life events (t(69) = 4.54, p < 0.01). No significant differences were found between the recreational loss and control groups, nor were there any indications that the physical health of any of the groups had been impaired by the disaster loss experience 1 year postdisaster.

The planned comparisons carried out to test the six hypotheses formulated for the first study question indicated that there were no significant differences between the two bereaved groups on any of the five outcome measures. Similarly, post hoc and planned comparisons revealed no differences between the property samples. Thus, it seemed advisable to determine whether the two bereaved groups and the two property groups could be combined prior to addressing the second study question. Combining the groups would result in an n = 69 sample size for the bereaved group and an n = 36 sample size for the property loss groups.

Inasmuch as the post hoc procedure (Scheffé) is a conservative test, one additional powerful statistical test was undertaken to determine whether the two bereaved groups could be combined and the two property loss groups could be combined. The groups were compared by pairwise discriminant function analysis on all outcome measures. For the bereaved group comparisons, the overall approximate F (5, 62) =0.99, (p = 0.43). For the property loss group comparisons, the overall approximate F (5, 30) = 4.85 (p <0.002). Based on these findings, along with the results from the first study question, the two bereaved groups were judged sufficiently similar to combine prior to further analysis. The two property loss groups were judged not similar enough to combine. Moreover, since the samples of the two property loss groups were small, the major focus for the second study question was on the combined bereaved group and the control group. See Table 3.3 for a summary of means, standard deviations, F ratios, and p values.

The Second Question

In order to examine the role of self-efficacy and social support as buffering negative effects of stress on health, Pearson correlations and hierarchical stepwise regression analyses were computed for the bereaved (n = 69) and control groups (n = 50) separately. Stress, self-efficacy, and social support were predictor variables, while depression, somatization, and physical health were outcome variables. Since the LES Negative Stress and Hassles scores were correlated (r = 0.77 p < 0.001), they were transformed to Z scores and then averaged to form a single measure of stress. In general, subjects having high levels of self-efficacy and high levels of social support expressed lower levels of depression than would have been predicted from their levels of stress. Nonetheless, stress accounted for 35 percent of the variance (p < 0.001). After statistically controlling for stress, together self-efficacy and social support accounted for a significant (p < 0.05) but low (7 percent) percentage of the additional variance. These findings suggest that when individuals are exposed to high rates of stress, belief in one's ability to adapt and external sources of support are helpful, but that both the quantity and quality of stressors experienced are more important in predicting health outcome.

TABLE 3.3. MEANS, STANDARD DEVIATIONS, AND OVERALL SIGNIFICANCE TESTS FOR DIFFERENCES BETWEEN MEANS FOR THE FIVE OUTCOME GROUPS

Outcome Measures	Group Means and Standard Deviations for Each Outcome					Overall F From ANOVA (df = 4, 150)
	Group 1 (BP)(N = 39)	Group 2 (BC)(N = 30)	Group 3 (PP)(N = 21)	Group 4 (PR)(N = 15)	Group 5 (C)(N = 50)	
Stress outcomes						
LES negative	10.67	15.63	16.10	7.47	5.94	9.52***
	(9.54)	(10.06)	(9.46)	(5.07)	(6.07)	—
Hassles	101.95	147.37	71.57	57.80	71.66	5.68***
	(97.25)	(93.73)	(51.44)	(57.34)	(68.40)	—
Health outcomes						
SCL Depression	1.16	1.39	0.93	0.65	0.74	6.70***
	(0.78)	(0.64)	(0.54)	(0.54)	(0.58)	—
SCL Somatization	0.63	0.88	0.69	0.38	0.42	4.05**
	(0.63)	(0.51)	(0.49)	(0.40)	(0.55)	—
Health	−0.03	−0.13	0.05	−0.08	0.11	0.77
	(0.62)	(0.86)	(0.51)	(0.62)	(0.55)	—

Abbreviations: BC, bereaved confirmed; BP, bereaved presumed; C, control; PP, property loss, permanent residence; PR, property loss, recreation residence.

Each mean and standard deviation pair are presented such that the top number is the mean. The bottom numbers of each pair enclosed in parentheses is the standard deviation.

**p < 0.01; ***p < 0.001

The Third Question

The third study question examined perceptions of the media. Since the disaster received widespread media coverage, an area of interest was whether the loss groups' perceptions of local newspapers, local television, national television, and national newsmagazines differed. All four loss groups were included in these analyses. No significant differences among the groups on the four forms of the media were obtained by one-way analysis of variance. Another important question was whether study subjects perceived the media as a help, hindrance, or not affecting their recovery. Differences did emerge in this area. The confirmed dead bereaved group viewed the media more negatively than did the other loss groups [F (3, 100) = 3.65, p < 0.01)]. Both bereaved groups perceived such media scale items as invasion of privacy, inaccuracies in news reporting, and extensive coverage, as factors contributing to the delay in their recoveries. By contrast, the property loss groups did not perceive the media as affecting their recoveries either positively or negatively.

Other Findings

The three areas of financial status assessed were change in income, adequacy of income, and satisfaction with financial settlement. Dissatisfaction with financial settlement was the predominant finding, but only among the permanent property loss subjects.

Perceived rate of recovery was measured by a nine-point Likert scale (1—not at all recovered, to 9—completely recovered). The mean rate of recovery for the bereaved groups was 5.90, indicating that the majority of subjects perceived they were only "somewhat recovered" 11 months following the disaster.

In order to answer the question, "Is disaster bereavement perceived most negatively by close relatives or intimate friends?", t tests were conducted to examine differences between the two groups on 14 study variables. Stress variables were negative scores from the LES and Hassles scales. Health outcome variables were SCL-90 subscale scores on depression and somatization, and scores from the Health Status Index. Support variables were size of network, contact with network, and perceived social support. Financial data were change and adequacy of income and level of satisfaction with disaster loss settlement. Loss variables were blame, comparative rating of the current death with other deaths experienced, the media scale score, and recovery rating. A priori, it was predicted that relatives would be "worse off."

Relatives indeed fared more poorly than friends of disaster victims on four variables: depression, t(66) = 2.30 p < 0.02; media, t(67) = −2.09, p < 0.04; comparative rating of the death experience,

$t(67) = -2.51$, $p < 0.01$; and recovery, $t(67) = -1.86$, $p < 0.05$. Differences approached significance on somatization and perceived overall social support.

Another area of interest was whether geographic proximity to the eruptive area would affect both loss and nonloss study participants on selected study variables. Three categories of geographic proximity were defined as follows: "immediate proximity"—living within a 15-mile radius of the designated danger zones (n = 34); "northwestern proximity"—living in Washington state but outside the 15-mile eruptive area and Oregon (n = 102); and "remote proximity"—living in the remaining United States and Canada (n = 19). One-way analysis of variance and planned paired comparisons were used to analyze the nine study variables: LES negative score, Hassles score, SCL-90 total score, SCL-90 subscale scores on depression and somatization, physical health, overall perceived social support, the media score, and recovery rating. Significant differences between the three groups when categorized by geographic proximity of the actively eruptive area emerged on two study variables: negative life events (LES negative score) and depression (SCL-90 subscale score). LES-$F(2, 152) = 3.99$, $p = < 0.02$, with those living in the immediate proximity reporting significantly more negative life events than the other two groups ($t(152) = 2.82$, $p < 0.006$). No differences were reported between the northwestern and remote proximities on negative life events. Proximity results must be interpreted with caution. Since property loss victims lived closest in proximity to the eruptive area, these variables may be confounded.

Regarding depression, the F ratio was not significant; however, pairwise comparisons indicated that those farthest away (remote proximity) were significantly more depressed than those living in the Northwest ($t(151) = -1.96$, $p < 0.05$). There were no significant differences on rates of depression between persons living within a 15-mile radius of the active volcano site and persons living in the remaining area of Washington and Oregon.

Structured interviews and open-ended questions regarding prior loss experiences and anger and blame corroborated statistical findings. Control subjects were excluded from open-ended questions since these items were specific to loss associated with the disaster. The ability to generalize these findings is limited because not all open-ended items were answered by all subjects.

The bereaved subjects who responded (78 percent) to the item regarding the extent to which past loss experiences helped them cope with the current loss generally indicated a lack of application of past coping mechanisms to the present situation. The predominant answer to "What past experience helped?" was "nothing" (48 percent of those responding). Other responses in order of importance were "prior death of a significant other" (29 percent) and "personal belief system" (23 percent).

In response to the question, "Are you angry at anyone at the present time for your loss?", response rates of the bereaved were lower than the permanent property loss group (20 percent to 52 percent). Bereaved respondents reported that immediately following the disaster, they were angry at God and at identification and rescue procedures for the deceased. A few of the bereaved were angry at the deceased victims themselves for being in the area. However, by the time data were collected, these same persons reported that information regarding the unexpected magnitude of the event helped them change their initial attributions that the deaths could have been prevented. However, 33 percent of the bereaved respondents believed the deaths were preventable, even though the disaster was not preventable. Both bereaved and property loss groups blamed government decision-making and inefficiency both pre- and postdisaster for their losses (63 percent).

The last open-ended question, "Is there anything else you would like to tell us to help us understand what you have been through?" was answered by 50 percent of the bereaved subjects. The major themes that emerged were: extreme stress during the waiting period of identification of the dead, no bodies for burial, no norms for distributing property and valuables. Many dead victims were middle-aged, thus both their parents and their children were bereaved. Furthermore, the large number of blended families (second and third marriages) made the decisions regarding deceased persons' belongings very sensitive issues among the bereaved. Themes of single young adults who lost both parents were: intense grief, seeing people who resembled their parents, nightmares, sensing sudden new responsibilities, being told by some unaffected individuals that their parents deserved to die for being in the area, and feeling abandoned by peers because they were "being forced to grow up quickly." Best friends reported an extreme sense of loss of talent among the dead, loss of their own youth and sense of identity, and urgency to reorder life priorities.

IDENTIFICATION OF HIGH-RISK POPULATIONS

Populations at risk can be defined as those individuals, groups, and families who are particularly susceptible to mental distress and physical illness by virtue of selected characteristics and exposure to unpredictable and uncontrollable factors in the environment, and who have inadequate resources with which to respond to environmental stressors.

The highly traumatic stressful events experienced by disaster victims appear to be related to a number of other subsequent stressors such as role function, inadequate outlets for expression of anger, lack of specific significant resources, and ongoing unpredictability in their respective situations.

Initially, it was expected that the presumptive death bereavement group would report the highest numbers of stressors, and the lowest levels of health and hence reflect the highest risk. Since findings did not substantiate these earlier beliefs, additional analyses for which the second author had major responsibility were conducted. Also, we wish to again call attention to the fact that our data were collected *11 months postdisaster*. The objective in identifying those at risk nearly a year following the disaster was to document levels of health in order to better understand disaster recovery processes. We were not attempting to evaluate prior services offered in the immediate geographical area nor trying to determine whether victims sought specific services. Rather, it will be recalled that the close relatives and friends of those who died as a result of the disaster lived in 10 U.S. states and two Canadian provinces, and therefore, did not experience a typical "sense of community" frequently discussed in disaster studies. The extent to which sense of community contributes to recovery, or the lack of it, has not been examined to predict high-risk status of disaster victims.

DELINEATION OF HIGH-RISK VARIABLES

Another look at the high-risk literature reported in Chapter 8 suggests that important high-risk variables could be analyzed individually and collectively across the entire bereaved study population (n = 69) since the presumed versus confirmed bereavement category did not identify a high-risk group. Moreover, the permanent property loss group experienced far different stress and health outcomes as well as differing considerably on demographic variables when compared to the recreational property loss group. Since the property loss groups were too dissimilar to combine, yet too small for many statistical analyses, the decision was made to focus specifically on the bereaved study participants as loss subjects and the intact control group (n = 50), which would serve as nonloss comparators.

The high-risk variables selected for additional analyses were age, gender, perception of social support, belief in preventability of the deaths, centrality of the relationship with the deceased prior to death, and negative scores on the LES. We did not include financial status which would ordinarily be important to include, based on the study finding that most bereaved subjects were satisfied with the status of their financial settlements.

Analysis of Individual High-Risk Variables

Hypotheses were made a priori regarding the effects of disaster bereavement losses on the three study outcome variables identified earlier: levels of depression and somatization as reported from the two subscales of the SCL-90-R, and level of physical health obtained from the *Physical Health Index*. The high-risk indicators were identified primarily by Pearson correlation. Also decided a priori, the criteria for acceptance of statistical significance of each individual high-risk variable was that at least two of the three outcome variables would need to be significant.

Age. It was predicted that bereaved persons less than 40 years of age would demonstrate lower levels of health, that is, the presence of depression, somatization, and disruptions of physical health when compared with those bereaved persons over 40. The hypothesis was supported. Pearson correlations for the bereaved group (N = 69) demonstrated that age was significantly correlated with two of three health outcome measures, SCL Depression ($r = -0.19$, $p < 0.05$) and physical health status ($r = -0.23$, $p < 0.05$). Age and somatization were not correlated ($r = 0.06$, NS). These correlations are shown in Table 3.4. For the control group (N = 50), Pearson correlations were significant only for the measure of depression ($r = -0.39$, $p < 0.01$) (see Table 3.4).

Gender. It was predicted that at this point in recovery, bereaved males would demonstrate lower levels of health than nonbereaved males. This prediction was not supported. Pearson correlations for the bereaved group (N = 69) demonstrate that bereaved males reported worse physical health than females ($r = 0.21$, $p < 0.05$). All other gender and health correlations for the bereaved group were nonsignificant. Likewise, for the control group (N = 50) being male was not correlated with health outcomes.

Social Support. It was expected that bereaved persons who reported positive perceptions of their social support system would demonstrate less negative health outcomes (depression, somatization, disruptions in physical health) than bereaved who viewed their support system negatively. This hypothesis was only partially supported by the data. For the bereaved group (N = 69) perceived social support and SCL Depression scores were significantly correlated ($r = -0.28$, $p < 0.01$) (see Table 3.4). Social support was not significantly correlated with the

TABLE 3.4. INTERCORRELATION MATRIX FOR RISK VARIABLES AND HEALTH OUTCOME MEASURES FOR THE BEREAVED AND CONTROL GROUPS

	Risk Factors						Health Outcome Measures		
	1	2	3	4	5	6	7	8	9
1. Gender[b]	B = 00 C = 00	-0.07 -0.27*	-0.24 0.20	-0.03 0.04	0.38*** —[a]	-0.09 —[a]	-0.40*** -0.03	-0.37*** -0.19	0.21* -0.12
2. Age		B = 00 C = 00	-0.18 -0.21	0.13 0.21	0.03 —[a]	-0.20* —[a]	0.06 -0.21	-0.19* -0.39**	-0.23* -0.06
3. LES negative (stress)			B = 00 C = 00	-0.08 -0.08	0.23* —[a]	0.24* —[a]	0.52*** 0.43***	0.49*** 0.44***	-0.48*** -0.38***
4. Perceived social support				B = 00 C = 00	-0.18	-0.17	-0.10	-0.28**	0.01 0.04
5. Importance of the deceased					B = 00 C = 00	-0.05 —[a]	-0.02	-0.12	-0.18 —[a]
6. Perceived preventability of the death[c]						B = 00 C = 00	0.21* —[a]	0.25* —[a]	0.02 —[a]
7. SCL Somatization							B = 00 C = 00	0.62*** 0.61***	-0.46*** -0.59***
8. SCL Depression								B = 00 C = 00	-0.25* -0.40**
9. Physical health status									B = 00 C = 00

Abbreviations: B, bereaved (N = 69); C, control (N = 50). [a]Not applicable to control group. [b]Coded 0 for females, 1 for males. [c]Coded 0 for unpreventable, 1 for preventable. *p < 0.05; **p < 0.01; ***p < 0.001.

other health measures. For the control group (n = 50), Pearson correlations demonstrated no significance between perceived social support and any of the health outcome measures (Table 3.4).

Preventability. Bereaved persons who viewed the traumatic circumstances of the death as preventable were expected to demonstrate greater degrees of morbidity (depression, somatization, physical health) when compared with bereaved persons who viewed the traumatic circumstances of the death as unpreventable. This hypothesis was supported by the data. Pearson correlations indicate significant relationships between belief of preventability and SCL Somatization ($r = 0.21$, $p < 0.05$) and with SCL Depression scores ($r = 0.25$, $p < 0.05$).

Prior Relationship. Bereaved persons who viewed their prior relationship with the decreased as central were expected to demonstrate lower levels of health (depression, somatization, disruptions in physical health) when compared with bereaved persons who viewed their prior relationship with the deceased as peripheral. This hypothesis was supported by the data. Pearson correlations between the importance of the deceased and SCL Somatization scores ($r = 0.28$), $p < 0.01$) and with SCL Depression scores ($r = 0.48$, $p < 0.001$) were significant.

Negative Life Stress. Bereaved persons who experienced higher amounts of stress were expected to demonstrate lower levels of health (depression, somatization, disruptions in physical health) when compared with bereaved persons who experienced lower amounts of stress. This hypothesis was supported by the data. Pearson correlations between LES negative scores (Stress) and all of the health outcomes were highly significant. SCL Somatization revealed a correlation of $r = 0.52$ ($p < 0.001$), SCL Depression a correlation of $r = .49$ ($p < 0.001$), and physical health $r = -0.48$ ($p < 0.001$) (See Table 3.4).

Analysis of Collective High-Risk Variables
In order to determine the extent to which the six risk variables *combined* could predict high-risk populations, multiple regression analyses were performed. The hierarchical stepwise procedure was selected because determining the amount of variance that could be accounted for by each predictor as well as in combination with the other predictors would be useful information. Several models based on theoretical concepts were developed to enter the six predictors into the regression equation. Only the one model which we retained is reported here (see Table 3.5).

At the first step, the predictor of stress was entered. At the second step, age and gender were entered in order of their statistical significance. At the third step, social support was entered. At the fourth step, importance of the deceased person and perceived preventability of the death were entered in order of their statistical significance. Six multiple regression analyses were completed, one for each of the three dependent measures (SCL Depression, SCL Somatization, physical health) for the bereaved and control groups separately. Results from the bereaved sample are reported first.

The significance of the overall F tests for the regression analyses ranged from $p < 0.05$ to $p < 0.001$. The stepwise contribution of each predictor of the total percentage of variance accounted for by each successive set of predictors are indicated in the percent of variance and adjusted R columns of Table 3.5. The F to enter each predictor, the multiple R, and beta-weights at the final step are also presented.

Stress was a highly significant predictor of the health outcomes in all three of the regression analyses for the bereaved. Stress accounted for 28 percent of the variance in somatization, 25 percent of the variance in depression, and 23 percent of the variance in physical health.

Once stress was entered as a predictor for the dependent variable of SCL Depression, three of the remaining five variables, female gender [$F(1, 66) = 6.35, p < 0.01$], perceived social support [$F(1, 64) = 5.09, p < 0.05$], and importance of the deceased person [$F(1, 63) = 9.33, p < 0.01$] contributed significantly to the remaining variance in depression. Neither age entered at the second step with gender nor perceived preventability of death, entered with importance of the deceased person at the fourth step accounted for significant variance as single variables. For the dependent variable of somatization, only gender contributed significantly to the remaining variance beyond stress [$F(1, 66) = 8.37, p < 0.01$]. Age, social support, perceived perventability, and the importance of the deceased did not account for any significant variance. For the dependent variable of physical health, only age (those under 40 years only) contributed significantly to the remaining variance beyond stress [$F(1, 66) = 10.97, p < 0.01$].

The same stepwise regression analyses were conducted with the control group ($N = 50$). Results of the regression analyses are presented in Table 3.5. Even though earlier results revealed that control subjects' mean stress and illness scores were much lower than those of the bereaved subjects, the stress-illness relationship is similar to that of the bereaved group. Results for the control group indicate that stress accounts for 19 percent of the variance in depression, 19 percent of the variance in somatization, and 9 percent of the variance in physical

TABLE 3.5. PREDICTING HIGH-RISK BEREAVED FROM VARIABLES: STRESS, AGE, SEX, SOCIAL SUPPORT, PREVENTABILITY OF DEATH, AND IMPORTANCE OF DECEASED PERSON: MULTIPLE REGRESSION RESULTS FOR BEREAVED AND CONTROL GROUPS[a]

Group	Predictor Variable	% of Variance Accounted for at Each Entry Step	F to Enter Predictor (DF)	Multiple R	Beta-Wt. at Final Step	Adjusted R^2	Overall F Statistic (DF)
			Outcome Measure: SCL Depression				
Bereaved (N = 69)	LES negative	24.5	21.77***(1, 67)	0.495	0.31	0.234	21.77***(1, 67)
	Sex	6.6	6.35*(1, 66)	0.558	-0.15	0.290	14.93***(2, 66)
	Age	2.0	1.95 (1, 65)	0.575	-0.11	0.300	10.74***(3, 65)
	SS	4.9	5.09*(1, 64)	0.617	-0.14	0.342	9.84***(4, 64)
	Importance DP[b]	7.99	9.33**(1, 63)	0.678	0.33	0.418	10.77 (5, 63)
	Preventability[c]	1.5	1.83 (1, 62)	0.690	0.13	0.425	9.40***(6, 62)
Control (N = 50)	LES negative	19.4	11.57***(1, 48)	0.440	0.43	0.177	11.57***(1, 48)
	Age	9.6	6.36*(1, 47)	0.538	-0.40	0.260	11.80***(2, 47)
	Sex	14.4	11.76***(1, 46)	0.659	-0.39	0.398	9.61***(3, 46)
	Social support	0.04	0.03 (1, 45)	0.659	-0.02	0.385	8.67***(4, 45)
			Outcome Measure: SCL Somatization				
Bereaved (N = 69)	LES negative	27.8	25.82***(1, 67)	0.527	0.44	0.267	25.82***(1, 67)
	Sex	8.1	8.37**(1, 66)	0.599	-0.24	0.340	18.52***(2, 66)
	Age	1.5	1.64 (1, 65)	0.612	0.15	0.346	13.01***(3, 65)
	SS	0.5	0.52 (1, 64)	0.616	-0.04	0.341	9.82***(4, 64)
	Preventability[c]	0.9	1.00 (1, 63)	0.624	0.11	0.341	8.06***(5, 63)
	Importance DP[b]	0.5	0.52 (1, 62)	0.628	0.08	0.336	6.75***(6, 62)

Control (N=50)	LES negative	19.1	11.38***(1, 48)	0.437	0.43	0.174	11.38***(1, 48)
	Sex	1.7	1.03 (1, 47)	0.457	-0.17	0.175	6.21** (2, 47)
	Age	2.6	1.57 (1, 46)	0.485	-0.17	0.185	4.71** (3, 46)
	SS total	0.16	0.09 (1, 45)	0.486	0.04	0.169	3.49* (4, 45)

Outcome Measure: Health

Bereaved (N=69)	LES negative	23.1	20.18***(1, 67)	0.481	-0.54	0.220	20.18***(1, 67)
	Age	10.9	10.97** (1, 66)	0.584	-0.31	0.321	17.08***(2, 66)
	Sex	0.2	0.28 (1, 65)	0.586	0.05	0.313	11.36***(3, 65)
	SS	0.01	0.01 (1, 64)	0.586	0.02	0.303	8.39***(4, 64)
	Preventability[c]	0.8	0.86 (1, 63)	0.594	0.09	0.301	6.87***(5, 63)
	Importance DP[b]	0.01	0.01 (1, 62)	0.594	-0.01	0.290	5.64**(6, 62)
Control (N=50)	LES negative	9.4	4.98*(1, 48)	0.306	-0.31	0.075	4.98* (1, 48)
	Age	1.7	0.89 (1, 47)	0.333	-0.16	0.073	2.93 (2, 47)
	Sex	0.97	0.51 (1, 46)	0.347	-0.10	0.063	2.10 (3, 46)
	SS Total	0.03	0.01 (1, 45)	0.348	0.01	0.043	1.55 (4, 45)

Abbreviations: DP, deceased person; SS, social support.

[a]After each F statistic the appropriate degrees of freedom are presented in parentheses.

[b]Importance of the deceased person.

[c]Perceived preventability of death.

*p < 0.05; **p < 0.01; ***p < 0.001.

health. By contrast to the bereaved group, the results for the control group demonstrated that both age and gender accounted for a significant amount of the variance for depression [$F(1, 47) = 6.36$, $p < 0.05$], [$F(1, 46) = 11.76$, $p < .001$], respectively. None of the other variables that were significant for the bereaved group were shown to be significant predictors for any of the three outcome variables for the control group.

Summary of High-Risk Analyses

When high-risk variables were correlated individually with three health outcome measures, all met criteria for significance except for male bereaved and perception of social support. However, these latter two variables were supported in part.

The selected set of six high-risk predictors were entered into the regression equation in the following order: negative life stress, gender, age, perceived social support, importance of the deceased person, and belief that death could have been prevented. Six multiple regression analyses were completed, one for each of the three dependent measures (SCL Depression, SCL Somatization, physical health) for the bereaved and control groups separately. The significance of the overall F tests for the regression analyses ranged from $p < 0.05$ to $p < 0.001$).

The suggestion that response to untimely death is a multivariate phenomenon was supported by the multiple regression analyses. Concurrent life stress was the highest predictor on all three health outcomes. However, when all six high-risk variables were used to predict outcome, 48 percent of the variance was accounted for with depression, 39 percent of the variance with somatization, and 35 percent of the variance with physical health. All six variables used concurrently, then, would be most predictive in identifying high-risk bereaved persons.

DISCUSSION OF THE STUDY FINDINGS

The Bereaved Groups

Findings from this study confirm reports from past disaster and bereavement studies: the death of a significant other has profound negative effects on the surviving bereaved (Ball, 1976–1977; Harvey and Bahr, 1980; Titchener and Kapp, 1976). Individuals bereaved by the volcanic eruption of Mount St. Helens experienced all three kinds of untimely death: premature, unexpected, and violent. Only four of the deceased were over 58 years of age, and all of the deaths were unexpected and calamitous. Age of both the deceased and bereaved has been shown to be both a high risk and rate of recovery bereavement indicator. Grief could be expected, and in fact, proved to be both acute and prolonged because relationships between the deceased and bereaved were central and many believed the deaths were preventable. Data collected nearly a year following the disaster supports intense and prolonged occurrence of grieving.

An intriguing finding was the high incidence of depressive symptoms and the low incidence of both professional help-seeking behavior and perceived recovery. In the current study, scores of the SCL-90 Depression subscale were significantly correlated ($r = -0.69$, $p < 0.001$) with rate of recovery for the combined bereaved group. However, depression scores and contacts with professionals were not significantly correlated ($r = 0.18$). Similarly, Ball (1976–1977) reported that only 4 percent of her sample sought help for depressive symptoms, yet 54 percent of the sample reported that they were only "somewhat recovered," and 11 percent reported that they were "not at all recovered" 7 months postbereavement. Similar findings were reported following the Buffalo Creek Disaster (Titchener and Kapp, 1976). A rival explanation to professional help-seeking might be that supportive networks fulfill this need. However, in the present study, depression and contact with one's social network for the combined bereaved group were not significantly correlated ($r = -0.08$) and no data regarding social support were included in either the Ball or the Buffalo Creek studies. Another rival hypothesis might be that the bereaved expected to be depressed, and hence, did nothing about feeling badly. This explanation also seems unlikely since the literature generally supports the notion that friends and relatives in Western cultures are uncomfortable with death and encourage short bereavements (Blauner, 1966; Weisman, 1973). Thus, this phenomenon deserves additional study.

An unexpected statistical finding was that the presumed dead bereaved did not report higher levels of stress and lower levels of health than the confirmed dead bereaved group. Factors that may account for the bereaved group similarities are characteristics of the event, sampling, time of measurement, and prompt legal resolution of presumptive death.

Characteristics of the Event. Relatives and friends of those presumed dead reported that information regarding the massive destruction of the area and conditions of the bodies of the confirmed dead helped them realize that only those rescued quickly or those outside the eruption zone could have survived. Thus, as time passed, hope for finding persons alive lessened. This factor appeared to strengthen the conviction that all persons in the area had died and may have reduced differences between the two bereaved groups. The major difference, however, was a lack of finality since bodies had not been found.

Sampling Effects. The bereaved of confirmed dead had a higher response rate than the bereaved of presumed dead (75 percent to 63 percent). In four cases, the closest relative of a presumed dead victim could not be contacted due to serious personal chronic illness and parents of four young adult victims of presumptive death refused to participate. Thus, it may be that the bereaved of those presumed dead did not participate because they were "worse off." Contrary to statistical findings, interview data suggest the presumed dead bereaved experienced the most devastating initial effects of the two groups. For instance, the bereaved of presumed dead reported waiting was "agony," "hoping, yet knowing they were dead," family distress in planning and carrying out memorial services, "It's hard to come to terms with no body," and difficulty giving court testimony to verify death.

Time of Measurement. While data collection 11 months postdisaster was a positive factor in substantiating the belief that those exposed to disasters suffer stress and health consequences beyond a few weeks duration, it may have inadvertently obliterated some differences between presumptive and confirmed death bereavement. Moreover, by the time data were collected, presumptive death status was legally resolved. That is, court testimony by a significant other that the presumed dead victim was either known or believed to be in the area, and that the person was indeed "missing," served as evidence of provisional death. These cases were then acted upon by a special legislative statute allowing beneficiary status on insurance policies and estates to be settled, even though official death certificates were not issued.

The current study findings suggest only modest support for the intervening role of social support. The *size* of an individual's network and level of depression was more highly correlated (r = −0.36, p < 0.001) than the contact with members of one's network with depression. This finding suggests that if individuals believe there are others to whom one can turn, perceptions of *potential* support change the labeling of the stressful event from overwhelming to manageable. Since perceived social support and actual social competence may be confounded, self-efficacy (the use of social competence) and social support were measured separately. Low scores on self-efficacy were correlated with high rates of depression (r = −0.35, p < 0.001), whereas the regression analyses indicated that, after controlling for stress, social support was higher for those experiencing physical illness. One possible explanation is that the level of social support increased due to needs for support during illness. Similar findings were reported by Andrews et al. (1978) and Coppel (1980). Perhaps depressive-prone individuals are more likely to exhibit depressive symptoms and perceive the environment as less supportive or drive others away. Moreover, if physical illness is sanctioned whereas emotional illness is stigmatized, depressed subjects may believe their behavior is inappropriate and not seek help from others. Thus, depression is likely to influence both intrapersonal and interpersonal supports.

Inasmuch as the media occupies a central role in the reporting of events, the effects of media coverage on the loss victims was of interest to the investigators. In addition to perceived hindrance to recovery, interview data also revealed high levels of dissatisfaction with all forms of the media among bereaved individuals. According to some study subjects, inaccurate identity of persons was shown on television, and dead victims' body parts were pictured in the newspaper without consent of next of kin. Further, some television reports of finding dead victims, while accurate, were reported to the public prior to notification of immediate relatives. Data regarding the effects of the media *following* a disaster are infrequently reported if gathered at all; yet, these findings raise important legal and ethical issues. The rapidity with which events are reported may contribute to both inaccuracy and insensitivity as was the case here.

No hypotheses were generated regarding how anger, blame, preventability, adequacy of financial settlement, past loss experiences, and perceptions of rate of recovery would affect the stress-illness relationship. The bereaved directed their anger primarily at identification and rescue procedures of their significant others. Some of the bereaved were angry at the deceased victims themselves for being in the area. However, by the time data were collected, these same persons reported that information regarding the unexpected magnitude of the event helped change their initial belief that the deaths could have been prevented. Nonetheless, 33 percent of the bereaved sample held onto the belief that the deaths were preventable. Forty-one percent of the subjects reported that there were no past loss experiences they could recall that helped them cope with their current loss. This finding reflects the relatively young study sample. Perceived rate of recovery was measured by a one- to nine-point Likert Scale. Subjects reported they were only "somewhat recovered" ($\bar{x} = 5.90$) 11 months following the disaster.

Finally, the therapeutic value of study participation, candor of response, and feelings of satisfaction toward research regarding grief and bereavement were reported by participants in this study as well as subjects participating in studies by Ball (1976–1977) and Malinak et al. (1979). In the current study, even those individuals who were not contacted for a personal or telephone interview wrote positive comments about participation in response to the final question. Subjects of all ages reported they "thought long and hard" about their responses. Further, some reported feeling better as a result of finally sharing their bereavement experience. About 95 percent of the participants in this study requested a report of the findings. These findings suggest that persons are willing to disclose sensitive information and apparently derived some therapeutic benefit from doing so.

The Property Loss Groups
The high levels of negative life events, anger, blame, and financial dissatisfaction reported by the permanent property loss group were not expected. Factors that might account for these results are geographic location of subjects, lack of resolution regarding property loss, and additional stressors, which could be reported on the LES.

Proximity to the Eruptive Area. With the exception of three subjects who moved away, the remainder of the subjects in the permanent property loss group (86 percent) reside close to or on the same property where their homes were destoyed by flooding of the Toutle River. Thus, these persons live with unpredictable and uncontrollable threat of recurring loss of homes, employment, and even significant others. This disaster phenomenon is called "stress as enduring" by Wilson (1972). By contrast, only 9 percent of the bereaved subjects live in the immediate area of Mount St. Helens. (Six additional bereaved families who also reside in the immediate area were invited to participate in the study, but declined.) While the death of a significant other is reportedly more stressful than loss of property, numerous stressful events that produce ongoing tension are an indication of concern. Proximity to the area was the highest stressor in one study of residents living near the Three Mile Island nuclear disaster site (Bromet and Dunn, 1981). In the current study, "immediate proximity" was also a factor that appeared to contribute to high rates of negative life events.

Financial Effects. Property loss had not yet been resolved financially at the time of data collection. Some property loss subjects have become both plaintiffs and defendants in lawsuits associated with property loss. Lengthy legal hassles appear to occur frequently following disasters (Singh and Raphael, 1981; Titchener and Kapp, 1976). The three areas of financial status assessed were change in income, adequacy of current income, and satisfaction with financial settlement. Dissatisfaction with financial settlement was the predominant finding, but only among the permanent property loss subjects.

Methodologically, the LES is an improvement over previous stress measures. However, it is possible that there are more events on the LES to which property loss subjects could respond. For example, moving, borrowing money, and changing schools are items applicable to property loss.

The permanent property loss group reported high rates of stress not significantly different from the bereaved groups. By contrast, stress scores from both bereaved groups were associated with high depression and somatization scores on the HSCL-90, whereas stress reported by property loss victims was related only to depression. This important finding may have been obscured had data from the four groups not been analyzed separately.

Identifying the High-Risk Bereaved

Our findings support findings from studies of other high-risk populations such as maternal/infant and the chronically mentally ill: Sociodemographic factors are important risk variables. However, the additional findings regarding closeness of relationship, belief of preventability, blame, concurrent life stress, and support, to our knowledge, have not been high-risk variables in prior disaster or bereavement research.

Sociodemographic Factors. In general, younger bereaved persons, under 40 years of age, demonstrated a greater amount of depression, poor health, somatization, and overall stress than bereaved persons over 40 years of age. It was also noted that the younger persons were more likely to view the death as preventable. Age was also highly significant for the control group in that it predicted depression, though not to the extent as measured for the bereaved (control = 18 percent, bereaved = 41 percent).

Bereaved females demonstrated the highest depression and stress ratings compared to males and the control females. Two of the health outcome measures, depression and somatization, were significantly correlated with being female. Additionally significant was the high correlation between females and the importance of the deceased person. In general, females had much higher levels of morbidity. A correlation was shown between bereaved males and physical health although there were no significant differences in the total health scores between either gender or group.

The literature suggests that social support is the most important factor in affecting the morbidity of bereavement (Maddison, 1968; Raphael, 1977; 1979–1980; Singh and Raphael, 1981). Social support was a significant factor in depression in this study, although the overall degree of significance with all of the morbidity measures was much less than was suggested by Singh and Raphael (1981). In the latter study, perceived social support was suggested as the prime risk indicator. Heller (1979) suggests too much importance has been given to social support as a factor in reducing morbidity. Heller suggests the depressed person in general is more likely to perceive the environment as less supportive, and suggests the need for differing degrees of support for different persons which would then make a single score on social support nonpredictive for individual needs. In our study, perceived social support was seen as a factor in depression for the bereaved group. Those persons who perceived they had poor social support demonstrated a greater amount of depression. To a lesser degree, perceived social support was an important factor for health and the amount of stress experienced for the bereaved group as compared with the control group.

Concurrent Life Stress. Stress was the most important risk factor. This finding has implications for the permanent property loss group who were not included in the risk analyses. For the bereaved, additional negative life events close to or at the time of a death of a significant other had been suggested as an important factor in a person's ability to cope with the presenting stress and the other event. The hypothesis to test this factor was supported. Conversely, concurrent stress was not found to be a significant factor in previous studies examining the risk factors for bereaved (Raphael, 1977; 1979–1980; Singh and Raphael, 1981). This may be due to the fact that the number of subjects was relatively small (N = 31) or with the procedure of identifying concurrent stresses. In this study, however, concurrent negative life events was the most important risk factor identified. Correlations were significant for all of the health outcomes as well as with the risk factors.

Rabkin and Struening (1976) suggest that when persons experience moderate stress they tend to believe they can handle the stress without additional support. In more severe stress and crises, persons do tend to require support as much of the other literature suggests, but in extreme stress nothing helps. The disastrous event experienced by some persons in this study may be considered an extreme stressor. This explanation seems plausible because control subjects who reported low social support did not report high rates of illness. It is clear that further research is required on this variable, perhaps separating social support from personality factors and levels of social competence.

Meaning of the Event. The personal meaning of the event was tested by two hypotheses dealing with the concepts of centrality/peripherality of the relationship and preventability/unpreventability of the circumstances of the death. This model of assessing risk was suggested by Bugen (1977). The study findings revealed younger persons more frequently viewed the death as being preventable and that females who had a central relationship with the deceased experienced increased stress, resulting in increased morbidity. As stated earlier, a central relationship coupled with a preventable death indicates an intense and prolonged grieving process. This concept was supported by the findings in this study as the data were collected 11 months after the disaster and thus found prolonged grief in subjects identifying these factors. Data appear consistent with the fact that 11 months following the disaster persons were able to process information regarding the magnitude of the event. Initially many of the bereaved individuals blamed their significant others for being in the area as well as authorities for not giving what was perceived as an adequate warning. Other recent disaster literature supports the notion that blame and preventability are significant factors in predicting outcome (Bromet and Dunn, 1981).

Finally, the suggestion of the interrelationship of the predictor variables was supported by the multiple regression analysis. When all six predictors are used to predict health outcome, 48 percent of the variance is accounted for with depression, 39 percent of the variance with somatization, and 35 percent of the variance with physical health. All variables used concurrently, then, would be most predictive in identifying high-risk bereaved persons. The concurrent use of the combined variables was confirmed by the correlation between stress and the recovery rates, which were also correlated with four of the risk indicators and all of the morbidity variables.

METHODOLOGICAL, CLINICAL, AND ETHICAL IMPLICATIONS

Methodological Implications

Several important methodological issues were addressed in this study. While both mental and physical illnesses following disasters have been reported in general, obtaining data from specific groups presents a difficult challenge for researchers. Subjects of past disaster studies have frequently been grouped together and described as "victims" of a given disaster. This is primarily because personal survival, loss of significant others, and property loss are seldom mutually exclusive conditions. Thus differential loss effects among victims of the same disaster have not been reported. Moreover, past studies examining bereaved persons under situations of confirmed versus persumptive death have been limited to family members of military men (McCubbin, 1976). Neither comparisons of bereaved family members and intimate friends of deceased disaster victims nor differential effects between the loss of permanent and recreational property have been reported.

In addition to the lack of sampling specificity in past research, much of the literature regarding human responses to catastrophic stress is based on anecdotal, case-by-case reports. Even when researchers are investigating the impact of larger scale disasters, such as fires in heavily populated buildings, airplane crashes, and earthquakes, the potential sample is still of finite size and frequently numbers less than 100. While the number of disaster studies that identify stress and health as outcome variables is increasing, many investigators have not used standardized measures to assess these variables. Consequently, neither researchers nor clinicians are able to compare the levels of impairment or evaluate interventions from study to study.

Specifically, consideration was given to measurement of negative life change instead of total change, utilization of a stress instrument that provided an opportunity for respondents to rate the impact of change (Sarason et al., 1978), and the inclusion of both social supports and self-efficacy as buffers of stress on illness (Coppel, 1980). The sample size of 155 subjects includes a control group and is larger and more representative than samples in some past disaster studies (Singh and Raphael, 1981; Titchener and Kapp, 1976).

Clinical Implications

Important clinical interventions should be directed toward: (1) recognition of the importance of such concepts of untimely death, centrality of the relationship and belief of preventability of the death, and endemic stress, in predicting the grief process; (2) encouragement of expression regarding the catastrophic circumstances of disaster loss; (3) rapid identification and access to the deceased with on-site crisis service; (4) assessment of loss victims for high-risk factors; (5) specific training for helping professionals and paraprofessionals; (6) backup consultation and support for mental health workers; (7) primary prevention teaching to local clergy, teachers, family practice physicians, and nurse practitioners, since these persons are likely to have early contact with loss persons; and (8) use of the media to inform people about appropriate coping mechanisms and available services.

According to Silver and Wortman (1980), professionals may underestimate what persons have been through. While listening may sound too simple for such a complex crisis, apparently it is not. Some study subjects mentioned that the interview and/or final open-ended questions, were their *first* opportunity to talk about the loss. Alternatively, beyond the immediate crisis, individuals have been shown to be reluctant to seek help (Lindy et al., 1981). See the chapters in Part Two for elaboration of clinical issues.

Ethical Implications

Ethical issues in both research and practice are far reaching; yet our analysis of such issues raises many questions. For example, risk-benefit ratios for *both* subjects and investigators, methods by which potential study subjects should be approached, destruction of initial data and potential subpoena in lawsuits, and involvement with the media are some of the ethical dilemmas we struggled with while carrying out this research.

SUMMARY AND CONCLUSIONS

The purposes of this chapter were to take the reader through the research process by using the volcanic eruption of Mount St. Helens in 1980 as a case example, and to exemplify in some detail a conceptual and research process for identifying high-risk populations.

Careful planning of research involving rare events such as earthquakes and volcanic eruptions has both risks and benefits. First, persons experiencing a rare event may be the targets of many researchers. A second risk regards a limited, highly vulnerable, research population that may not be found, or if found, may refuse participation. The benefits in this case were many. Careful attention to media coverage provided information regarding the nature of disaster losses (i.e., confirmed and presumed dead bereaved, permanent residence and recreational property loss) as well as important information such as processing of death certificates. Finally, an intensive and somewhat prolonged planning period allowed an exhaustive literature search, investigation of standardized measures of stress, illness, and support, tool development and pilot testing, as well as planning the "linked pairs" sampling strategy and locating study participants.

Inasmuch as many study participants who enjoyed a "central" (important personal) relationship with the deceased lived in locations *not* geographically close to the eruptive area, a combination of data-gathering options were used: self-report of standardized, mailed questionnaires, telephone interviews, and personal interviews.

The study results are important not only because significantly high levels of stress and illness were documented but also because the control group was of sufficient size (N = 50) and was compared with the loss subjects on a number of important variables. Since the original study prediction that presumed death bereavement would identify the high-risk population did not hold up, a series of secondary analyses to identify bereavement risk was undertaken. Six variables—age, gender, centrality of the relationship, belief of preventability, social support, and stress when taken together, accounted for nearly 50 percent of the variance, with stress being the most important high-risk variable for all health outcomes. Longitudinal data collected three years postdisaster are currently being analyzed.

SUGGESTIONS FOR FUTURE DISASTER RESEARCH

More research is needed on both the conditions of loss (i.e., bereavement, property) and at different points in recovery. Short-term recovery studies should gather data that aid in identifying those at-risk, suggest early interventions, and promote efficiency of helping operations. Long-term recovery data are needed to formulate policy and clarify issues on which litigations are based. Furthermore, instruments that successfully measure disaster variables need to be reported. At present, no two studies have used the same measures to assess stress and health outcomes. Until there is some consistency across studies, researchers and clinicians alike have no way to compare "victims" of one study with those of another. Finally, comparative conditions of untimely death need to be studied so that questions regarding whether accidental death bereavement as it occurs, case-by-case is similar to violent death bereavement resulting from mass emergencies. Evidence appears to suggest an affirmative answer, but generalizations cannot be made on the limited data currently available.

REFERENCES

Andrews, G., Tennant, C., Hewson, P., Vaillant, G. Life event stress, social supports, coping style and risk of psychological impairment. Journal of Nervous and Mental Disorders, 1978, 166, 307.

Ball, J. Widow's grief: The impact of age and mode of death. Omega, 1976–1977, 7, 307–333.

Bandura, A. Self-efficacy: Toward a unifying theory of behavioral change. Psychological Review, 1977, 84, 191–215.

Blauner, G. Death and social structure. Psychiatry, Journal for the Study of Interpersonal Processes, 1966, 29, 378–394.

Bromet, E., Dunn, L. Mental health of mothers nine months after the Three Mile Island accident. Urban and Social Change Review, 1981, 14, 12–15.

Bugen, L. Human grief: A model for prediction and intervention. American Journal of Orthopsychiatry, 1977, 47, 196–206.

Cohen, R.E., Ahearn, F.L., Jr. Handbook for Mental Health Care of Disaster Victims, Baltimore: Johns Hopkins University Press, 1980.

Coppel, D. The relationship of perceived social support and self-efficacy to major and minor stresses. Unpublished doctoral dissertation, University of Washington, 1980.

Derogatis, L., Lipman, R., Rickels, K., et al.: The Hopkins Symptom Checklist (HSCL): A measure of primary symptom dimensions. Psychological measurements in psychopharmacology. Modern Problems of Pharmacopsychiatry, 1974, 7, 79-110.

Harvey, C., Bahr, H. The sunshine widows: Adopting to sudden bereavement. Lexington, Ky., Heath, 1980.

Heller, K. The effects of social support: Prevention and treatment implications. In A. Goldstein, F. Kanfer (Eds.), Maximizing Treatment Gains: Transfer Enhancement in Psychotherapy. New York: Academic Press, 1979.

Horowitz, M. Diagnosis and treatment of stress response syndromes: General principles. In H. Parnd et al. (Eds.), Emergency and Disaster Management. Bowie, Md.: The Charles Press, 1976.

Kinston, W., Rosser, R. Disaster: Effects on mental and physical state. Journal of Psychosomatic Research, 1974, 18, 437-456.

Lazarus, R., Cohen, J. The Hassles Scale. Stress and coping project, Berkeley, Calif.: University of California, 1977.

Lifton, R.J., Olson, E. The human meaning of total disaster: The Buffalo Creek experience. Psychiatry, 1976, 39, 1-18.

Lindy, J., Grace, M., Green, B. Survivors: Outreach to a reluctant population. American Journal of Orthopsychiatry, 1981, 51(3), 468-478.

Maddison, D. The relevance of conjugal bereavement for preventive psychiatry. British Journal of Medical Psychology, 1968, 41, 223-233.

Malinak, D., Hoyt, M., Patterson, V. Adults' reactions to the death of a parent: A preliminary study. American Journal of Psychiatry, 1979, 136, 1152-1156.

McCubbin, H. Coping repertoires of families adapting to prolonged war-induced separations. Journal of Marriage and the Family, 1976, 38, 461.

Murphy, S. Coping with stress following a natural disaster: The volcanic eruption of Mt. St. Helens. (Doctoral dissertation, Portland State University, 1981.) Dissertation Abstracts International, 42, 10B p 4014 (University Microfilms No. 82-07, 736.)

Murphy, S., Stewart, B. Linked pairs of subjects: A method for increasing the sample size in a study of bereavement. Omega. In press.

Powell, J., Rayner, J. Progress notes: Disaster investigation July, 1951-June 30, 1952. Edgewood, Md.: Army Chemical Center, Chemical Corps Medical Laboratories, 1952.

Rabkin, J., Struening, E. Life events, stress, and illness. Science, 1976, 194, 1013-1020.

Raphael, B. Preventive intervention with the recently bereaved. Archives of General Psychiatry, 1977, 34, 1450-1454.

Raphael, B. A primary prevention action programme: Psychiatric involvement following a major rail disaster. Omega, 1979-80, 10, 211-226.

Sarason, I., Johnson, J., Siegel, J. Assessing the impact of life changes: Development of the life experiences survey. Journal of Consulting and Clinical Psychology, 1978, 46, 932-946.

Silver, R., Wortman, C. Coping with undesirable life events. In J. Garger, M. Seligman (Eds.), Human Helplessness: Theory and Application. New York: Academic Press, 1980.

Singh, B., Raphael, B. Post disaster morbidity of the bereaved. The Journal of Nervous and Mental Disease, 1981, 169, 202-212.

Titchener, J., Kapp, F.T. Family and character change at Buffalo Creek. American Journal of Psychiatry, 1976, 133, 295-599.

Weisman, A. Coping with untimely death. Psychiatry, 1973, 36, 366-379.

Wilson, R. Disaster and mental health. In G. Baker, D. Chapman (Eds.), Man and Society in Disaster. New York: Basic Books, 1972.

PART TWO

Clinical Applications for Disaster Populations

4

The Impact of Traumatic Injuries on Disaster Recovery

Martin E. Silverstein

Injury and death constitute a major potential component of all catastrophic events. One would expect that an ethical, humane society would concentrate its concerns on the protection of life and the rescue of the injured in both limited and massive disasters, yet the management of acute traumatic injury has only recently become one of the priorities of our society. This chapter will introduce readers to the issues and problems associated with traumatic injury following disaster.

Until a bit more than two decades ago, the prevention and management of bodily injury in civilian situations was the concern of a handful of medical professionals and industrial safety specialists. By the 1960s the rising highway accident toll could no longer be tolerated, nor could other quotidian accidents. The success of military surgical systems and the potential utility of technological advances in the aerospace and other research fields promised new approaches to prehospital rescue and trauma care. In 1966 all of these factors culminated in the dissemination of the now-famous white paper, *Death and Disability: A Neglected Disease* (National Academy of Sciences, 1966). That landmark publication led to a concerted administrative, legislative, and private sector medical attack on traumatic injuries in the United States. The major thrust of those activities eventuated in the establishment of medical rescue and care systems designed to cope with highway accidents.

It is fewer than 4 years ago that a much smaller but rapidly growing movement began attempts to analyze and mitigate the acute human injury resulting from civilian mass casualty events. The basic characteristics of this new trend in disaster medicine resemble those of the decade-old assault on highway and urban accidents such as the application of scientific traumatology and the development of extra-hospital emergency medical systems. Mass casualties resulting from disaster, however, represent a qualitatively different problem; one which, to a large extent, remains minimally approached and largely unsolved (Brutman, 1982; Disaster Research Center, 1977).

The reasons for societal neglect of the problem and for the failure to apply resources to solve management problems regarding the acute trauma patient injured in the course of disasters are both historical and social. Civilian mass casualty events tend to occur sporadically in scattered areas around the globe and the causes are multiple. Because of the infrequency of any single type of disaster in a locality, group memory tends to be short and it is difficult for a community to apply the energy and other resources requisite for preparation for disaster casualties. Society has other priorities for its limited resources and tends to postpone or minimize preparations.

Until recently, and perhaps even now, science and technology have been slow to develop the predictive methodologies so necessary to save lives. Even with satisfactory prediction and warning systems, the multiple pathologic problems presented by acute injury make the mobilization of adequate resources difficult.

There are authorities in the field of disaster who believe that sufficiently rapid mobilization of medical resources for the salvage of life and the minimization of crippling is impossible in mass casualty events. Examination of the history of the solution of medical problems, however, reveals that this nihilistic attitude tends to exist initially toward all major medical puzzles. Ingenious research scientists supported by public commitment have overcome the obstacles.

THE TOLL

The magnitude of the problem of human injury and death in some disasters demands a concerted approach to rescue and recovery. Accidents of all sizes cost the United States a total of 87 billion dollars in 1981. Public accidents, a category that excludes motor vehicle crashes, work-related accidents, and injuries incurred at home accounted for 6.6 billion dollars while fire disasters alone resulted in a 6.7-billion dollar cost. Unfortunately, death counts are much more available than are the numbers of injury victims. Nevertheless, they do provide an indicator of the human cost of trauma and a hint of the numbers who might have been saved. Accidents are the fourth highest cause of death, accounting in 1981 for 105,561 fatalities in the United States alone (National Safety Council, 1982).

Individual disasters vary greatly in the quality and quantity of physical injury to human beings as opposed to other aspects of suffering. It is perhaps for this reason that the suggestion has been made that the other components of disaster recovery—the restoration of the fabric of society, the replacement and repair of property, and the care of the dislocated but uninjured—receive higher priorities than treatment of the injured. This is a societal decision which should be made consciously by the polity rather than by default. There is insufficient information describing the consequences to society of disaster-incurred disability and death to allow a reasonable assessment of priorities. The human injury consequences of many disasters may be surprisingly low, but this is not always true. At least 500,000 people died as a result of a cyclone that struck East Pakistan in 1970. By no means were all the victims killed immediately. Wind-collapsed structures trapped many who, for lack of rapid rescue, were drowned by the ensuing 15-m-high waves or were lost to traumatic shock and blood loss. This cyclone illustrates, in the extreme, a dreadful problem of disaster rescue. Vitani of the League of Red Cross Societies reported that there were "no medical problems" remaining "hours later" (Vitani, 1980, p. 190). The earthquake in Friuli, Italy in 1976 gave some indication of the probable consequences of the expected California earthquake of the next decade which will be much larger. Friuli was remarkable for the rapid medical response to it. Thus, its ratio of 300 injured to 100 dead is significant and illustrates what might be accomplished by adequate advance planning.

In the United States acute technological disasters are a relatively common, if geographically dispersed, form of disaster. For example, the traveling public is particularly subject to disaster injury. There were 10,500 hotel and motel fires in the United States in 1981. One hundred and thirteen persons died in the structural hotel collapse in Kansas City, Missouri in that same year while 1,300 people died in air transportation accidents (National Safety Council, 1982).

The hospitalization costs for all trauma patients may be estimated from the 1978 data in which 3,738,000 patients were admitted with the diagnosis of traumatic injury out of a total of 36,000,000 hospital admissions (National Safety Council, 1982).

The highest cost of traumatic injury with survival is not measured in dollars but in sociopolitical terms. The United States has seen a steady trend which has shifted the public conception of responsibility for protection, rescue, and recovery from disaster away from private organizations toward governmental agencies. There is considerable evidence from foreign examples that the perceived mishandling of a disaster is a costly experience for public officials. More important is the consequent loss of confidence in the structure of society and in the immediate government.

CHANGES IN DISASTER AND SOCIETAL ATTITUDE

In the United States, disaster response and attitudes toward disaster response have changed with each historical period. When the country was basically agricultural and the population density generally low, disasters were regarded largely as unpredictable acts of God. Aside from individual prudence—"wilderness wise"—within the vanguard of a westward-moving society, there was no organized attempt to predict and prepare for disaster. The distinction between the knowledgeable scout and the tenderfoot was basically the ability to avoid geographical, meteorologic, and malicious human disasters. A study of the technology of building construction and wagon and water-borne vehicles reveals an early awareness of technological disaster and skillful methods of avoidance. During the same period, public opinion accepted reliance on local neighborliness and on extended volunteerism as the sources of rescue, recovery, and reconstruction.

Federal responsibility was considered to be protection of the nation's borders against foreign military invasion and later, in the second half of the 19th century, protection against invasion of epidemic microbes. The United States Public Health Service was the rescuer of last resort in the San Francisco earthquake of 1906. There is considerable evidence that public opinion began a conversion during the Great Depression which continued during and after World War II (Silverstein, 1977).

The United States has become a complex interdependent nation with an increasing population density. The American citizen from the time of the Roosevelt era has begun to look to the state and Federal governments as the protector against and rescuer from natural, technological, and conflict disasters.

With the recent increases in urban population, the wisdom of the early agricultural American society has to a large extent been lost. Residential and industrial building have invaded known flood plains, tectonic, or active volcano areas and has, in some cases, created the substance for natural hazard by unthinking or unknowing destruction of protective ecosystems. The potential for increasing numbers of technological and conflict disasters has increased, in part, for the same reasons.

Concurrently, the attitude of American public opinion has, perhaps necessarily, changed to a belief and a demand that society as a whole, and government in particular, provide for the safety of inhabited areas. In the event of a disaster, government is held culpable and responsible for prediction, warning, prevention, rescue, recovery, and reconstruction. These trends as well as the actual increase in numbers and extent of catastrophes involving human injury are increasing the public demand for students and managers of disaster preparation and response.

THE GENERAL TRAUMA MODEL

The cost and difficulty involved in rescue and recovery of traumatized victims of disasters is best illustrated by the common model of single-accident–single-victim trauma. Our present emergency medical system and trauma center arrangement are structured to cope with a small number of severely injured persons. The highway injury epitomizes the model. Almost all vehicular accidents are deceleration events with the transfer of kinetic energy to portions of the victim's body. Accompanying thermal burns may or may not occur. One or two persons each suffers a collection of injuries within ground ambulance- or helicopter-transportable distance from a hospital which contains a trauma center. The elasped time between the occurrence of the accident, the response of the emergency vehicle and personnel, and the return to the trauma center is often a matter of minutes.

Beyond extrication of the victim from the collasped vehicle and rapid transportation, relatively little is done at the site to treat traumatic injuries. The concept of stabilization of the victim at the site prior to transportation is now generally regarded as disadvantageous (Bodai et al., 1983). The inelegant order to pre- or extrahospital personnel is "scoop and run." Resuscitation and treatment of multiple injuries in the hospital emergency department requires a minimum of three to five professionals plus large amounts of stationary and expendable equipment. The next step, the trauma operating suite with its specialized team demands anesthesiologists, three or four surgeons, nurses, technicians, blood supplies, gases, and medications. The more severely injured, and this is the typical case, is then moved to a unit in a characteristically 12-bed specialized critical care unit where medications, dressings, special life support equipment, and special personnel are expensive. The patient is then moved to a standard hospital unit at a cost of several hundred dollars a day, and eventually psychologically and physically rehabilitated. Throughout the entire process, ancillary services, including various laboratory and radiological facilities are required. The survival of one multiple injury patient commonly costs tens of thousands of dollars. Burn patients follow the same essential model, except that they require larger numbers of skilled personnel, multiple operations, specialized burn units to which they are immediately admitted, and longer hospitalizations with consequently even higher costs. The treatment of the trauma victim is a labor-intensive and capital-intensive skilled process.

TRAUMA IN DISASTER VICTIMS

There are occasions when disaster victim care follows the same model but there are usually significant differences and additional elements. The precipitating event, such as a chemical explosion, a flood, or a hurricane may provide an element of injury which is common to most of the victims. A common injury among a large number of victims stresses the specialized facilities for the treatment of that type of injury. In some cases such as chemical explosions, fires, and volcanic eruptions, the dominant injury pattern may be unfamiliar to the medical rescuers.

The large number of casualties slows the extrication process. The limited resources available require a sorting, or triage, decision process. Delay in transportation caused by the circumstances of the disaster or simply by the number of casualties prohibits the "scoop and run" procedure.

Thus, the need for temporary on-site care frequently is a unique characteristic of early disaster medical recovery. There is strong suspicion that many victims are lost or doomed for lack of necessary extrication, resuscitation, and specialized care at the site and before transportation to hospitals. It is this single aspect which demands the attention of disaster response planners at this time. Extensive community preparation is required in preparation for general and specific disasters if recovery of the trauma victim is to be successful. West (personal communication, 1982) in his studies of California trauma resources has found strong indications that communities tend to overestimate their capability and the expertise available for the management of patients at the site of disasters and the number of hospital units available for long-term recovery. Research has not been conducted regarding the relationship between physical injury, other concurrent losses, and recovery outcome.

THE FINANCIAL COST

There is no standard for financing systems for the recovery of disaster trauma victims. On-site recovery costs tend to be born largely by the local political jurisdiction through their police, fire, and emergency medical services and the state by way of its emergency medical services system, if one exists, and by activation of the National Guard. Federal mobilization is usually too slow to provide early input of resources. In the United States, the Federal military medical apparatus participates only under special circumstances at the present time. The Department of Health and Human Services, the Department of Defense, and the Federal Emergency Management Agency are in the process of organizing a National Disaster Medical System which hopefully will provide long-range transportation of victims and permit the allocation of distant hospital facilities (Beary, 1983).

The cost of the long recovery period in hospitals is primarily a cost to the victim and eventually to the community. Often hospitals and the communities which support them bear an inordinate burden of the costs for care of trauma victims. The general trauma model described above indicates the variables of the postsite medical cost equation: the number of victims, the multiplicity of injuries, the type of injury, and, perversely, the success of the initial recovery process. A small community may be crippled by the short- and long-term loss of skilled workers in the public and private sectors during the recovery period. The Buffalo Creek Flood in Pennsylvania and the subsequent United States Supreme Court decision and monetary award set a precedent which may influence the future reimbursement of costs generated by necessary medical care and permanent disability. The Court in that case determined the liability of a private corporate entity. In some cases property owners and providers of transportation services are insured against loss. The Federal Emergency Management Agency administrates a program of reinsurance for special cases of victim reimbursement.

HUMAN COSTS

It is difficult, if not impossible, to quantify the human suffering of complex disaster, destruction, and recovery. Communities are disrupted and the breadwinners of families may be injured at the same time that worksites and homes are lost. A number of people in a single community handicapped by the same disaster represent a significant change in the emotional and financial configurations in that community.

DEATH AND COMMUNITY RECOVERY

Disaster trauma may result in mass death. The process of victim location, retrieval, and identification, and determination of cause of death is traditionally carried out by law enforcement agencies. Families usually bear funeral expenses. The periods of public anxiety, grief, and adaptation are long and painful. Chapters 3 and 11 in this book address bereavement loss.

THE REVOLUTION IN DISASTER TRAUMA MANAGEMENT

While there have been valid arguments against the allocation of resources for early trauma care in disaster-prone localities in the past, the increasing capability for prediction, the global communication systems, and especially the accelerating pace of advances in resuscitation and in operative trauma surgery are changing societal responsibilities to the disaster victim. A policy of denial of early rescue is now inhumane. Detailed predictive studies such as *The Physical and Social Consequences of a Major Thames Flood* (International Research Institute, 1981) will allow the rescue community to make its preparations. Our greater understanding of specific injuries of special disasters such as smoke deaths from fires and ash deaths from volcanism will contribute to sophisticated preparatory measures. The global establishment of regional trauma centers is placing pressure on disaster rescue organizations to utilize the medical state of the art. The survival of more victims after each disaster and the consequent need for long-term recovery care is likely to be the net result of the changes.

SUMMARY

Acute mass casualties represent a critical problem for disaster managers which is yet to be adequately approached in this era. The number and configuration of injuries present unique problems to trauma surgeons. The potential for large numbers of casualties and of deaths will influence the long recovery period. The individual and societal costs in monetary and human terms mandate efforts to achieve maximum prevention and early care of acute injuries.

REFERENCES

Beary, J. National Disaster Medical System. Paper presented at the Annual Meeting of the American College of Surgeons Committee on Trauma, San Antonio, March 1983.

Bodai, I.M., Smith, J.P., Frey, C.F. Pre-hospital stabilization of critically injured trauma patients: A failed concept. Presented at the American Association for the Surgery of Trauma, Chicago, October 1983.

Brutman, A.F. Responding to the Mass Casualty Incident. New Britain, Conn.: Emergency Training, Inc., 1982.

Disaster Research Center. The Delivery of Emergency Medical Services in Disasters. Columbus, Ohio: Disaster Research Center, 1977.

International Research Institute. The Physical and Social Consequences of a Major Thames Flood. London: Foxcombe Publications, 1981.

National Academy of Sciences, National Research Council. Accidental Death and Disability: The Neglected Disease of Modern Society. Washington, D. C., 1966.

National Safety Council. Accident Facts. Chicago, 1982.

Silverstein, M.E. Medical preparation for terrorism. Terrorism, 1977 , 1.

Vitani, J. The role of resuscitation in global disasters. In R. Frye, P. Safar (Eds.), Types and Events of Disasters: Organization in Various Disaster Situations. Berlin: Springer-Verlag, 1980.

5

Selected Foci in the Spectrum of Posttraumatic Stress Disorders

Calvin J. Frederick

Along with an increased understanding of psychosomatic disorders, presently termed psychophysiological reactions, within the last few decades it has become clear that a broad spectrum of measurable effects of psychological stress could become manifest in humans at all age levels. A special component of this phenomenon, namely, psychic trauma, was probably first recognized per se, in the early 1940s. This has developed into a significant condition called Post-Traumatic Stress Disorder (PTSD) which was officially listed for the first time in the third edition of the Diagnostic and Statistical Manual (DSM III) of the American Psychiatric Association (1980) (see Table 5.1). Following the notion of "shell shock" in World War I, where it was believed that the noise of explosives could bring on an observable behavioral and physical condition in military personnel, it became apparent that such a disorder had a psychological basis which was later called "war neurosis" (Titchener and Ross, 1974). It has long been suspected that these disturbances might have both acute or long-term effects. The specific range of stressors which could evoke such disturbances has been recognized only within the last couple of decades. In addition to the existence of a recognizable stressor which would be likely to evoke symptoms of distress in the majority of persons, typical symptoms include reexperiencing the traumatic situation; a difficulty in experiencing normal feeling, that is, an emotional anesthesia or reduction in being involved with the world around oneself; and an avoidance of situations that symbolize or represent the traumatic event.

The stressor that evokes a PTSD is beyond the range of ordinary experiences such as bereavement from deaths by natural causes, marital conflicts, illness, and business losses. The psychological injury can

110

be experienced when the victim is alone such as in the case of physical battering, or witnessing a violent death, or as part of a group of other people, for example, being an earthquake victim or being in military combat. The stressors that produce this disorder encompass a range of events including natural disasters (floods, tornadoes), fortuitous disasters (airplane crashes, explosions, fires), and planned, human-induced, so-called man-made disasters (hostage-taking, bombings, sniper shootings into crowds). Although a variety of subjective responses are experienced by victims of PTSD, some of the most common are recurrent thoughts of the trauma, fitful sleeping and nightmares, phobic-like reactions, and avoidance of stimuli that evoke recollections of the event. While it is clear that children as well as adults experience the disturbance, it remains to be seen whether some significant differences can exist between these groups and if so, how they manifest themselves.

By definition, a disaster must comprise a catastrophic situation in which a number of people are involved. When deaths occur, the probability increases for the development of psychic disturbances but loss of life is not a sine qua non for the event to be defined as a disaster or for the appearance of PTSD as a sequelae. In practical terms a major disaster is one that causes sufficient physical damage to property

TABLE 5.1. DIAGNOSTIC CRITERIA FOR POSTTRAUMATIC STRESS DISORDER

A. Existence of a recognizable stressor that would evoke significant symptoms of distress in almost everyone.

B. Reexperiencing of the trauma as evidenced by at least one of the following:
   1. Recurrent and intrusive recollections of the event
   2. Recurrent dreams of the event
   3. Sudden acting or feeling as if the traumatic event were reoccurring, because of an association with an environmental or ideational stimulus

C. Numbing of responsiveness to or reduced involvement with the external world, beginning some time after the trauma, as shown by at least one of the following:
   1. Markedly diminished interest in one or more significant activities
   2. Feeling of detachment or estrangement from others
   3. Constricted affect

D. At least two of the following symptoms that were not present before the trauma:
   1. Hyperalertness or exaggerated startle response
   2. Sleep disturbance
   3. Guilt about surviving when others have not, or about behavior required for survival
   4. Memory impairment or trouble concentrating
   5. Avoidance of activities that arouse recollection of the traumatic event
   6. Intensification of symptoms by exposure to events that symbolize or resemble the traumatic event

American Psychiatric Association. Diagnostic and Statistical Manual of Mental Disorders, (3rd Ed.). Washington, D.C.: American Psychiatric Association, 1980.

and persons as to warrant major assistance by the state and Federal
governments. However, the importance of psychological trauma was
recognized by the United States Congress in establishing P.L. 93–288,
the Disaster Relief Act of 1974 when such terms as "mental health problems," "adverse effects upon families and individuals," and "human
suffering" were used in the hearings formulating this piece of legisla-
tion. A separate portion, Section 413 addressed the "Crisis Counseling and Training" aspects of major Presidentially declared disasters.
The basic notion is that outside assistance must be provided to persons who have become victims due to events over which they had no
control.

The author (1983) has personally validated the presence of this phenomenon in both research and treatment realms covering a wide variety of trauma situations. Extensive discussions can be found over an
established range of stressors, for example, the accounts of hostage-taking by Mulder (1983) and Van der Ploeg (1983); aircraft accidents by
Frederick (1981); natural and human-induced or man-made catastrophic
events by Melick et al. (1982) and Frederick (1983); physical assault
and battering by Sadock (1980) and Groth and Burgess (1980); human
torture by Daly (1980); political siege by Fields (1977), McWhirter
(1982), and McWhirter and Trew (1981); prisoners of war, and the Holo-
caust by Eitinger (1965, 1971, 1983); refugees by Krumperman (1983);
and military combat by Figley (1978), Foy et al., and Yager et al. (1984).

Although the prescribed 6-month time period with respect to the
development of chronic or delayed PTSD is somewhat arbitrary, the
author's experience has tended to confirm this temporal period. The
development of long-term conditions appears to persist from the point
of the traumatic event to a period of 6 months or more afterward or
to display the symptoms that have lain fallow for a similar time period
and which surface 6 months or even years later. In retrospective
examination, these long-term signs and clues have often been observed
by other persons close to the victim. Signs such as irritability and lack
of concentration begin to disclose themselves over time before becoming fully recognizable. The author will delineate selected types of situations where such stress disorders have been clearly manifest in the
development of measurable psychological sequelae. Without appropriate treatment this disorder can persist almost indefinitely. In Veterans
Administration (VA) Medical Centers many, if not most, of the symptoms of chronic or delayed PTSD have now become apparent in some
World War II and Korean War veterans more than 30 years after their
war experiences.

It is important to know that children, like adults, can suffer from
PTSD. The author has shown that PTSDs occur as a highly frequent
response among both children and adults roughly in the order shown

in Table 5.2 when classifying common psychiatric disturbances as listed in DSM III. This order of occurrence is not immutable and may vary with circumstances. It can serve as a guide, however, in what to look for when traumatic events develop. For children the most prominent disorders are: (1) avoidant anxiety response, (2) separation anxiety, (3) sleep disorders, (4) overanxious reactions, (5) simple phobias, (6) agoraphobias, (7) PTSDs, and (8) attention deficit disturbances. Startle responses and adjustment reactions both at home and at school have been found to be very common among children. This has been confirmed internationally by my European colleagues Mulder (1983) and Van der Ploeg (1983). Among adults the following relative frequency of prominent disorders obtains: (1) generalized anxiety, (2) simple phobias, (3) PTSDs, (4) agoraphobias, (5) depressive reactions, (6) paranoid responses, (7) somatization reactions, (8) inhibited sexual desire, (9) overuse of tranquilizers, and (10) substance abuse.

A profile on the Minnesota Multiphasic Personality Inventory (MMPI) clearly reveals an acute disturbance among persons with PTSD where there are peaks indicating anxiety, irrational thinking, and low personal identity and self-esteem. The profile is so markedly distressed that in the absence of other information and diagnostic skill these cases might be mistakenly diagnosed as an initial fulminating psychotic reaction. Figure 5.1 shows these aspects clearly. While certain variations in the profile may occur, of course, this general picture has been present with striking consistency.

NATURAL AND HUMAN-INDUCED CATASTROPHIC EVENTS

Posttraumatic Stress Disorders can affect persons of all ages, from all walks of life. This seems to be especially so in disastrous situations of both a natural and man-made or human-induced kind. Experiences from more than 25 catastrophic events including hurricanes, tornadoes, floods, earthquakes, nuclear accidents, and airplane crashes have borne this out in the author's experience. Early symptoms to which the clinician should be alert are physical complaints such as headaches, stomach pains, sadness as a precursor to depression, isolation and withdrawal, and conduct disturbances, including night terrors or occasional withdrawal into prolonged sleep. Even though such disturbances appear temporary, they may persist and can be noticed by astutely observant family members, close friends, or school personnel. Victims of major disasters go through various phases as a result of the experience as outlined in the previous chapter.

The phases that occur in a man-made or human-induced disaster

TABLE 5.2. COMMON PSYCHIATRIC DISTURBANCES FOUND IN DISASTERS RANKED IN RELATIVE FREQUENCY OF OCCURRENCE

Adults			Children and Adolescents		
Rank		DSM III Disorder[a]	Rank		DSM III Disorder[a]
1	300.02	Generalized anxiety disorder	1	313.21	Anxiety disorder, avoidant disorder
2	300.29	Simple phobia	2	309.21	Anxiety disorder, separation anxiety disorder
3	308.20	Posttraumatic stress disorder, acute	3	307.46	Sleep terror disorder
4	309.81	Posttraumatic stress disorder, chronic or delayed	4	313.00	Over-anxious disorder
5	300.21	Agoraphobia, with panic attacks	5	300.29	Simple phobia
6	300.22	Agoraphobia, without panic	6	300.22	Agoraphobia, without panic
7	296.2	Major depression, simple episode	7	308.20	Posttraumatic stress disorder, acute
8	296.3	Major depression, recurrent	8	309.81	Posttraumatic stress disorder, chronic or delayed
9	298.30	Acute paranoid disorder	9	314.01	Attention deficit disorder with hyperactivity
10	300.81	Somatization disorder	10	314.80	Attention deficit disorder, residual type
11	302.71	Inhibited sexual desire	11	309.40	Adjustment disorder with mixed disturbance of emotions and conduct
12	304.6	Other specified substance, tranquilizing agents	12	300.23	Social phobia
13	307.60	Alcohol abuse	13	305.0	Functional enuresis
14	305.4	Barbiturate or similar sedative abuse	14	312.21	Conduct disorder socialized nonaggresive
15	305.7	Amphetamine or similar sympathomimetic	15	307.70	Functional encopresis

[a]Classification codes from the third edition of the Diagnostic and Statistical Manual of the American Psychiatric Association (DSM III).

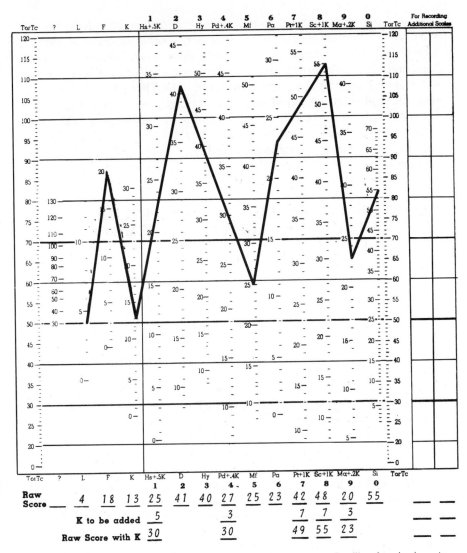

	Raw Score	K to be added	Raw Score with K
L	4		
F	18		
K	13		
Hs+.5K (1)	25	5	30
D (2)	41		
Hy (3)	40	3	30
Pd+.4K (4)	27		
Mf (5)	25		
Pa (6)	23		
Pt+1K (7)	42	7	49
Sc+1K (8)	48	7	55
Ma+.2K (9)	20	3	23
Si (0)	55		

Figure 5.1. Minnesota Multiphasic Personality Inventory Profile of typical acute case showing effects of stress in Posttraumatic Stress Disorders in adults.

vary somewhat, although the psychological symptoms of anxiety, insomnia, phobias, and depressed feelings are similar. Resentment against the cause is differentially focused since natural disasters are frequently viewed as acts of God while human-induced catastrophes focus upon human culpability. In the latter case, the phases usually found are: an *initial impact* period quite similar to that of natural disasters, *ac-*

ceptance and/or apparent respect for the perpetrators (although this will vary with circumstance), *victim and perpetrator interaction* during which feelings may run high but be suppressed, *disintegration* or termination of the perpetrators' control, and *resolution* which may be satisfactory only to the parties involved. The Three Mile Island incident illustrates one aspect of such a catastrophic event while the Hanafi Muslim takeover of the B'nai B'rith building in Washington, D.C. represents another. In any case, being alert to the likelihood of psychological and emotional disturbances and the need for treatment are cornerstones needed for building effective intervention programs.

DISASTERS COMPARED WITH THE PSYCHIC TRAUMA FROM HOSTAGE-TAKING, COMBAT, AND POLITICAL SIEGE

The reader may note from Table 5.2 the noticeable effects of disaster and other selective traumatic events from psychosocial and psychophysiologic processes. The clear presence or absence of these observable aspects of the human condition may be helpful to crisis teams in the field. With regard to the phases that occur, recognizable similarities and differences appear. Each traumatic event has its own kind of initial impact which may be of short duration (minutes or hours, e.g., natural disasters) or of a longer time span (days or weeks, e.g., military combat and political siege). In a tornado, for instance, the impact frequently lasts only a matter of minutes, whereas in military combat or political siege the initial impact occurs with greater duration. Even though combat or political siege may continue for months or years, by definition the impact per se occurs in a traumatic sense in a shorter time frame. Another component that cuts across most traumatic events is that of ego decompensation. The pervasiveness of disappointment and disillusionment in natural disasters is related to but not identical with ego decompensation which appears in a more obvious fashion in other types of catastrophic situations. The final period of reorganization is related to trauma mastery and recovery in the other situations noted. A cohesiveness tends to develop in the heroic period early on and continues somewhat into the honeymoon phase. This is characterized by altruistic comments and the need to engage in constructive activity and share experiences. Although such activity helps to delay the onset of disillusionment and feelings of depression, the latter inevitably appear when individuals are heavily engaged or strongly effected by the catastrophic situation. Anger and resentment, coupled with frustration, appear during the disillusionment phase in natural disasters and may last from a few weeks to a year or more. The victims tend to examine their neighbors' plight or absence of it and contrast it with their own lives. Often when one's neighbors have fared relatively well, resentment and envy are evoked and may be expressed overtly as well as covertly. The cohesiveness and cooperative spirit that were present previously disintegrate and become overridden by feelings of anger and annoyance. The annoyance with government officials tends to generalize and spill over onto one's own neighbors. These phenomena, in part, are related to the phases which occur in other traumatic situations, namely, interaction, resistance and denial, acceptance and repression, and decompensation. Many of these phenomena are noted in Table 5.3 where a relationship is noted between specific behavioral responses and a given stressor. As stated in Chapter 1, additional research is needed to substantiate these findings.

Psychological/behavioral symptoms which have been observed in a wide variety of stressful situations are delineated in Table 5.3. The appearance of anxiety, phobias, feelings of depression, and some form of substance abuse manifest themselves as common psychological responses presenting themselves in numerous traumatic situations. The appearance of flashbacks, mounting hostility, and substance abuse have appeared more prominently among Vietnam veterans than among persons in other wars. The debilitating aspects of these psychological responses must not be underestimated. Feelings of helplessness, self-abnegation, irritability, and unchanneled anger can result in seriously disturbed acting-out behavior. When this happens, of course, the likelihood of serious injury to self or others must be recognized. The appearance of suicide is not as great in most natural disasters as it is in the other stressful events noted. Victims of the stress of military combat, by contrast, appear to be more likely to commit suicide than act out against other persons. Intrusive thoughts manifest themselves almost universally in these situations as well.

The psychophysiologic symptoms which are listed in Table 5.2 present an important commonly observed response, namely, insomnia accompanied by nightmares. This is expressed in the form of reliving of the traumatic disturbance in some manner during sleep. In addition, hyperalertness or startle responses are very marked. There are occasions when most victims are noticeably jumpy and others when they are somewhat less so. However, this edgy quality is related to the appearance of irritability as a clear psychological symptom. Gastrointestinal disturbances are prominent in the form of upset stomachs, anorexia, diarrhea, and vomiting. Hypertension should be checked and observed, even among the teenage population. The appearance of essential hypertension, in contrast to malignant hypertension tends to

TABLE 5.3. COMPARISON OF EFFECTS OF DISASTER AND OTHER SELECTED TRAUMATIC EVENTS UPON PSYCHOSOCIAL AND PSYCHOPHYSIOLOGIC PROCESSES[a]

	Natural Disasters	Hostage-Taking	Military Combat	Political Siege
Phases	1. Initial impact 2. Heroic 3. Honeymoon 4. Disappointment 5. Reorganization	1. Initial impact 2. Interaction 3. Acceptance/acquiescence 4. Decompensation 5. Trauma mastery/recovery	1. Initial impact 2. Resistance/denial 3. Acceptance/repression 4. Decompensation 5. Trauma mastery/recovery	1. Initial impact 2. Denial/assertive 3. Acceptance/repression 4. Decompensation 5. Insight/recovery
Psycho-logical/ behavioral symptoms	Anxiety Insomnia Depression Anorexia Phobias Hostility Resentment Loss of concentration Paranoid reaction Substance abuse Intrusive thoughts	Anxiety Anorexia Phobias Helplessness/depression Anhedonia Memory deficit Loss of concentration Substance abuse Intrusive thoughts Marital discord	Anxiety Phobias Feelings of failure Helplessness/depression Self-abnegation Paranoid reactions Flashbacks Irritability Hostility/anger Intrusive thoughts Loss of concentration Substance abuse Marital discord	Anger Hostility Irritability Anxiety Paranoid reactions Intrusive thoughts Alcoholism
Psycho-physio-logic symptoms	Insomnia/nightmares Inhibited sexual response Enuresis/encopresis (children) Anorexia Hypertension Hyperalertness/startle	Insomnia/nightmares Skin disorders Vomiting Inhibited sexual response Trembling Hypertension Diarrhea Hyperalertness/startle	Diarrhea Trembling Vomiting Insomnia/nightmares Skin disorders Stomach problems Hypertension Hyperalertness/startle	Insomnia/nightmares Stomach problems Diarrhea Hypertension Hyperalertness/startle

[a]Listed in approximate rank order of occurrence.

118

abate as the recovery period ensues and the stressors become less manifest.

The presence or virtual absence of the responses listed in Table 5.4 will be of value to those working directly with victims of disaster and other traumatic events. It is useful to be aware of the fact that guilt, which is a criterion listed in the evaluation of PTSD, displays itself as different types. A feeling of guilt about not preventing the event appears in persons who have become hostages while this does not usually appear in the other calamitous situations listed. Guilt about not becoming more active during the crisis and helping other persons to survive or become effective in some degree is shown clearly in all of the areas listed except for political siege. The feeling that one could have done more to help prevent the plight of neighbors or friends is a common component. Having feelings of avoidance of situations, direct or symbolic, that represent the trauma, relates, in particular, to a fear of returning to the scene. This is especially marked in victims who have been hostages. Similar situations, such as having been victims of sniper fire in civilian life, are related to the stressors noted herein. In other kinds of situations there may be a desire to return to the scene of the event, even though there is some fear of it. Curiously, however, there is an avoidance of symbolic activities which represent the catastrophic stimulus. Heavy rains or thunderstorms may serve as recurrent negative stimuli to victims of flooding whereas scenes of military combat can evoke the avoidant response in traumatized victims of combat. The appearance of aberrant characterologic acts, such as looting, is found in victims of natural disasters but not in victims of hostage-taking or in victims of combat other than in Vietnam veterans in whom conduct disturbances have developed. Rejection, humiliation, doubt about the seriousness of complaints or indications of malingering, and the belief that the plight of the victims was self-precipitated did not appear for the most part in natural disasters or in many combat veterans (Vietnam excepted) but are present as correlates of other traumatic events. It is interesting to note the responses of crisis workers in terms of burnout. Worker burnout occurs early in natural disasters but late in most other calamitous events.

PSYCHOLOGICAL ASSESSMENT

In the assessment of adolescents between the ages of 16 and 18 years old, the author has found an MMPI profile which seems to be indicative of PTSDs which is similar to that found among adults only less acute. Moreover, the presence of conduct disturbances appears more

TABLE 5.4. CORRELATES OF BEHAVORIAL RESPONSES WITH DISASTER AND OTHER SELECTED TRAUMATIC EVENTS

	Natural Disasters	Hostage-Taking	Military Combat		Political Siege
			Vietnam	*Other Military*	
Event prevention guilt	0	+	0	0	0
Nonactivity guilt	+	+	+	+	0
Reprisal desire	+	0	+	0	+
Fear of returning to scene	0	+ +	0	0	0
Avoidance of symbolic activities	+	+	+	+	+
Aberrant acts	+	0	+	0	+ +
Rejection by others	0	+	+	0	+ 0[a]
Humiliation	0	+	+ +	0	+
Doubt by others about genuine complaints	0	+	+	0	+
Victim precipitated	0	+	+	0	+ +
Enduring group cohesiveness	0	+	0	+	+
Anger with officials	+	0	+ +	0	+ +
Early worker burnout	+	0	0	0	0
Late worker burnout	0	+	+	+	+

Abbreviations: + +, strong relationship; +, moderate relationship; 0, little or no relationship.
[a]Rejection by others +; by one's own group 0.

clear-cut along with an identity crisis in terms of sexual orientation (see Fig. 5.2 for details). As the reader may note, there are peaks indicating depression and neurotic-like symptoms along with irrationality and feelings of suspiciousness and persecution. In addition, the subjects appear to be sitting upon an emotional lid, as it were, and to be readily volatile in terms of acting-out behavior. The symptoms peculiar to

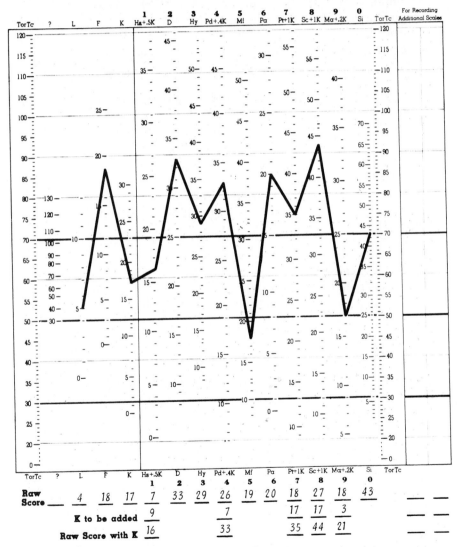

Figure 5.2. Minnesota Multiphasic Personality Inventory Profile of a typical case of the effects of stress in Posttraumatic Stress Disorders in late adolescents.

adults: when adults have PTSD, one of the most pervasive symptoms, in addition to the basic criteria for classification, is an extremely acute emotional state. This may not appear on the surface in cases of delayed stress but it can be tapped through psychological examination and testing. A striking appearance of irrationality and withholding of tension and acting-out tendencies is striking. The results indicate superficially that the scores are so acutely high that the records might be invalid. In point of fact, this simply accentuates the seriousness and acute quality of the psychological condition. While not all adults are explosive in terms of constituting an acting-out hazard to those around them, there are those whose irritability is such that this kind of behavior is clearly present and to some extent can be predicted. The MMPI profile of a typical acute case among adults is illustrated in Figure 5.1.

In selected individuals, a number of seemingly bizarre and violent past experiences are present such as: mutilation of the enemy, killing of innocent women and children, throwing the enemy out of aircraft, and firing at random at nonmilitary populations. This behavior existed in all wars but was apparently much more common in the Vietnam era and the Korean conflict.

Exposure to an overt experience with combat appears more likely to exacerbate such symptoms and adds to the likelihood of a marked PTSD of a severe and long-term type.

Individuals suffering from PTSDs from other causes such as major catastrophic events of both a natural and man-made type, rape, and being held hostage are far less likely to engage in such violent acts and needs for retribution. In part, this is no doubt due to training for combat in armed conflict and the attending psychological orientation to carry out such acts. The notion of "kill or be killed" is frequently imprinted into the thoughts of combat troops.

TREATMENT AND RECOMMENDATIONS

These illustrations will serve to emphasize the special problems encountered in long-term delayed stress reactions for both diagnostic and therapeutic purposes. One caveat which is especially significant for the clinician is to be aware of the possibility that such conditions exist. Unfortunately, the occurrence of these conditions is frequently confused with the development of borderline states. Such a misdiagnosis frequently contributes further to the problem due to lack of understanding and inadequate or improper treatment. Because this phenomenon is relatively new but has occurred with increasing frequency, it is all the more reason for the present-day clinician to become astutely vigilant and alert to the possibility that the condition exists. The author has encountered numerous persons who have suffered from PTSDs of both the acute and chronic varieties who have not received appropriate treatment.

It is a sine qua non for effective resolution of the difficulties inherent PTSDs to achieve *trauma mastery*. This is usually accomplished in severe cases only if the victim becomes deconditioned or desensitized to the traumatic stimuli involved. Unless this occurs the symptoms may continue for years with the individual functioning at varying levels of efficiency both personally and in the workplace. Some persons who function marginally take positions requiring less pressure and therefore work at a much lower level than their inherent capabilities might allow. Others attempt to work closer to their optimal levels of functioning and experience failures which may result in dismissal from the position and thus add insult to injury. Moreover, marital and interpersonal difficulties are pronounced and continue to worsen as time goes on. This situation may be accompanied by problems of substance abuse and acting-out behavior in a violent vein. The latter phenomenon is much more likely to occur, as has been noted, among persons who experience severe traumatic incidents. The victim will never forget the trauma but mastery of it can and must occur in order to allow the individual to function effectively in daily life.

For years, anxiety neurosis was listed as the most prominent service-connected disability among victims of catastrophic situations whether they were victims of war [prisoners of war (POWs) or traumatic combat], hostage-taking, or human-induced or natural disaster. Inasmuch as the term "anxiety neurosis," as used prior to DSM III, was relatively broad in scope, it failed to address the specific components inherent in PTSDs. Treating an individual for anxiety took a different avenue and failed to focus upon the necessity for desensitizing the individual to specific traumatic stimuli. The unfortunate result has been that many persons who have been suffering from PTSD have not been diagnosed accurately and in addition have not received appropriate treatment. At a conference held in the Netherlands in 1981, which was cosponsored by the World Health Organization and the Dutch Ministry of Welfare, Health and Cultural Affairs, authorities from all over the world addressed the need to make recommendations for the treatment of persons who had suffered from violent traumatic disturbances, including disasters. The working definition of the term "traumatic disturbance," adopted by that conference, was "the interhuman infliction of significant and avoidable pain and suffering." The reader can readily note that all of the phenomena selected for this chapter fit that criterion. With proper preparedness and planning even many catastrophic situations that appear to be natural disasters are avoidable, and appropriate steps should be taken on the parts of all governments throughout the world to address the needs of their citizens and preclude or lessen these traumatic sequelae. As noted earlier, in catastrophic situations the U.S. government has emphasized the need to help those whose plight arises from events that are not of the victims' own making.

Frequently there are second injuries or second wounds, as described by Symonds (1980) and Daly (1980). The point is stressed that often individuals who presumably are trying to help, even professionals, are insensitive to the real needs of the victim and thereby add to the problem through lack of understanding and acceptance, or by outright rejection. Long-term adverse effects on mental health should be expected in persons experiencing serious traumatic incidents when symptoms appear or continue after several weeks duration. This expectation should always be taken into account when physical and psychological assessments are made. Individual differences can contribute to the problem, such as: age, gender, personality structure, social environment, support systems, type of trauma experienced, and severity and duration. In every instance treatment should evaluate the nonmedical needs of the individual as well as the medical ones. Following an effective deconditioning and desensitization period, direct guidance and behavior control can be useful in a group situation, although the clinician should be alert to the fact that timing is of the utmost importance. Some individuals may not be able to function in a group until after specific individual treatment has been provided. In certain instances, relatively long-term psychotherapeutic treatment may be of value but its usefulness will be blunted at best if deconditioning and desensitization have not occurred earlier.

Vietnam veterans in several treatment groups in which the author has been a consultant have been obvious victims of PTSD of a chronic type. Their strong negative feelings need to be understood and dealt with while at the same time these victims must be assisted in focusing upon how to become effective in everyday living situations. The need to learn ways of becoming more effective in the job market is an essential component in the treatment of these persons who may be psychologically immature at the time of the traumatic event. They have frequently been unable to get or hold jobs, maintain effective marriages, or become efficient productive members of society for the variety of reasons noted. Victims of PTSD may find it difficult to remain seated during the usual psychotherapy process and may walk about the room due to the tension and frustration which they are experiencing. Thus it is necessary to employ relaxation techniques and decondition these individuals to distressing stimuli. The employment of psychotropic medication may be useful with some victims but certainly its use should not be viewed as an alternative to understanding, deconditioning, ventilation, and appropriately timed psychotherapy. Although antidepressants and phenothiazenes may be of use it should be remembered that many if not most victims of PTSDs are essentially normal, healthy, functioning people regardless of their socioeconomic status. In most cases medication should be withheld because of its possible interference with effective psychotherapeutic and desensitization endeavors. This should be fully explained to the subjects. They should not be treated as patients in the traditional sense unless they wish it and clearcut medical indications warrant it.

Child abuse and the maltreatment of children may become manifest, especially in younger children. Each program should be tailored to fit the individual needs of the subject, since feelings of self-worth and self-esteem are of cardinal importance in victims of PTSD. Every effort should be made, therefore, to avoid the phenomenon of the second injury or second wound which can only complicate the problem and drive the person further away from effective help-seeking avenues. Even well-meaning friends and family will often remark or suggest that victims have contributed to their own difficulties and have brought such difficulties on themselves in some manner. The idea is stated or implied that had they been more alert, prudent, and constructive in their actions they would have been able to avoid it. Children may be accused of being "bad" and making matters worse for adults. Such lack of acceptance is insensitive and is perceived by the victim as damaging rejection. When adults suffer from PTSD their disturbance spills over onto children and becomes contagious, in effect. Knowing of this possibility ahead of time can lead to its prevention by appropriate actions on the part of nonprofessional and professional persons alike.

A POSTTRAUMATIC STRESS DISORDER REACTION INDEX

A measurement procedure was developed by the author patterned after the criteria for PTSD that are listed in DSM III. This procedure, which is essentially in checklist form, allows the clinician to ascertain the presence or absence of PTSD and assess some measure of its degree of severity (see Appendix to Chapter 5). The term "reaction index" alone is used on the form itself to minimize suggestion or a plus or minus "halo effect," in case subjects themselves fill out the form.

It is preferable for the clinician to administer the form orally, but if the subject fills it out the clinician should always examine the answer and question further for needed clarification.

A score of seven or more specific items listed between numbers 1 through 22 indicate the presence of the disorder. The following items are particularly significant: 1, 2; any item 3 through 6, any item 7 through 10, any two items 10 through 17, and any item 18 through 22. At least moderate severity is shown if 7 to 12 items are checked and more than a dozen items reveals that the PTSD is marked in its severity. As the reader will note, items 18 through 21 simply determine whether or not the disorder is acute or chronic. The other items, particularly items 23 through 26, provide additional information for use by the clinical worker.

This measurement procedure has been used by the author in determining PTSDs in a broad spectrum of stressful events, including major disasters, hostage-taking, physical battering, suicide, and homicide.

The scale correlates at +0.95 with persons diagnosed in clinical settings in hospitals as compared to those persons diagnosed officially by mental health personnel as having PTSD. Additional psychometric properties are yet to be established. This is not surprising since the measurement procedure was developed directly from the criteria used in DSM III, which is that customarily used by trained mental health professionals, who are knowledgeable about the occurrence of PTSD. It may be worth noting, at this juncture, that because of the recent appearance of this disturbance in its present form, as noted in DSM III, there are still a number of mental health workers in all disciplines who are not as current in their knowledge of diagnostic procedures relating to PTSD as they no doubt will be in the near future. Because of its resemblance to anxiety states, borderline states, and some kinds of character or conduct disturbances, the diagnosis of PTSD may not be employed when it is applicable. Of course, it is possible for individuals to have "double psychopathology," so to speak. In other words, an individual can possess a character disorder or a neurosis and still be suffering from PTSD overlaying some basic personality disturbance. It must be emphasized, however, that the disorder can and does occur with great frequency in individuals who are essentially normal and the presence of premorbid psychopathology is not a sine qua non for diagnosis.

It is hoped that the material contained herein will enable health and mental health professionals to become more cognizant of the pervasive aspects of PTSD and realize that it may mimic or be associated with other disorders. More accountable treatment, training, and research should flow from heightened consciousness raising and increased awareness of the problems inherent in traumatic disorders.

REFERENCES

American Psychiatric Association. Diagnostic and Statistical Manual of Mental Disorders (3rd Ed.). Washington, D.C.: American Psychiatric Association, 1980.

Daly, R. Compensation and rehabilitation of victims of torture. Danish Medical Bulletin, 1980, *27*, 245–248.

Eitinger, L. Concentration camp survivors in Norway and Israel. Israel Journal of Medical Sciences, 1965, *1*, 883–895.

Eitinger, L. Accute and chronic psychiatric and psychosomatic reactions in concentration camp survivors. In L. Levi (Ed.), Society, Stress and Disease. New York: Oxford University Press, 1971.

Eitinger, L. Psychological consequences of war disturbances. In H. van Guens (Ed.), Helping Victims of Violence. The Hague, Netherlands: Ministry of Welfare, Health and Cultural Affairs, Government Printing Office, 1983.

Fields, R. Society Under Siege: Psychology of Northern Ireland. Philadelphia: Temple University Press, 1977.

Figley, C.R. Stress Disorders Among Vietnam Veterans. New York: Brunner/Mazel, 1978.

Foy, D., Sipprelle, R., Rueger, D., Carroll, E. Etiology of post-traumatic stress disorders in Vietnam vets: Analysis of premilitary, military and combat exposure influences. Journal of Consulting and Clinical Psychology, 1984, *52*, 79–87.

Frederick, C. (Ed.) Aircraft Accidents: Emergency Mental Health Problems. Department of Health and Human Services, Washington D.C.: Publication No. (ADM) 81–956, 1981.

Frederick, C. Violence and disasters: Immediate and long-term consequences. In H. van Guens (Ed.), Helping Victims Of Violence. The Hague, Netherlands: Ministry of Welfare, Health and Cultural Affairs, Government Printing Office, 1983.

Groth, A., Bergess, A. Male rape: Offenders and victims. American Journal of Psychiatry, 1980, *137*, 806–810.

Krumperman, A. Activities of the Health Centre for Refugees in the Netherlands. In H. van Guens (Ed.), Helping Victims of Violence. The Hague, Netherlands: Ministry of Welfare, Health and Cultural Affairs, Government Printing Office, 1983.

McWhirter, L. Growing up in Northern Ireland: From "Aggression" to the "Troubles." In A.P. Goldstein, M.H. Segall (Eds.), Aggression in Global Perspective. New York: Pergamon Press, 1982.

McWhirter, L., Trew, K. Social awareness in Northern Ireland children. Bulletin of British Psychological Society, 1981, *34*, 308–311.

Melick, M., Logue, J., Frederick, C. Stress and disaster. In E. Goldberger, S.

Breznitz (Eds.), Handbook of Stress. New York: Free Press, 1982.

Mulder, D. From hostage to victim of violence. In H. van Guens (Ed.), Helping Victims of Violence. The Hague, Netherlands: Ministry of Welfare, Health and Cultural Affairs, Government Printing Office, 1983.

Sadock, V. Rape. In H. Kaplan et al. (Eds.), Comprehensive Textbook of Psychiatry. Baltimore, Md.: Williams & Wilkins, 1980.

Symonds, M. The "second injury" to victims. Evaluation and Change, 1980, Special Issue, 36–38.

Titchener, J., Ross, W. Acute or chronic stress as determinants of behavior, character, and neurosis. In S. Arieta, F.B. Brody (Eds.), American Handbook of Psychiatry. New York: Basic Books, 1974.

Van der Ploeg, H. Identification of victims. In H. van Guens (Ed.), Helping Victims of Violence. The Hague, Netherlands: Ministry of Welfare, Health and Cultural Affairs, Government Printing Office, 1983.

Yager, T., Laufer, R., Gallops, M. Some problems associated with war experience in men of the Vietnam generation. Archives of General Psychiatry, 1984, *41*, 327–333.

APPENDIX TO CHAPTER 5: REACTION INDEX

Please answer each question by placing a check mark in either the "Yes" or "No" space provided. Please be sure to answer all questions.

1. Do you believe that your exposure to (event)* was an extreme stressor that could cause emotional problems?   Yes ____   No ____

2. Do fears of personal experiences with (event) continue in your mind regularly?   Yes ____   No ____

3. Have you reexperienced any disturbing scenes about your exposure to (event) in any way, physically or emotionally?   Yes ____   No ____

4. Do uncomfortable thoughts about your experiences in (event) seem to invade your mind in spite of efforts to keep them out?   Yes ____   No ____

5. Do dreams about your (event) experiences keep coming back?   Yes ____   No ____

6. Do you sometimes see or think of something that makes you feel as if your (event) experiences are about to happen again?   Yes ____   No ____

7. Are you as interested as ever in nearly all activities that were important before (event) experience, such as sports (e.g., bowling, golf, going to football games, and so forth) or playing cards with a group, reading, or going to the movies?   Yes ____   No ____

8. Have your fears with regard to (event) exposure ever left you numb or emotionally unfeeling?   Yes ____   No ____

9. Are you now more detached and less involved with other people than you were before exposure to (event)?   Yes ____   No ____

10. Can you express your emotions and feelings as freely as you could before your exposure to (event)?   Yes ____   No ____

11. Are you jumpy, edgy, and more easily startled than before you were exposed to (event)?   Yes ____   No ____

12. Do you sleep well most of the time?   Yes ____   No ____

13. Do you feel guilty that you came out better or perhaps went through less trauma than others?   Yes ____   No ____

14. Is your memory as good as it always was?   Yes ____   No ____

---

* Wherever (event) appears the applicable traumatic event term is used, for example, "combat," "flood," "battering," "injury," "airline crash," and so forth.

15. Can you concentrate as well as you always could?   Yes _____ No _____

16. Do you avoid activities which might make you re-
    member your (event) experiences?   Yes _____ No _____

17. When something resembles (event), or reminds you
    of it, do your feelings of distress increase.   Yes _____ No _____

18. Did symptoms of distress begin within 6 months
    of the time your exposure to (event) took place?   Yes _____ No _____

19. If yes, did the last of these symptoms disappear
    within 6 months following (event) exposure?   Yes _____ No _____

20. Were any symptoms of distress present for more
    than 6 months following (event) exposure?   Yes _____ No _____

21. Have you noticed any distressing symptoms which
    were delayed and appeared at least 6 months after
    your exposure to (event)?   Yes _____ No _____

22. Have you talked with a crisis worker or received any
    professional assistance resulting from the (event)? Yes _____ No _____

23. If yes, circle the letters noted for all areas which
    apply:
    a. Medicine
    b. Psychological
    c. Pastoral (religion)
    d. Social welfare
    e. Financial (loans, housing, property loss)

24. Has a close friend or family member been affected
    in a negative way by your exposure to (event)?   Yes _____ No _____

25. If yes, circle the letters noted for all areas which
    apply:
    a. Medicine
    b. Psychological
    c. Pastoral (religion)
    d. Social welfare
    e. Financial (loans, housing, property loss)

6

Children as Victims of Disaster

Connie J. Boatright

A natural disaster is a phenomenon which is always a surprise and never welcome. It is something that always happens to "the other guy," and by its very nature, finds us unprepared and leaves us with various aspects of retrospective thought and "what ifs." After a disaster, we generally, in a somewhat haphazard and impromptu fashion, discover some things which we should have known before. Such was the case with this writer.

Having been reared in the Midwest, I was familiar with tornadoes and aware that they occur in spring as sure as the snow falls in winter. As a child, I participated in and rehearsed the annual tornado drills at elementary school. I had been near to and witnessed devastation to others and their property, but felt secure that I lived in a city which had never experienced a tornado. As an adolescent, I worked in a hospital which treated hundreds of victims of the infamous "Palm Sunday Tornado" of 1965.

None of my limited experience prepared me for the "real thing" which happened in the spring of 1974. As county health nurse, I was making rounds to the rural community schools. One of the schools on my agenda was about to experience an unforgettable trauma.

The day began as uneventful and routine for most of the residents of the community. Overcast skies progressed to sprinkling then heavy rain by afternoon.

The school day completed, the children boarded the school buses. As they were about to depart to their destinations, the proverbial "calm before the storm" was evident. One very alert bus driver sited not one, but two funnel clouds which appeared

to be purposely descending on the community with the school
as their major target. The driver quickly and calmly alerted
the other drivers and the faculty members who hurried the children to the school basement where they assumed the "duck
and cover" position.

First there was quiet, then intense roaring and an overwhelming feeling of resistance, of being sucked up and swooped
away. Within minutes, which seemed like eternity, the damage had been done. While little hands brushed dirt and debris
from clothing and hair, eyes gazed upward and saw the sky.
What was a school building just moments before was now unrecognizable rubble. One boy said that he thought maybe he
had died and gone to heaven.

No one was seriously injured. There was an eerie feeling
apparent among the mass of children as they began emerging
from the piles and saw yellow strips of twisted metal where
school buses were just moments before. The school that was—
the town that was—would never be the same again.

The remainder of the day involved recovering from the major shock and encountering new ones. The emotions were intense: bewilderment and despair on faces of people as they
viewed what had once been their homes; the horror and panic
among parents who had just returned from their jobs in the
city to find their homes demolished and then assumed that the
children were home from school and buried under the bricks
and wood; the confusion of having no communication within
the community or to the rest of the world; the utter futility
and frustration of attempting to piece together "something"
and not having a starting point.

As days progressed, the myriad of government, secular,
community, and health agencies organized and administered
various levels of care and assistance. Weeks later, the residents
were living in makeshift houses and government-provided trail-
ers and had returned to their jobs. Children were relocated at
nearby schools. Everything was returning to normal—so it
seemed.

Occasionally, parents of child victims shared concerns regarding their children's behaviors—I heard accounts of fear
of storms, fear of sleeping alone, nightmares, of not wanting
to go to school.

Not long after the disaster, I moved from the community
to return to graduate school. It was there that I had the op-

portunity to investigate my questions regarding disaster recovery. I explored then and have continued to examine issues of children and disaster and formulated a basis to share with others who may find themselves in a position which demands knowledge of disaster and postdisaster intervention.

Children, as a category, have been neglected in disaster research. Some clues to the areas where children suffer most can occasionally be cited in the literature. The San Fernando Valley Child Guidance Clinic, after working with children in the 1971 Los Angeles earthquake, reported that children frequently develop specific fears as a result of the disaster situation. Some children may develop school phobia and may be afraid or reluctant to go to school (Coping with Children's Reactions to Earthquakes and Other Disasters, 1971). Kingston and Rosser (1974) reported that those children "most at risk" are those in the 8- to 12-year-old age range.

As research on children in disaster is scarce and research on school phobia and disaster is virtually nonexistant, there is a need for more knowledge which can be utilized in maintaining or restoring mental health in children succumbing to the trauma of disaster.

School phobia has been repeatedly referred to in the literature as a potential problem of postdisaster children but there is little research to support a correlation of these two variables. This study was done in an effort to bring new knowledge to the field and validate the anecdotal accounts reported in the literature.

PURPOSE

The purpose of this study was to determine the psychological effect of disaster on children, reflected in absenteeism from school at $1\frac{1}{2}$, 8, and 14 months postdisaster.

Hypotheses
   H_1: At $1\frac{1}{2}$ months postdisaster, there will be no difference between the school absenteeism of students who experienced the disaster and absenteeism of students who did not experience the disaster.
   H_2: At 8 months postdisaster, there will be no difference between the school absenteeism of students who experienced the disaster and absenteeism of students who did not experience the disaster.

H_3:   At 14 months postdisaster, there will be no difference between
the school absenteeism of students who experienced the
disaster and absenteeism of students who did not experience
the disaster.

H_4:   At $1\frac{1}{2}$ months postdisaster, there will be no difference between the school absenteeism of girls who experienced the
disaster and absenteeism of boys who experienced the disaster.

H_5:   At 8 months postdisaster, there will be no difference between
the school absenteeism of girls who experienced the disaster
and absenteeism of boys who experienced the disaster.

H_6:   At 14 months postdisaster, there will be no difference between
the school absenteeism of girls who experienced the disaster
and absenteeism of boys who experienced the disaster.

BACKGROUND

Stress and Coping in Children

According to Murphy (1974), children experience normal expected stress
as they move from preschool into the school setting, where rigidities
and pressures mount through the school years. Added stresses (specific or combined pressures, frustrations, pain) differ with different children, depending on constitutional and acquired thresholds, affective
and automatic lability, consequences of previous trauma, conflict, anxiety, subjective or objective mitigating factors, and effectiveness of defenses. (For instance, two children may become exposed to the same
trauma, but one emerges "sick" and the other "well," depending on
the aforementioned variables.)

With undue stress, the need for coping evolves. Coping includes
all those efforts to deal with the environmental pressures that cannot
be dealt with by reflexes or organized skills, but involves struggles,
trials, and persistent focused energy toward a goal. Coping involves
responses to threats, dangers, frustration, losses, defeat, obstacles, and
strangeness to new and unknown demands. Murphy (1974) adds that
in the coping process, effort is put forth to solve a problem with built-
in adaptational mechanisms, that is, reflexes, on one end of the con-
tinuum, and complete mastery with competence at the other end. The
resulting coping depends on many factors, including how the situation
is appraised.

There are three aspects to the appraisal, according to Lazarus et
al. (1974)—primary, secondary, and reappraisal. Primary appraisal concerns the judgment that some outcome may be harmful, beneficial, or
irrelevant. Secondary appraisal is the perception of the range of cop-

ing alternatives through which harm can be mastered or beneficial results can be achieved. Primary and secondary appraisal are very closely
related. Reappraisal is a change in the original perception, for example, from benign to threatening or vice versa. Coping changes in quality and intensity as new information and previous outcomes are
appraised. After the appraisal process, the individual chooses his coping method. Lazarus et al. (1974) identified two classes of coping. One
is action tendencies which attempt to eliminate or mitigate the threat
and the other is cognitive maneuvers where appraisal is altered without action directed at changing the situation. The second class is more
commonly referred to as defense mechanisms and involves behaviors
such as denial, avoidance, rationalization, and so forth. School phobia
falls into the second class.

In the framework of White (1974), securing adequate information
is fundamental in successful coping and adaptation. There can be too
much or too little information received. Too little will cause underload-
ing, leaving the individual with no way to decide a course of action.
Too much information, or overloading, can create cognitive confusion.
The amount of information is not as important as the meaning of information, however, in terms of potential benefits and harm. Once the
"correct" amount is secured, the cognitive field can incorporate it and
take a course of action.

The cognitive field alone does not guarantee adaptive behavior if
internal organization is not balanced. The internal disorganization could
be from illness or fatigue, but also from strong and unpleasant effects,
such as anxiety, grief, and shame.

Murphy (1974), cited energy reserves as another prerequisite to coping. The "second wind" phenomenon, of having a capacity to mobilize
resources under stress, to be strained and still put out extra energy,
could well fall under the internal organization category. Murphy (1974),
too, sees the importance of a healthy state in the coping process. Resti-
tution by sleep, rest, and food is required after a struggle. Food, and
the gratification it provides, also contributes to the child's valiant struggle. Equally important is the capacity to evoke help, use help, relate
to new objects, and accept support. As Murphy (1974) concluded, the
struggle for mastery depends on expectation and trust in future gratification.

A discussion on coping and adaptive behavior cannot be complete
without consideration of maladaptive behavior. According to Wolff
(1970), maladaptive behavior is a symptom of communication which
tells something about underlying disturbances. Symptoms are not usually obvious. They have no general meaning but are personal and specific to each individual.

Behavioral disorders in children may be categorized as: (1) anxiety disorders, and (2) conduct disorders. Behavioral disorders following a disaster would fall under the first group, for example, excessive anxiety following the trauma. When anxiety occurs, defense mechanisms (regression, denial, and the like) come into play. These mechanisms help protect the individual from behavioral disorganization.

For the parents and teachers, with any child experiencing emotional problems, it is important to (1) allow the child free expression of feelings, (2) help correct misperceptions of the environment, and (3) provide insight, helping the child understand the feelings, to increase mastery over the emotions. It is axiomatic that in any situation of stress, children should be allowed to talk out their true thoughts and feelings (Wolff, 1970).

School Phobia. Rivlin (1936, p. 36) was one of the first to explore the concept of school phobia. He described phobia as "a fear reaction to a stimulus which, among normal people, does not result in fear. The same act may indicate a rational habit, a fear, or a phobia; the distinction is made on the basis of motivation and not its over-manifestation." He added, "by resorting to fears and phobias, the youngster seemingly avoids contact with the forces that threaten, or that did threaten in the past, his precarious emotional equilibrium." He believed that as a child grows and matures, fears and phobias lessen as the fears and situations which caused them disappear and the child learns to overcome the difficulty rather than avoid or run away. Unfortunately, some fears continue to persist in spite of increased maturation, intelligence, and experience.

According to Mussen (1974), occasional mild reluctance against going to school is common among children in "middle childhood" and many children have "physical" illnesses which disappear as soon as they are allowed to stay home. A persistent morbid fear, however, is significant, and represents a dread of some aspect of the school situation, concerns about leaving home, or many times, both.

From a more contemporary source, the *Diagnostic and Statistical Manual of Mental Disorders* (DSM III) (American Psychiatric Association, 1980), what was once listed as school phobia is now in the general category of separation anxiety disorder. The diagnostic criteria for this particular disorder include, but are not limited to:

A. Excessive anxiety concerning separation from those to whom the child is attached as manifested in at least three of the following:
    1. Unrealistic worry about possible harm or abandonment by major attachment figures

2. Unrealistic worry that an outward calamitous event will separate the child from a major attachment figure
3. Persistent reluctance or refusal to go to school in order to stay home or with attachment figure
4. Persistent reluctance or refusal to go to sleep unless child is next to attachment figures—or child will not sleep away from home
5. Persistent avoidance of being alone in the house and emotional upset if child cannot follow attachment figure around the home
6. Repeated nightmares about separation
7. Complaints of physical symptoms on school days
8. Signs of extreme distress upon separation from attachment figures
9. Social withdrawal, apathy, sadness, difficulty concentrating if not with major attachment figure

B. Duration of disturbance of at least 2 weeks
C. Not due to other disorder (e.g., psychotic disorders)

Wolff (1970) also affirms that school phobia children display shyness, fears, and physical symptoms, such as abdominal pain and vomiting when it is time to go to school. She too adds that the children want to go to school, but cannot bring themselves to go. They have a great deal of anxiety about leaving their mothers. Nevertheless, these children usually have the potential to be good students.

It is difficult to determine who may experience school phobia. Kessler (1966) found that although boys outnumber girls as clients in most child guidance clinics, it is reported that more girls experience school phobia. Wolff (1970) believed that part of the difficulty in determining emotional disturbances in children is due to the differing attitudes of teachers and parents. The differences are partially due to the real differences in the behavior of children at home and at school. This indicates that one cannot rely on data only from teachers or parents, but must include both groups.

It is assumed that school phobia interferes with learning. According to Mussen (1974), failure to attend to information, an obvious cause of memory failure, can be the result of many factors, most frequently being interfering thoughts and distracting stimuli. There is a negative relationship between memory and anxiety. Anxious children have poorer recall, and, therefore, poorer learning than less anxious children. The anxiety creates distracting stimulation that interferes with attention and incoming information, and impairs memory. It seems likely, then, that the anxious children's grades would be lower than other children's.

Whether maladaptive behavior is labeled school phobia, separation anxiety or some other category, it is important that differential diagnosis be employed. A child whose behavior seems irrational to observers may be misdiagnosed as retarded, psychotic, characterological, and so forth, when perhaps the single irrational behavior exhibited is the only element which is abnormal, in an otherwise normal functioning child. In the situation of a postdisaster child victim experiencing school phobia kind of behavior, the child can be assisted through the crisis by a collaborative effort between significant others at home and school. Together, parents and teachers can provide support, firm limits, and an atmosphere which demonstrates to the child that the school day has returned to "business as usual."

If a child persists with an overabundance of fear and avoidance of school behavior, professional intervention should be initiated. Through psychological testing, using the DSM III, behavioral history and assessment, the appropriate diagnosis and treatment can be derived.

Of recent interest to psychiatric/mental health practitioners is the diagnosis of posttraumatic stress disorder. Frederick, in Chapter 5 of this volume, describes the disorder. Although it is generally utilized in diagnosis of adults who have experienced a traumatic event (disaster, war, unique personal experience, and so forth) a postdisaster child victim with prolonged school phobia or pronounced anxiety symptoms could very well be appropriately diagnosed with this disorder.

Again, it is important that differential diagnosis be utilized in order to establish the most appropriate interventions.

Reaction of Children to Disaster. The majority of maladaptive behaviors and inappropriate emotions among children who survive a traumatic natural disaster surface within hours. In addition to regressive behaviors such as enuresis and fear of being alone, some children regress to earlier fears of going to sleep. This can result in insomnia and somatic complaints. Young survivors may also manifest behaviors characterized by docility, lack of responsiveness, inhibition of activity, and absence of emotions (Crabbs, 1981).

Children may be unable to adjust to their disaster experience immediately and initial reactions may persist for months or even years after the event. Since the majority of a child's waking hours are spent in the school setting, it is of particular importance to determine whether the maladaptive behaviors are manifested in the classroom. It is not uncommon for young disaster victims to exhibit increases in fighting, crying, school phobia, daydreaming, and cognitive errors. It is speculated that educational achievement and school attendance diminishes among school-age victims, but this has not been well researched and validated (Crabbs, 1981).

Following the February 1971 earthquake in Los Angeles, the San Fernando Valley Child Guidance Clinic published a pamphlet entitled *Coping with Children's Reactions to Earthquakes and Other Disasters.* The pamphlet was designed to assist parents, teachers, and other adults who may be in contact with children who are victims of natural disasters. It states that fear and anxiety are normal reactions to any danger which threatens life or well-being and that children, after a disaster, are afraid of recurrence, death, or injury; of being separated from their families; of being left alone. It suggests that parents may help a child by reassuring him or her, listening to his or her fears, explaining about the disaster, and maintaining discipline. The most frequently reported problem that parents encounter occurs at bedtime. The child may refuse to go to bed alone, may have difficulty falling asleep, may wake up during the night, or may have nightmares. It is advised that parents be more flexible at first with these specific circumstances, but that things should return to normal within a few days. Sometimes regressive behavior, such as thumb sucking, occurs. The parent should be patient, as this behavior will probably disappear within a few days. Irrational fears, such as fear of beds, houses, or darkness, or school phobia (refusal to go to school), sometimes occur. With school phobia, the parent and teacher must be firm and let children know that they expect them to attend school. If fears and unusual behaviors continue or become worse, professional psychiatric help should be sought.

A study conducted by Dohrenwend et al. in 1979 following the Three Mile Island nuclear accident, revealed that somatic symptoms such as stomach aches and nightmares were especially common among girls and children in the low grade levels. The highest levels of distress were experienced by children with preschool siblings, those living within 8 km of the plant, and those whose families had evacuated the area. Many of these children continued to experience distress above the expected level 2 months after the incident (Logue et al., 1981).

McIntire and Sadeghi (1977) emphasize that children tend to respond in an egocentric manner to any threat to emotional security with anxiety, denial, distortions, displacement, or reversal of feelings. Since disaster can certainly be viewed as "a threat to emotional security," it can be expected that children will respond with one or more defensive measures.

Children have been described as having problems for as long as 4 years after a natural disaster. The bulk of studies have relied on general-opinion surveys of observers or parents. Some investigators have reported that, after a natural disaster, many parents deny their children have problems. Because of this denial, children's reactions to natural disasters may be underestimated (Burke et al., 1982).

Kingston and Rosser (1974) reported the effects of disaster on mental and physical states. They cited that although there is much literature on various aspects of disaster, there has been no comprehensive review of its psychiatric consequences. They view disaster as a situation of massive collective stress which is a combination of individual stress reactions and changes in the social milieu. They gave brief attention to children, advising that the predominant fear of children following disaster is separation from the parents. A high incidence of regressive behavior occurs, especially in a tense atmosphere where the disaster had to be "forgotten." They concluded that children rarely need psychiatric treatment, but do need an opportunity to ventilate anxieties to a sympathetic adult. Those most at risk are between 8 and 12 years old with a previous history of physical or emotional illness and come from unstable homes.

Consideration of children following a disaster is found in the *Training Manual for Human Service Workers in Disaster* (1976). Particularly noteworthy is their summary of behavioral symptoms and treatment options for ages 1 through 18. This table has been included in the appendix of the present book.

METHOD

Sample

The sample population consisted of second through sixth grade children. The experimental sample was composed of second through sixth grade students whose parents granted permission for review of school records. The children were enrolled at School X when the April 3, 1974 tornado occurred. The school building in which the children were located was at that time destroyed, but no one was seriously injured. The children have since merged into the student body at School Z, 9 miles from School X. All School X children commuted to this school by bus.

The control sample was composed of second through sixth grade students whose parents also granted permission to review school records. They were enrolled at School Y, which is approximately 14 miles from School X. These children were not involved in the tornado or other known disaster.

Both the experimental and control groups represent children from the same school system. Both groups were exposed to the same basic educational philosophies and both groups attended school for the same number of days and over the same period of time. The communities of both samples were rural, midwestern towns with agriculture and industry as the primary means of parental income.

Permission to conduct the study was obtained from the superintendent and school board of participating schools and principals of Schools X, Y, and Z. In addition, each parent was asked to sign a release and consent form granting permission for the researcher to look at individual student files.

Data Analysis

Days absent, recorded on each subject's file, were noted at $1\frac{1}{2}$, 8, and 14 months postdisaster. Those temporal points reflected the termination of Spring 1974, Fall 1974, and Spring 1975, respectively. The mean numbers of days absent were calculated for the experimental and control groups for the times designated in the hypotheses. Two-tailed t tests were performed and standard deviations were computed to determine deviations from the norm.

Two tailed t tests were also conducted between boys and girls in both study groups to determine if there was a significant difference between gender.

RESULTS

Table 6.1 specifies the number of boys and girls in each grade for both the experimental and control groups. Since each student was required to submit parental permission in order to be included in this study, the figures do not represent 100 percent of the actual subjects involved in the disaster.

The actual numbers represented include 47 of a possible 102 experimental subjects, or approximately 46 percent of the total experimental population, and 75 of a possible 200 control subjects, or approximately 38 percent of the total control population. Therefore, the eight-percentage point difference indicates greater study coopera-

TABLE 6.1. GROUPS BY GENDER AND GRADE

Grade	Experimental (N = 47)		Control (N = 75)	
	Girls	Boys	Girls	Boys
2	8	6	9	9
3	2	2	10	3
4	8	6	9	6
5	4	6	7	7
6	2	3	7	8

tion by the experimental group. There was no remarkable difference between numbers of girl or boy subjects who participated in the study. The greatest percentage of participation was by the second grade control subjects; the least percentage of participation was by the sixth grade experimental subjects.

Results are presented with each hypothesis.

H_1: At $1\frac{1}{2}$ months postdisaster, there will be no difference between the school absenteeism of students who experienced the disaster and absenteeism of students who did not experience the disaster.

The null hypothesis was rejected at the 0.01 level of probability. As shown in Table 6.2, absenteeism at $1\frac{1}{2}$ months postdisaster was significantly higher in the control group ($\bar{x} = 4.2$ days) than in the experimental group ($\bar{x} = 2.0$ days). It was expected that absenteeism would be higher in the experimental group than in the control group. Although the null hypothesis was rejected, results were in reverse of the predicted direction.

H_2: At 8 months postdisaster, there will be no difference between the school absenteeism of students who experienced the disaster and the absenteeism of students who did not experience the disaster.

The null hypothesis was rejected at the 0.05 level of probability. Table 6.2 summarizes t test results for H_2. At 8 months postdisaster,

TABLE 6.2. ABSENTEEISM AT $1\frac{1}{2}$, 8, AND 14 MONTHS POSTDISASTER

Group	N	$\bar{x}$	Standard Deviation	t
$1\frac{1}{2}$ months				
Experimental	47	2.0	2.3	
Control	75	4.2	4.4	3.1**
8 months				
Experimental	47	4.4	4.1	
Control	75	2.7	3.7	− 2.5*
14 months				
Experimental	47	4.6	3.6	
Control	75	3.0	3.3	− 2.5*

*p < 0.05; **p < 0.01.

the experimental group experienced a greater degree of absenteeism ($\bar{x}$ = 4.4 days) than the control group ($\bar{x}$ = 2.7 days). The results were in the predicted direction.

H_3: At 14 months postdisaster, there will be no difference between school absenteeism of subjects who experienced the disaster and absenteeism of subjects who did not experience the disaster.

The null hypothesis was rejected at the 0.05 level of probability. Table 6.2 summarized t test results which indicate that at 14 months postdisaster, the experimental group experienced a greater degree of absenteeism ($\bar{x}$ = 4.6 days) than the control group ($\bar{x}$ = 3.0 days). The results were in the predicted direction.

H_4: At $1\frac{1}{2}$ months postdisaster, there will be no difference between the school absenteeism of girls who experienced the disaster and absenteeism of boys who experienced the disaster.

The null hypothesis was not rejected. Results of the t tests (Table 6.3) show no significant difference between absenteeism and gender at $1\frac{1}{2}$ months postdisaster.

H_5: At 8 months postdisaster, there will be no difference between the school absenteeism of girls who experienced the disaster and absenteeism of boys who experienced the disaster.

The null hypothesis was not rejected. Table 6.3 summarizes t test

TABLE 6.3. ABSENTEEISM AT $1\frac{1}{2}$, 8, AND 14 MONTHS POSTDISASTER BY GENDER

	n	Mean	Standard Deviation	t
$1\frac{1}{2}$ months				
Girls	24	2.2	2.8	
Boys	23	1.8	1.5	− .54
8 months				
Girls	24	4.1	2.8	.58
Boys	23	4.8	5.2	
14 months				
Girls	24	4.5	3.6	
Boys	23	4.7	4.2	.12

results which indicate no significant difference between absenteeism and gender at 8 months postdisaster.

H_6: At 14 months postdisaster, there will be no difference between the school absenteeism of girls who experienced the disaster and absenteeism of boys who experienced the disaster.

The null hypothesis was not rejected. As shown in Table 6.3, results of t tests reflect no significant difference between absenteeism and gender at 14 months postdisaster.

The experimental and control groups were also compared by grade levels, although not statistically analyzed due to the small N. Grades two, three, four, five, and six all held greater absenteeism in the control group at $1\frac{1}{2}$ months postdisaster. The greatest difference was in grade two with a mean of 2.3 absent days for the experimental group and a mean of 5.9 absent days in the control group.

Inspection of the raw data revealed in the experimental group a range of 3.1 mean days absence for the fourth grade to 6.4 mean days for the fifth grade at 8 months postdisaster. In the control group, the range was from 0.6 in grade five to 3.4 in grade two. The small N per grade was too small for statistical analysis.

At 14 months postdisaster, the lowest mean number of absenteeism was in grades four and five, 3.4 each, in the experimental group, with 8 days for the eighth grade students. The range of mean days absent in the control group was 1.8, fifth grade, to 5.1 in the sixth grade.

DISCUSSION

It is interesting to note that the absenteeism from school at $1\frac{1}{2}$ months following the disaster was significantly greater in control subjects than in experimental subjects. The clue may be in the *low* absenteeism of the experimental group compared to the control group. Keeping in mind that the population studied was rural in nature, it can be considered that the experimental group felt more secure at school after the disaster. In rural communities, the school and church are frequently the focal points of community activity and fellowship. Most families were acquainted with, if not friends with, the students and faculty at the "new" school. In addition, on a pragmatic level, many subjects had literally lost their homes and, at $1\frac{1}{2}$ months postdisaster, remained in the process of locating new residences. Therefore, the school was a convenient and stable place for the subjects to spend their days.

The results at 8 and 14 months postdisaster were as predicted. These results reflected absenteeism during the fall semester, after the subjects had been at home with their families for the summer months. They had most likely spent the summer months continuing to restore their homes to predisaster states. Subjects and their families had much time to reflect on the devastating events which had occurred in the spring of the year. Returning to school may have been very difficult for the children. One can imagine that leaving home and family to board a bus would be very difficult, particularly on days that were dark, rainy, and windy.

The results comparing male and female subjects' absenteeism showed no statistical significance. Socioculturally, however, the fact that males and females responded the same may be very significant. The societal norms pertaining to males and females are in the process of alteration. Perhaps the effort for equality of the sexes applies more to emotional responses now than before. Parents and teachers alike may not be distinguishing one set of behavioral expectations for boys and another set for girls. From the results of this study alone, one can observe that boys and girls responded similarly in their behaviors of being absent from school. To discover the specific causative factors in each case would involve further study.

Review of absenteeism according to grade levels indicated that second grade control subjects had a much higher degree of absenteeism at $1\frac{1}{2}$ months postdisaster. These subjects were in kindergarten at the time of the disaster. It is possible that control parents were very cautious with their young children who were in their first year of school. It seems natural that hypervigilence would be most evident in parents of children who were in the process of being "weaned" from home to school; therefore, the parents may have kept the children out of school in the name of protective parenting.

At 8 months postdisaster, the fifth grade experimental subjects exhibited the highest degree of absenteeism. As previously cited in this chapter 8- to 12-year-old subjects would have the greatest difficulty adjusting to a postdisaster phase. The fifth grade subjects were in the third grade at the time of the disaster. The usual age of a third grader is 8 to 10 years old. The literature thereby supports the findings in this study which report an elevated rate of absenteeism among fifth grade subjects at 8 months postdisaster.

This study indicates that at 14 months postdisaster, second and third grade victims had a much higher degree of absenteeism than the control group. These children were kindergarten and first graders, respectively, at the time of the disaster. The investigator can offer no plausible explanation for these results except to repeat the possibility that parents of younger (5- and 6-year-old) children may be more protective and therefore keep children home from school more frequently.

Some questions raised by the study include: How does distance traveled to school affect results? After the disaster, experimental subjects were required to be transported to a new school setting, 9 miles from their school, which had been destroyed. In addition, the 8- and 14-month points included many days of icy, snowy, cold weather, which could have an effect on traveling. How much was this reflected in absenteeism? Another question which comes to mind is: were there any incidents of communicable disease (chicken pox, mumps, measles, and the like) evident in the schools? This could account for a portion of the absenteeism. While these factors would be expected to occur randomly among students in both schools, the samples may have been too small to reflect other reasons for absenteeism.

Although absenteeism was higher at 8 and 14 months in the experimental subjects than in the control subjects, it remained at the same level of significance for the experimental subjects at 8 and 14 months. This indicates that experimental subjects had reached a "leveling-off" period of absenteeism at 14 months postdisaster. Further investigation of absenteeism of the same subjects at temporal points later than 14 months would be of interest.

A study of this type is always inhibited by the design—an ex post facto design indicates that data regarding predisaster conditions were not available. A study utilizing predisaster information would be beneficial in showing if the absentee patterns of the involved subjects are occurring only since the disaster, or if the control group and experimental group absentee patterns have always been different from one another.

Absenteeism is only one small area of children's behavior which deserves investigation. Through review of the literature, it is evident that academic grades and psychosomatic complaints are also involved in school phobia and its related stressor. A study of academic grades and/or types and numbers of psychosomatic complaints of experimental and control subjects would enhance the theory body of postdisaster emotional trauma.

CONCLUSIONS AND SUGGESTIONS

From what has been learned about children and disaster, discussion can be generated among health care providers, educators, and parents in order to formulate plans for the "just in case" situation. Direction can be extracted.

It is of ultimate importance to realize that children have higher order needs such as belonging, love, information and understanding. Frequently, these needs go unmet while parents, volunteers, and other adults assume responsibility for securing basic needs, such as food, clothing, safety, and shelter. When the higher-order needs go unfulfilled and are combined with intense emotional and behavioral responses to a disaster, maladaptive effects will often emerge (Crabbs, 1981).

Crabbs (1981) outlined the following guidelines to be considered when working with students from a disaster-stricken community:

1. Maintain focus on the most "at-risk" population. The victims and those demonstrating problems should be given priority attention.
2. Encourage the victim-children by mobilizing them, involving them in activities, and returning at least some aspects of their lives to normal.
3. Get support from adults and encourage them to be open and honest with the children.
4. Confront the crisis which has actually happened. Do not reinforce denial of reality.
5. Give honest appraisals, not false assurance. Do not play fortune-teller and assure the victims when things will return to normal. Be honest and offer help.
6. Develop support systems. Generally disaster disrupts social ties. Match victims with nonvictims, and so forth.
7. Consult with teachers. Serve as a resource by providing materials, information and ideas. Capitalize on classroom activities by assisting teachers in leading group discussions and other activities.

Some specific classroom activities which involve feelings about the disaster may be utilized and include unfinished sentences, artwork, graffiti board, magic box, music, and community speakers.

McIntire and Sadeghi (1977) advise the pediatrician to assume a role, applicable to any health care provider, by addressing the following:

1. For all age groups: Since all disaster victims feel uncomfortable, it is imperative, especially for infants and young children, that the family remain together.
2. For parents with young children:
   a. Since your children may have difficulty expressing disquieting feelings, encourage them to talk about their feelings and work toward resolution and acceptance of what has happened.
   b. It is always sad to lose possessions, so parents should pay

close attention, listen, and share their feelings. It may help
to do drawings and "play tornado."
c. Even if they get in the way, the children should take part
in the cleanup.
d. Parents should be made aware that their children may
demonstrate some regressive behavior such as clinging, not
wanting to sleep alone, and the like. Encourage parents to
employ firm, but understanding discipline, especially after
a few days.
3. For parents with older children and teenagers:
a. Accept older children's comments and do not imply a sense
of guilt.
b. Direct teenagers' energy toward cleanup.
4. Parents of emotionally disturbed children should realize that
their children are at greater risk, may experience more severe
problems, and may require professional help.
5. Practically all parents are capable of helping children cope with
fears and anxieties. If problems persist, parents should be encouraged to seek counseling from the pediatrician, mental
health clinic, and other sources of help.

To place the health care providers' role with disaster (or children
in disaster) in perspective, it can be equated with learning cardiopul-
monary resuscitation; hopefully it will never be needed, but it is vital
to know and practice the techniques.

Disasters will continue to occur, and health care providers will be
expected to perform. Preparedness is the best resource.

REFERENCES

American Psychiatric Association. Diagnostic and Statistical Manual of Mental Disorders (3rd ed.). Washington, D.C.: American Psychiatric Association, 1980.
Burke, J.D., Jr., Borus, J.G., Burns, B.N., et al. Changes in children's behavior
after a natural disaster. American Journal of Psychiatry, 1982, 139,
1010-1014.
Coping with Children's Reactions to Earthquakes and Other Disasters. Van
Nuys, Calif.: San Fernando Valley Child Guidance Clinic, 1971.
Crabbs, M.A. School mental health services following an environmental disaster. Journal of School Health, 1981, 51, 165-167.
Dohrenwend, B.P., Dohrenwend, B.S., Kasl, S.V., Warheit, G. J. Technical staff
analysis report on behavioral affects to President's Commission on the Ac-

cident at Three Mile Island. Washington, D.C.: President's Commission on the Accident at Three Mile Island, 1979.

Glass, G., Stanley, J. Statistical Methods in Education and Psychology. Englewood Cliffs, N.J.: Prentice-Hall, 1970.

Kessler, J.W. Psychopathology of Childhood. Englewood Cliffs, N.J.: Prentice-Hall, 1966.

Kingston, W., Rosser, R. Disaster: Effects on mental and physical state. Journal of Psychosomatic Research, 1974, *18*, 437–465.

Lazarus, R.S., Averill, J. Opton, E. The psychology of coping: Issues of research and assessment. In G. Coelho et al. (Eds.), Coping and Adaptation. New York: Basic Books, 1974.

Logue, J.N., Melick, M.E., Hansen, H. Research issues and directions in the epidemiology of health effects of disasters. Epidemiologic Reviews, 1981, *3*, 140–162.

McIntire, M.S., Sadeghi, E. The pediatrician and mental health in a community-wide disaster. Clinical Pediatrics, 1977, *16*, 702–705.

Murphy, L. Coping, vulnerability, and resilience in childhood. In G. Coelho et al. (Eds.), Coping and Adaptation. New York: Basic Books, 1974.

Mussen, P. Child Development and Personality. New York: Harper and Row, 1974.

Rivlin, H.N. Educating for Adjustment. New York: D. Appleton-Century Co., 1936.

Training Manual for Human Service Workers in Major Disasters. Washington, D.C.: Department of Health and Human Services, 1976.

White, R. Strategies of adaptation: An attempt at systematic description. In G. Coelho, et al. (Eds.), Coping and Adaptation. New York: Basic Books, 1974.

Wolff, S. Children Under Stress. London: Penguin Press, 1970.

7

Emotional Consequences of Disasters

Jerri Laube

There are few systematic evaluations of the nature, scope, and duration of psychological stress responses of disaster victims. However, there is abundant evidence in reports from various health agencies and disaster relief organizations that sociopsychological problems occur as a result of disasters.

Chapter 1 of this book uses Powell and Rayner's conceptual framework as an organizing theme. These time periods typically evoke general characteristic patterns of behavior, but in addition, there are distinctly different reactions to disaster. Psychological responses to disaster vary according to the phase of disaster (warning, threat, impact, inventory, rescue, remedy, and recovery) to the disaster event (unexpectedness, suddenness, intensity, and duration) and other intrapersonal psychosocial variables (age, concurrent life stresses, perception of the imact of the loss, and past loss experience).

This chapter describes each of the time phases identified by Powell and Rayner, followed by the unique stresses a disaster poses.

STAGES OF DISASTER

Warning
Warning, the first stage, indicates the presence of danger with specification to time and place. The warning period may vary from as short a period as a few seconds or minutes, as in a tornado, to as long as several days as in the event of a hurricane. National Weather Service advisory messages and announcements of a "watch" fall in this time period.

People vary widely in their attention and response to the warning period according to their perception, interpretation, and implications to self. Warnings may not penetrate the person's awareness—or, because of varying dissemination processes, the warnings may be out of the person's range. For example, during the 1974 tornado in Xenia, Ohio, there were no warnings by sirens or loudspeakers. The morning newspaper had issued a severe storm warning for up until 3 P.M., but this was not seen by nonsubscribers nor by those people who delay reading the newspaper until after work in the evening. One local radio station disc jockey did broadcast, between playing records and talking, that a storm was predicted. At 4:10 P.M. he began reporting that there was an immediate threat of a tornado and that people should take cover. However, a large portion of the adult population of Xenia would not have been tuned in. Individuals who reported that they had heard the warning admitted that they only "stored" the warning. As they said, they had become conditioned to disregard the message for in the past many similar warnings did not culminate in disaster. They had become complacent. In their complacence they behaved as if tornadoes only happen in "other places"—anywhere else but Xenia!

One television station also carried the tornado warning, interrupting the regular programming. The program, however, was a rerun of "Leave it to Beaver" with an audience composed chiefly of children. Of the adults at home at the time, most reported that they were out of television range. A large proportion of adults in Xenia were on their way home from work at the time of the tornado. The time was 4:40 P.M.

It is paramount to disseminate the warning in the best possible mode in order to accomplish the goal of alerting people to danger. There is only a limited time between the awareness of a predicted disaster and the expected event. Disaster warnings should be directed to reach individuals by at least two sensory systems. For example, if the warning is broadcast on television the viewer can see the message as well as hear the words, and thus the viewer is more likely to actively receive the messages than if it were by radio only. Reaching persons through two senses may be accomplished by policemen patrolling streets (visual) and announcing the warning via loudspeaker (audio). Authorities should use every means available to them to spread the warning.

Threat

The second stage of disaster, threat, may evolve gradually out of the warning stage or may occur without warning. Threat is constituted by a change in condition indicating that danger is imminent. The length of time varies from a few minutes to up to 24 hours in cases of hurricane and flood warnings. The threat period is included in what is officially termed a warning when issued by the National Weather

Service—such as a tornado or hurricane warning. People are more likely to comply with emergency directives in the threat stage than they are in the first stage of warning. It is in this stage that people are urged to take protective shelter or, if the event demands, evacuate.

Impact

The third stage, the period of impact, is the entire period of destructive activity by the agent. It may be instantaneous or last several days. During this period the individual is bolted into action in a self-preservation attempt for self and family (if in close proximity). This is the period of the body's automatic response to threat, the activation of the sympathetic nervous system, commonly called the "fight or flight reaction."

While impact refers to a single event, in disaster there may be one or more events in an impact period. An illustration of a one event impact period is a tornado; the winds hit and then are gone. By contrast, the period of impact from a hurricane includes two events—the great wind, the calm of the eye, and then the second force. Floods and earthquakes produce a number of impact events with the upheaval of earth and buildings and washouts of bridges and roads.

Inventory

The victim of disaster becomes aware of the extent of destruction for the first time in the inventory phase. This is the period in which the individual finds out what has happened, what is left, and what must be done. Searching for one's own family is urgently begun. Persons reportedly have unusual strength and drive during this period.

Stories are told of how one individual single-handedly lifted a heavy beam to free a victim and another individual moved a heavy appliance. Under normal circumstances, such feats are impossible.

Activity in the inventory phase, while goal directed, may not always be to the advantage of the individual. Depending on the person's perception of what has happened, rescue may even be impeded. It is very probable that the person will revert to a prototaxic type of thinking process during this acute stage. For example, if a person becomes aware of gas in the room at the same time he or she has just performed a particular action, the person may assume that performing this action has caused the gas escape and spend precious minutes trying to "undo" the act (Fig. 7.1).

Rescue

The rescue phase brings in outside help as well as professional mobilization from the community. The community swarms with disaster workers (official and voluntary), consultants, government officials

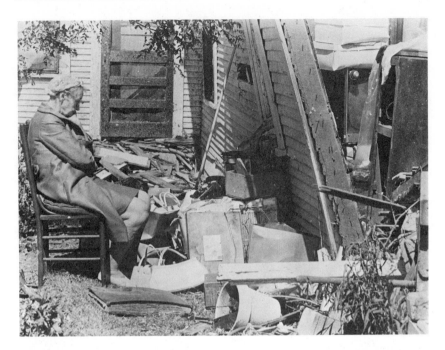

Figure 7.1. A 76-year-old woman of Lubbock, Texas survived the May 11 tornado which tore through the heart of the city by hiding in the closet of her home, almost the only part of the structure left undamaged. *(Photo courtesy of the American Red Cross)*

(which may even include the President of the United States), sightseers, and frequently tons of supplies are donated which must be sorted and distributed.

Volunteer activity is a natural relief for tension and emotions which have heightened the impact. It is most important for people's mental health that they be permitted to help during this period. If they are not assigned by an authority, however, they probably will find something to do on their own (Figure 7.2). As one registered nurse recounted, when told her services were not needed at a Red Cross First Aid Station following a tornado, she picked up a broom and started sweeping! (Fig. 7.3).

It is during the rescue period that the survivors begin to bury their dead. This may be done through individual or mass funerals with little or with much ritual. In the event of large number of deaths, particularly in underdeveloped countries, the bodies may be buried in a common grave.

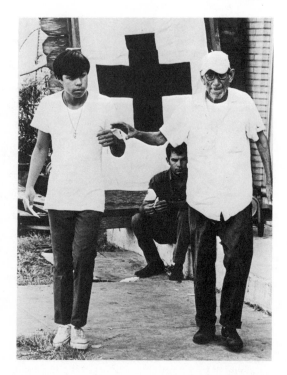

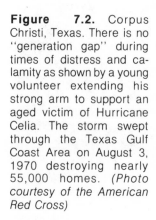

Figure 7.2. Corpus Christi, Texas. There is no "generation gap" during times of distress and calamity as shown by a young volunteer extending his strong arm to support an aged victim of Hurricane Celia. The storm swept through the Texas Gulf Coast Area on August 3, 1970 destroying nearly 55,000 homes. *(Photo courtesy of the American Red Cross)*

Remedy

Long-term rebuilding and grief work make-up the sixth stage, the remedy period. This stage may last a year or longer. Typically, insurance claims are filed, the debris is cleaned up, building plans are submitted and approved, contracts awarded, and construction completed. In respect to grief work, the survivors must grieve their losses, both the tangible and intangible. The amount and time of grief work is positively correlated to the significance of the loss (Fig. 7.4).

A strong community morale is said to evolve in this period. Evidence of camaraderie behavior can be observed in interesting ways in the disaster communities. For example, slogans are posted on car bumper stickers. In Xenia, Ohio following the 1974 tornado, bumper stickers read, "Xenia lives!" The stickers in Wilkes-Barre, Pennsylvania, following the 1972 flood read, "The Valley with a Heart Coming Back Better Than Ever," the bumper stickers in Biloxi, Mississippi, after Hurricane Camille read, "Together We Build," and stickers in Monroe, Louisiana, following the 1983 flood stated, "Maybe We Should Build An Ark."

Another example of high community spirit was observed in Biloxi, Mississippi after Hurricane Camille in 1969 when *The Daily Herald* ran

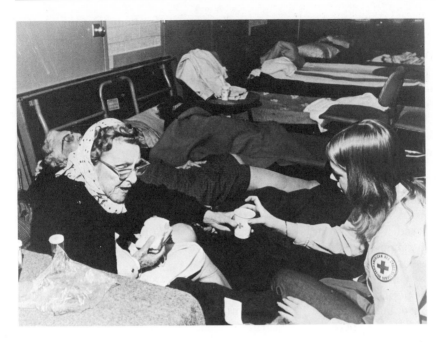

Figure 7.3. Xenia, Ohio, April 1974. A young Red Cross volunteer gives coffee and solace to one of the hundreds of victims left homeless when a tornado devastated large sections of the city. *(Photo courtesy of the American Red Cross)*

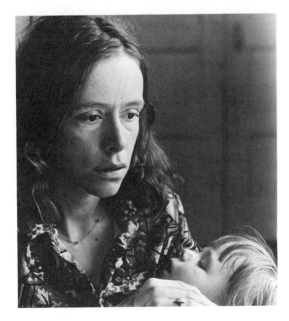

Figure 7.4. Grundy, Virginia, April 22, 1977. Worry and despair are etched on the face of this flood victim as she holds her exhausted child. *(Photo by George Chitty courtesy of the American Red Cross)*

a six-column picture on page one of a partially destroyed home with an American flag fluttering on a bent pole in front of the wreckage. An accompanying editorial suggested that people who intended to remain on the Coast and rebuild, could fly the flag in front of their ruined homes and businesses as a symbol of the will to recover. The editor of *The Daily Herald* bought 600 flags at cost from a distributor, with the thought of being able to probably sell most of them. In less than 2 months, he had sold all of those plus 5200. Nearly six thousand flags were erected and flown in front of damaged and destroyed buildings!

Recovery

The last phase, the recovery period, is technically the remainder of the survivors' lives and the area's existence. The victim's grief work is completed. The survivor is emancipated from the bondage to the deceased. The time needed for individual recovery, however, is not confirmed by research.

One is struck with the accuracy of the statement that the recovery period is the remainder of one's life when residents commonly refer to Beulah or Celia or "The Storm" as reference points. Life events are recalled as "before The Storm" or "after The Storm."

CASE ILLUSTRATION

The following is a transcript of an interview which took place between the author and a young woman seven years after she had experienced the San Fernando Valley earthquake in 1971. The interview is included to illustrate the phases of disaster, as perceived and recalled by one individual.

> JL: You said you lived in San Fernando Valley?
>
> YW: Yes.
>
> JL: And the earthquake, that was in '70?
>
> YW: '71.
>
> JL: How old were you at that time?
>
> YW: 24.
>
> JL: That occurred early in the morning, right?
>
> YW: Yes, it was at 6:00 in the morning.
>
> JL: Were you asleep when it occurred?
>
> YW: Yes, we were all in bed. It was still dark outside. It was just beginning to get light but it was still dark in the rooms, in the bedrooms. It started—well I had felt earthquakes before,

you know little small ones and it had always been kind of exciting. At the time it woke me up I thought someone was shaking my bed trying to wake me up. That was the first impression I had. Then the shaking just kept getting stronger and stronger, and I realized what it was. I really felt at the time that the intensity was such that the house would not be able to stand up. It was just incredible. I didn't think that the house could withstand that, so I got out of bed. I tried to stand up but I couldn't. The ground was shaking that much that I could not stand, and so I got down and tried to get under my bed as much as I could to get something over me. I felt something fall on me and I thought that the roof was caving in.

JL: Were you in the room by yourself?

YW: Yes.

JL: Did you call out for anybody?

YW: I don't remember. I remember somebody yelling. I lived with my family and I remember somebody screaming, but I don't think I yelled out to anyone. All I can remember thinking was that the house was coming down. They said, I think, it lasted for a minute. A little more than a minute.

JL: How long did it feel like to you?

YW: Oh, a lot longer than that. Like I said, the ones I experienced before were a couple of seconds, you know, just a little tremor.

JL: You said something fell. What fell?

YW: A lamp fell and hit me and when it stopped—

JL: Off the ceiling, you mean?

YW: No, off my bedside table. When it actually stopped there was nothing really damaged in the house. The books had fallen out of my bookshelf. Things had fallen off of tables and that kind of thing, but we all ran outside.

JL: What did you have on?

YW: Just a nightgown or something.

JL: You ran out like that?

YW: Yes. I might have put a robe on, I can't remember that much. It was very warm. It was a beautiful day. It was just getting light and we all ran outside and there was water rushing down the street. We couldn't figure out for a long time what that was, but it was water that had overflowed from swimming pools. It mustn't have been—well it couldn't have been more than a couple of minutes after the first major shock that there were other ones. All that day they were just constant. In fact, I remember my dad and I going out to the backyard right after the first earthquake. In our backyard we looked toward the mountains and up toward San Fernando, the small city where I worked, and all we could see was what looked like smoke. We thought that there were fires. It turned out that there were a couple of fires that had started off, but later, reading about it, I found that it was just dust rising from the mountains and around where the major part of the earthquake was. I was standing in the backyard with my dad when another earthquake hit. This was within an hour or so. They all feel a little bit different. That one, I just felt like the whole patio we were standing on just dropped. We had electric wires going across our backyard and they just started whipping around in circles and immediately dad and I decided that that was not the place to be, in the backyard; so we got out of there.

JL: Did you run back in the house?

YW: All that morning I was afraid to be in the house. I guess people had always said that the best place in an earthquake is to be out in the open some place where you have nothing over your head, away from buildings. I was very much afraid to be in the house all that morning. When we were in, we had the door open ready to run out.

JL: What did you hear on the radio or the news media at that time?

YW: I don't remember exactly when we turned on the television or whatever, but we did hear that the area that we were in was the area that was hardest hit. Even Los Angeles people had definitely felt it in Los Angeles, but there wasn't any great damage. The first thing that we heard was that this dam that was right north of us, it is an earthen dam, that it had been badly damaged and might give way at any time. They started to drain this dam and about a couple of hours after the earthquake police came around to our neighborhood, just on motorcycles, telling everybody to get out.

JL: That's how you got warned then?

YW: Yes.

JL: Did they knock on the door or use a loud speaker down the street or . . . ?

YW: I can't remember. I think we were outside. The thing that they were telling everybody, that if the dam broke our neighborhood would be under 6 feet of water. They told us to get out immediately. They didn't give us any time, they just said "Get out." So, we had to start packing things into cars. We had three different cars at the time. My family were all at home and we had to decide what we wanted to pack in the cars and where we were going. We had a dog. So, we took all three cars and everybody drove a car.

JL: And packed as much as you could? What kinds of things did you take, do you recall? In general.

YW: I remember taking, it's kind of funny, a few clothes and I remember taking a blanket, wrapping a blanket up, thinking that I might be some place where I'd need it, you know need a blanket. I didn't know where we were going. I had like a, kind of like a scrapbook, not a scrapbook exactly, kind of a box that I had saved all kinds of mementos and newspaper clippings, and all kinds of things that were really important to me. I remember I just grabbed that and I took that. That's something I didn't want to lose, and it was real important to me. There wasn't time to take anything else, really.

JL: Did you drive one of the cars away?

YW: Yes, I think I did.

JL: Can you remember the level of emotion in your home at that time? Was it panicky?

YW: No, there really wasn't panic. I think I was the one that was most affected, myself and my younger brother. I guess there was some amount of—there was a lot of fear. I was very much afraid, especially when they had been talking about the dam breaking. I was impatient, I remember, with my parents, they were trying to gather things together and all I wanted to do was get out. I was very much afraid. I think that a lot of the fears developed later. At that time we were so busy doing so many things.

JL: Did you recall looking around the neighborhood? Were other people in your neighborhood doing the same kind of thing you were?

YW: Oh yes, everybody had to be out. It was really a spooky feeling when we finally got out on the street and it was just bumper to bumper traffic. Everybody was just leaving the neighborhood. It was really kind of an eerie feeling.

JL: You didn't know if your homes were going to be there when you came back.

YW: That week that we stayed, we went to Santa Monica which was down near the ocean, and we stayed with friends a couple of days and then in a motel for the rest of the time. It was a week that we were away. I later found out that where I worked, in San Fernando, the whole city was practically closed and there was a lot of damage on the main street and to the buildings in town. You couldn't go into the town at all. So, my office was damaged to the point you couldn't go into it. I think my dad and my brother, who worked down in Los Angeles, went to work to least the last few days.

JL: Did you find out about your work at that time?

YW: I think I called somebody and found out.—They told us to report to another office I think, but they said that in the situation that I was that I wouldn't have to come back until I could get back into our house. I can remember the days that we were in Santa Monica. I think the first thing that I noticed was that my family stayed as a group, none of us wanted to be alone. We would sit on a couch together and the people that we were staying with didn't have any idea of our fear. You know, all that week there were constant aftershocks. It was just all the time.

JL: Could you feel them in Santa Monica too?

YW: Oh yes. The people that we were with, it didn't bother them that much, you know. It really bothered us a great deal. When we went back to the house, I think that's when I first started feeling afraid. We went back in an afternoon. It was light. We were one of the first ones back into the neighborhood and the neighborhood was just empty. There were just no people. When we went back into the house everything was exactly as we left it. The books were out of the bookcases. There were dishes that were broken on the floor. On our mantel we had a clock that was my grandmother's. It was a very ornate clock with a pendulum. During the earthquake it had slid back and fallen against the wall and had stopped. So, we walked back into the house and the clock was lying against the wall and it said 6:00 on it.

JL: Were there National Guard men stationed around to prevent looting?

YW: Police—police were there guarding the neighborhood. They had set up road blocks and everything and we had to show them, or tell them where we lived, or some kind of proof that we belonged in there because they were there to prevent looting and all of that.

JL: So you didn't have any looters in your neighborhood?

YW: No. The first few nights we were back in the house—well, first of all I didn't want to go to bed at all. I was very frightened when it was dark.

JL: Now, did that just happen after you got back in the house or did that happen also in Santa Monica?

YW: It was more so when I got back into the house. It was, like in Santa Monica, I was in a different place a whole different environment and it didn't happen there. So it was when I got into the house. The first night back into the house my whole family stayed up all night. My mother and dad had a king-size bed, and we all sat on the bed and played cards all night.

JL: You were just going to do that for the rest of your life, yes?!

YW: At that point I felt like we were going to because nobody wanted to turn the lights off, nobody wanted to be alone in their room to go to bed. Eventually everybody got back to normal except me. I really think that for a long time I was frightened. I slept in my parents' room for awhile with them.

JL: I don't know what you mean by with them? You mean in the king-size bed with them?

YW: No. I think I set up a cot or something. I felt very much like I was regressing somehow in my childhood. I felt very much like a child. I was ashamed of it because I'm supposed to be an adult but I felt like I wanted to be with somebody, particularly my parents. It must have taken me at least a week, maybe two weeks to even get to the point where I could go back into my bedroom by myself. Even in the daytime to be there alone. Finally, when I did go back to sleeping in my own room, I slept with the light on, and I didn't sleep really. I layed awake all night waiting for the next earthquake. I think what sacred me more than anything was the fact that there was never any warning. It seemed like the shocks were completely irrational. You didn't even know what it was; you couldn't see anything. The earth under your feet, that you thought was something secure and stable, you felt like was giving away.

JL: I've heard that, what you have just said, so frequently from people. Particularly about staying in somebody else's room at night, whether it was a parent or friend.

YW: It was a major inconvenience as far as my life was concerned. My whole life changed. I completely quit doing things on my own away from other people. I had to be with someone else at all times. I can remember evenings and even when I started going back to work I couldn't stand to be alone. I'm trying to remember all this. Obviously everybody was affected more than I'm remembering. I wasn't the only one because my older brother took off work, took some vacation time and moved to another state with my younger brother.

JL: That's how they took care of it. They moved out of the area?

YW: Yes, they just left. I wanted to do the same thing. So my mom and dad and I left for awhile. I think maybe it was only a week. But we went to Arizona. We had some friends in Arizona, we just went there. I can remember the first night when we left California and I think we stayed in Yuma or something like that the first night. I can remember, it was the first sleep that I had had. I could relax and feel like I could let down my guard. It wasn't going to happen here. Well it could have, I mean, you know, there's no guarantee, but I felt like it.

JL: How long was that after the quake?

YW: A couple of weeks. So, at that point I told the people at work that I was leaving. It was a matter of my mental health. I think I even went to our family doctor and I know he prescribed some kind of tranquilizers for me at that time. He also wrote a note for me to be off work for a week or two. But at that point I felt like I had to leave and if it meant losing my job I would leave anyway. You know, the job was not that important to me at the time. I was desperate. I had to get out of there. When we came back, I think it was like three weeks or so that they needed to repair the damage to our office, and that was a big step. I remember going back into the building. Even though it had been repaired, that was something, going into that area of San Fernando. There was still so much damage.

JL: You're talking about damage, was there a change in how the environment looked? For instance, trees down?

YW: Not so much trees down. A lot of damage to the streets. A lot of places where the streets had buckled or collapsed. There were, in San Fernando, there were buildings that were badly damaged. One apartment building, I remember, was practically destroyed. You know, buildings where there would be big cracks in the walls, or the walls would have fallen down. In San Fernando, its an older section of town, and on the main street some of the buildings' walls just gave way and you could see the rooms in there, you know, the chairs and tables sitting in there.

JL: Like the front of a dollhouse?

YW: Yes, and there were a number of people killed in San Fernando in that area. I think there were 50 some total from the earthquake. The Veteran's Hospital in San Fernando collapsed. It was a very old hospital. I think there were 40 some people killed there. There was another hospital, L.A. County Hospital, all of which was brand new. It had been dedicated a month before and it was destroyed. It was right near the center of the earthquake.

JL: Do you remember sharing your feelings about your scared feelings, or talk about any of this to people?

YW: I didn't, with my family, yes. I mean, they were all very aware of how I was affected. I don't think I talked to anybody else too much, I think I was really embarrassed to show how afraid I was. I felt like it was very childish. It was a bad time in my life to begin with. I was out of college. I had dropped out of student teaching and I felt like it was very much of a failure kind of a thing. I was in a job that I did not enjoy. I took the job because I needed work and I felt at that point that my life was just going nowhere. I didn't know what I wanted to do. I was just really at loose ends. I just was lost. I felt like I had lost contact with a lot of people I had gone to college with. I didn't have any friends particularly. There were just a lot of things, a lot of worries, kind of anxieties going on. The earthquake brought all these things to a head again. I hadn't been in any kind of counseling or anything like that for quite awhile and it just brought all these things back; all the kinds of fears and so that kind of pushed me. I went to talk to a priest, the only person I could think of that I could go and talk to. He referred me to a counselor at Catholic Social Services and I went to see him probably not more than three or four times and made the decision to leave Los Angeles, to get out. This was a real major decision for me because of the closeness of my family. It would mean leaving home for the first time.

JL: So in a time span, how long was that from the earthquake, do you know?

YW: From the time, to the time I actually left, was from February until July.

JL: That's when it occurred, in February?

YW: Yes.

JL: So when you were in counseling, by the time you saw this person about two or three times, that was what month? About?

YW: I'm not really sure. I can't remember.

JL: You stayed in San Fernando Valley?

YW: Yes, I stayed a little while. I remember, I left the job 1 year from the time that I had taken the job. I had decided I was going to stay on the job for a year. That was part of the reason for leaving in July. I think it was June that the year was up. My parents had decided that they wanted to visit my brothers, and so we coincided my moving with their visiting so that they could help me and drive back with me. So there were various reasons why I waited for a little while.

JL: And how you talked about this to your family, about your moving, was what? What did you tell them as the reason you were moving?

YW: Because of the earthquake.

JL: They wanted to come with you?

YW: No, not really. My mother wanted to leave Los Angeles. They were tied there a little bit because of my dad's job and he had just a year or so more to go before he could retire and various other reasons. I don't think he was really that affected. All of a sudden I saw my father as a very strong figure. It was like he was kind of the rock.

JL: And you wanted to be close to him.

YW: Yes, I really did.

JL: So, he had a quiet strength and it showed during this emergency.

YW: Yes. He was very calm throughout the whole thing.

JL: So after you moved how long before you went back to your home in California?

YW: I think I went back two years later.

JL: And how was that?

YW: I don't remember having any great fear going back. I think being removed from it for that length of time helped. It was really a dramatic change.

JL: Did you have nightmares or dreams about the earthquake then?

YW: No. Not really. I can't remember. When I went back to Los Angeles I didn't feel any earthquakes. You know, they didn't have any the few days I was there. I don't know how I would react if I went through one again, you know, or if I felt it. I did feel one here.

JL: It's been a few years.

YW: Well, occasionally, but this has been maybe three years ago. I remember very vividly because I was talking on the phone to a friend at the time and it was a day when we had tornado warnings and storms and everything. I felt the bed shake, and she was saying "What's that?" We both felt it at the same time, and I knew what it was. She didn't. And I said "That's an earthquake," and she said "You're kidding." But again, I don't know. It was small enough and it just didn't really evoke the fear.

JL: You said that your life style changed dramatically after the quake because you wanted to be with people, that you had changed from being alone in solitary activity to having to be with people. Did that continue the whole time you were in California?

YW: Yes.

JL: And then you came here and it wasn't so important?

YW: No it wasn't at all important.

JL: As you think about yourself now, are you thinking that your behavior is different than postearthquake in California? Have you "gotten over it"?

YW: Yes. I don't think there were any really long lasting effects. The major effect I would say is that it brought about major changes in my life. It forced me to do some things that I might never have done. But as far as lasting emotional effects, I don't know. The only thing, I was thinking as a result of that, like I said, a lot of the things I experienced made me feel kind of ashamed of my behavior, you know the way I couldn't be alone. I felt kind of disappointed in the way I reacted in a crisis, so to speak.

JL: How do you feel about that now?

YW: I don't know. These are things I haven't really thought about for a long time. And the kinds of feelings and everything that I had. I don't think I'd behave the same way now.

JL: How do you feel about the way—?

YW: About the way I behaved?

JL: Yes.

YW: It doesn't bother me now. It really doesn't. I don't feel ashamed about anything now or the way I behaved. I really think that probably all those kind of fears that I expressed, I think it was really a healthy kind of thing to get all that out.

JL: OK.

YW: That's something, you know, I've never thought about that before. Because I've never given much thought to what effect it had on me other than the fact that it made me move here. You know, the kind of physical effect in that sense. But as far as emotional effect, I guess it provided kind of a catharsis, in a way.

JL: I notice your anxiety increasing part of the time we were talking and then decreasing again. That is not surprising because you recalled some experiences that you hadn't thought about in detail. With your talking about it, were you aware of some increased feelings?

YW: Yes. One thing I was thinking, you asked me if I had talked to other people at that time about my fears and all. I guess I did a little bit to some of the people I worked with because I remember someone telling me I did (someone who was totally unconcerned with the whole thing, and there were many people like that). I think that gave me a great deal of anxiety, feeling that those people were somehow better than I. Why is it affecting me like this? Am I a coward? "It's your time to go, you know, and you don't have any control. You might go in an automobile accident, you know, why be so afraid of the earthquake or whatever?" And another person saying that my problem was a fear of death and to try to work on that. And I was trying to explain to them, "Well I suppose, yes, I do have a fear of death, but I don't think about it in regards to other things." I think there are two things that I have a major fear of and it was not a fear of dying so much as fear of the earthquake itself or a fear of possibly dying that way. It was that specific kind of fear. The other things I have a fear of are airplanes and airplane crashes. It's those specific things that the fear is and not just death.

JL: You felt like you had to defend your position though.

YW: Yes.

JL: Now, as you look back, were there any things that were funny? As you think back about it? The kind of behavior you laugh about now?

YW: I think it's extremely funny, about how we handled the light at night. My brothers slept together in a bedroom and our bedrooms were divided by a hallway where the bathroom was. Eventually, as we got a little bit stronger, we could turn the lights off in our bedrooms but we had to leave the bathroom light on. The only person I ever talked to about the earthquake was my younger brother. We don't see each other that often anymore. Now he, next to myself, was the one that was most affected. We get together every once in awhile and will just talk about the earthquake.

JL: Still?

YW: We still do. I don't know how he reacts because I know he feels them now. I know that they have earthquakes all the time where he lives.

JL: Do you find yourself dating your experiences by pre- and postearthquake?

YW: Yeah. I mean a lot of people that—that's another thing, my brother and I you know are very aware of the date that it happened, you know. A lot of people have completely forgotten, you know, even what year it was. We're very aware of that. I still think about it every February 8. I'm very aware that that's the anniversary, that's the date. I talked to people here and they are vaguely aware that they read about it. My brother and I refer to The Earthquake, my whole family does—The *Earthquake*. There was only one, you know, and other people don't understand.

JL: I know. Thank you for talking with me about your experience.

STRESSORS

Next, this chapter will focus on the unique stressors of disaster and their consequences. Specific destructive factors have been identified in disaster and these are nearly always present, whatever type of disaster occurs:

1. EXTREME SENSE OF URGENCY. The immediate crisis excludes at-

tention to other matters. The victims entire world revolves around his or her losses. The person perceives an immediate, severe danger and engages in self-preservation behavior. Once the person is in a safe position, this sense of urgency is transferred onto those for whom the person is responsible. This may be family, employees, or a patient/client group. All of the individual's actions result from this sense of urgency. As the saying goes, it is "brawn rather than brains." High tension prevails which in turn creates greater tension and turmoil. This in turn decreases scope of awareness and delays normalcy.

2. GUILT. Guilt of the survivor has frequently been described in disaster literature. Lifton (1967), in his study of the psychological effects of the atomic bomb in Hiroshima, found that survivors experienced the open eyes of corpses as evoking guilt. It was as if the eyes were communicating, "Why me, why not you?"

Survivors question if they have done enough toward saving others during the disaster. If the survivor knew the victims (or if the victim is similar to someone he or she knows) the guilt gets compounded through concerns that the survivor may not have done enough for the deceased during the latter's lifetime. Or, the survivor will obsess over a wrong doing (real or imagined) toward the deceased.

Guilt has a deeper origin than the spoken concerns of the survivor. The dynamics of guilt may be due to ambivalent feelings experienced in early childhood toward a parent. This is successfully held in the unconscious until a traumatic situation creates pressure sufficient to bring these feelings to the conscious awareness in the form of guilt. In "normal" grief responses, the guilt will dissipate, although no time frame has been established through research.

3. SUDDEN DEATH OR INJURY. Survivors may have to deal with this emergency on their own, for a short while. Medical personnel will not be immediately on site, as these people are having to deal with their own reactions to stress and also, means of travel is frequently impeded. Being required to administer first aid and manage rescue operations is sufficient to evoke great anxiety in the survivors. Medically untrained survivors feel propelled by a sense of urgency yet must keep alert to their limitations. Moreover, survivors are frequently faced with multiple deaths of close relatives and friends.

4. DESTRUCTION OF HOMES AND PROPERTY. Property damage creates a changed physical environment for the survivors (Figs 7.5, 7.6). This sudden change provokes a disturbance in the psychological equilibrium which is particularly disruptive to the aged. As people grow older there are fewer significant persons in their lives. This loss of significant people is compensated by their material possessions.

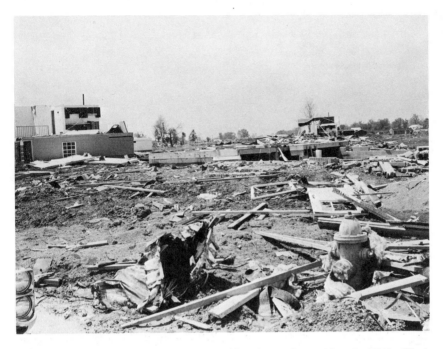

Figure 7.5. Scenes from the Mother's Day tornado on May 8, 1972. *(Photo courtesy of the American Red Cross)*

The following responses, from tornado victims, to Laube's (1974) questions about what affected them most illustrate the impact of property damage.

"Loss of antiques and old homes"
"Seeing all the damage in Xenia"
"Losing all of those beautiful old trees,
     Xenia will never be the same."
"The courthouse clock stopped, I miss it so much."
"Homes demolished, those lovely old homes"
"Seeing all the destruction"
"Xenia won't ever be the same. We'll have a lot
     of new buildings, but it won't be the same."
"The massive destruction; it's hard to comprehend."

5. INTERFERENCE WITH MEANS FOR SATISFYING BASIC NEEDS. With electricity, water, and gas supplies interrupted, the person must strug-

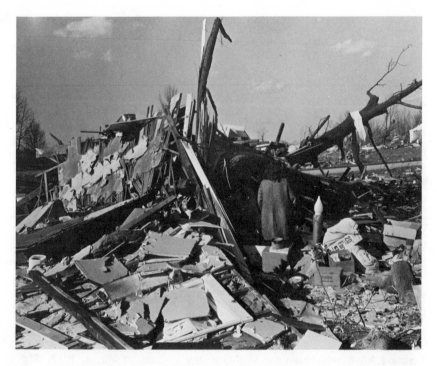

Figure 7.6.   Demolished home of Berlin Gross family, Grant City, Indiana, resulting from April 3, 1974 tornadoes. *(Photo courtesy of the American Red Cross)*

gle with alternative means for satisfaction of thirst, hunger, and elimination (Fig. 7.7). With destruction of homes and impeded travel, the victim must also contend with protecting him- or herself against the elements of wind, rain, cold, and/or heat. Basic physical and security needs must be met for survival of life. If there is destruction or interruption in the usual ways of obtaining or securing these needs, then there will be a decrease in satisfaction of higher-level needs. As physical and emotional security of the individual is threatened, psychological disequilibrium will result.

6. INJURY, DEATH, AND DESTRUCTION OF EMERGENCY PERSONNEL AND EQUIPMENT. Emergency personnel who live in the disaster-struck community are as vulnerable to destructive forces of disaster as any other individual. They too have to protect their satisfaction of basic needs. They have families and are subject also to the emotional impact of loss. Thus, as listed above in point 3, the survivors may have to deal with the emergency on their own for awhile. Backup emergency personnel and equipment is nearly always available, however, from surrounding areas and certainly from distant areas. With the advancement

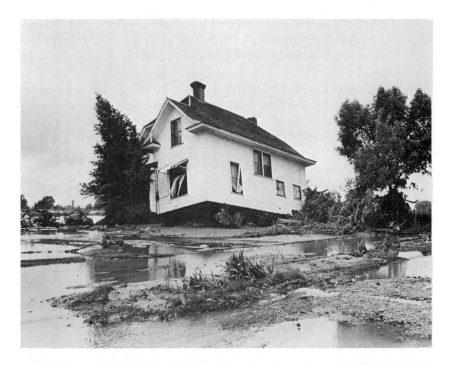

Figure 7.7.   Blackfoot, Idaho, June 1976. This home was knocked off its foundation by the wall of water that swept through this community when the Teton Dam burst. The dam disaster destroyed or damaged more than 4000 dwellings in the resulting flood. *(Photo by Phil Gibson courtesy of the American Red Cross)*

in air travel, help is quickly available. At the time of the disaster impact, however, this is not so easily recognized by the victim.

7. DESTRUCTION OF ROADS AND VEHICLES. With the highways obstructed, transportation of the injured, and movement of supplies is impeded. The likelihood of this occurring in both natural and man-made disasters is high. This intensifies the considerations described in points 3 and 5 above.

Disaster workers have had to resort to extraordinary means in order to make their way through the debris. One man told of walking, climbing, and crawling an approximate distance of 8 miles to reach an elderly couple in their home, a house which was less than 2 miles distance if the streets had been cleared. Even if the streets were not obstructed with debris, travel by auto would become difficult with the gasoline shortage due to pump failure created by the electric power failure. In addition, the absence of street and traffic lights would create more problems for vehicle and pedestrian travel.

8. BREAKDOWN OF COMMUNICATION SYSTEM. Disruption in com-

munication is one of the major factors in isolating individuals thus resulting in major disturbance of the social environment. When communication is established between the victim and the rescuer, anxiety is diminished.

Another aspect of communication breakdown is the impact rumors have on the rescue operations. With people's heightened fear and anxiety, they are most vulnerable to suggestion and consequently aid unwittingly in the spread of rumors. Rumors are probably the greatest source of anxiety.

9. THREAT AND FEAR. According to Janis' research (1958), an optimal amount of anxiety as a result of fear from threat of body harm, along with the successful experience of handling it, is necessary for effective behavior in later phases of disaster. Too much anxiety, however, is inhibiting and will preclude constructive behavior.

In the event of a disaster, the objective reality is that there is potential danger. How people feel in relation to their power to cope determines the threat they experience.

REACTIONS TO DISASTER

Based on extensive study of psychological effects of stress and disaster, Lifton and Olson (1976) described a "survival syndrome" which is composed of five categories. These are: death imprint and anxiety, death guilt, psychic numbing, counterfeit nurturance and unfocused rage, and the struggle for significance—the capacity of survivors to make significant meaning of their experience with death and destruction.

Individual mental stress has taken various forms in past disasters. Persons under the great stress of disaster react in one of five general ways according to the nature and magnitude of the disaster (American Psychiatric Association, 1966). These are: (1) normal reaction to disaster (showing signs of disturbance, but regaining composure soon after the first impact), (2) individual panic, (3) depressed reaction, (4) overactive response, and (5) bodily reaction.

Menninger (1952) reported two sets of psychological responses in individuals following the Kansas River flood according to whether or not the person was directly affected by the flood. For those persons whose property was not directly affected the following reactions were observed:

1. Vague feeling of personal threat with desire to do something
2. Frustration
3. Feeling of relief with assignment to any kind of work

4. Social status disappeared entirely—bank presidents and laborers worked side by side
5. Exhilaration during the emergency
6. Increased griping, following the immediate danger.

For those persons who were victims of the flood, the following observations were made:

1. Disbelief—would not move from house until forced to evacuate
2. Apathy, confusion—became overly concerned with trivia
3. Relief with talking about the flood
4. Less inclined to volunteer for work. Even those in shelters were reluctant to assist in any way.
5. Frequent use of first aid stations for very minor or inconsequential complaints
6. Unique responses to personal loss. Those that lost the most in the flood, and had the least in the form of resources, asked for less help than did those who had lost much less.
7. Scapegoating. Although not evident during the emergency, afterward it became very common.
8. The refugees became overly dependent.

The San Fernando Valley earthquake of 1971 was highly destructive and left psychological consequences particularly to the children. It was very frightening to the children to have their homes shake, and then find themselves plunged into the darkness due to disruption of electric service. Many children suffered fears, phobias, sleep disturbances, and nightmares long after the incident. Hundreds of parents and children called the Child Guidance Clinic for help (Howard, 1971). Parents were concerned because their children were clinging excessively to them. Children were frightened and unwilling to leave their homes. They reacted with alarm to noises. Other common complaints of parents were that they were reverting to earlier behaviors such as enuresis and encopresis. Children were afraid to go into rooms alone, afraid to sleep in their beds alone, and begged to sleep with their parents.

Other symptoms of emotional difficulties one should be alert to in children are: increased irritability, resumption of earlier speech habits such as "baby talk" or stuttering, increased sibling rivalry, thumb sucking, either withdrawal from playmates or increased arguing and fighting, and loss of interest in usual toys, games, and hobbies.

The following problems were reported by Whalen (1972) in the Greater Harrisburg area in Pennsylvania following the flood caused by

Hurricane Agnes. Of 2000 families reached through door-to-door contact, 2 percent of the families needed referral for emotional support. Emotional upsets seemed to appear chiefly in physical symptoms such as backaches, poor appetite, loss of sleep, fatigue, and tenseness. Other indications of problems, although seldom reported, were apathy, irritability, anger, and withdrawal. For a number of people, the resultant losses were just one more difficulty added to other existing ones with which an individual could not cope.

The largest group needing emotional support was the elderly. As described by Whalen (1972) the emotional response among the aged was one of depression and despair from having lost homes and being uprooted from familiar surroundings. For many of the elderly, who by virtue of their advanced age had already lost primary relatives and friends, all they had were their Bibles, pictures, and keepsakes. Loss of these sentimental items then resulted in feelings of hopelessness and helplessness.

Disorientation and memory loss may also be expected in the aged population. If they become disoriented they are likely also to exhibit anger, agitation, and suspiciousness. As cited in Chapter 1, however, these findings have not been fully supported by more recent disaster studies. Thus, the aged may not present the major management problems inferred.

It is not unusual to find scapegoating following a disaster. Although some families resort to their usual pattern and find a scapegoat in their own members, a large number make disaster relief agencies and assistance providers their target. The following observations by Laube (1974) exemplify scapegoating behavior.

In the 3- to 4-day period following the tornado in Xenia, Ohio, people were busy taking inventory of their losses and going about in a rather dazed-like condition. They professed over and over how thankful they were that their family members had been saved. They could not say enough for the assistance offered by the various agencies. The general emotional climate was one of closeness. As was frequently heard, the people had come up sharply against the meaning of life and their own mortality. However, by the end of only 1 week, complaints were beginning to erupt against the helping agencies and people. The complaints ranged from the number of forms needed to be completed, to the Red Cross taking over and doing everything or doing nothing, depending upon who was talking to whom and when. The insurance agents took their share of the criticism also, being complained against if they were more than 5 minutes late for appointments.

A common misconception of behavior following disaster is that panic is natural and commonplace. Quite the contrary, mass panic has seldom been found. According to Quarantelli and Dynes (1971), the frequency of panic has been overexaggerated. They attribute the major impressions people have about behavior in disaster to the news media and fiction.

Based on data from 11 disasters (Quarantelli, 1954), panic is always oriented with reference to the threatening situation, as in running away from a collapsed building. However, one may run toward danger if escape lies in the same direction, as in running through a sheet of fire to an exit. Panic is seen as an adaptive action without consideration of alternative courses of action. If a crisis situation has been defined as likely to cause panic, such as with a fire in a crowded place, then the probability of panic is increased. The probability is further increased when there is immediate, severe danger with no apparent escape.

Fogelman and Parenton (1959) observed no evidence of serious emotional disorders that could be directly associated with disaster in their study of Hurricane Audrey. Behavior was primarily family oriented, including outward to the extended family. They reported that a number of the people thought the end of the world had come but appeared reconciled to their fate.

Moore (1958) found residual emotional effects of disasters. Four months following the Waco tornado, which 85 percent of the black families and 53 percent of the white families in his study reported some members of the family showing abnormal fear of unusual weather conditions. When the subjects were asked if "emotional upset" was observed in any member of the family, 17 percent of the black families and 30 percent of the white families surveyed replied affirmatively.

Various people have proposed ideas as to why people cope adaptively or maladaptively with stress. According to Hocking (1969), constitutional factors and childhood experiences are important when considering the reactions of people to the ordinary stresses of life. These factors may influence an individual's tolerance, but if the stress (such as a community disaster) is great enough, all individuals will develop neurotic symptoms. The "great enough" is the key concept in his theory.

The tsunami study of Lachman et al. (1960) ruled out, or at least relegated to a minimum role, education and previous disaster experience as determinants of adaptive behavior. The major influencing factor they identified was ambiguous communication with respect to the danger.

Nutritional status has sometimes been linked to the individual's psychological coping ability. It was found that the prisoners-of-war in Japanese camps during World War II had the most difficult psychological problems during periods of malnutrition (Hocking, 1969). The severity of symptoms was also found to be related to the hardship of imprisonment, head injuries, and physical illnesses.

Lifton and Olson (1976) identified five major characteristics that may be found in some type of combination in all disasters. Psychological difficulty is likely if all five are found in a single disaster, as in the Buffalo Creek flood. The five characteristics are: suddenness of event, human callousness in causation (man-made rather than natural), continuing relationship of survivors to the disaster, isolation of the community, and totality of destruction.

There is no single lineal causality of maladaptive response in disaster. Individuals and families react differently because of their previous coping experiences, their physical and emotional health, resources available, characteristics of the disaster event, and the efficacy of crisis intervention. It is known, though that the different phases of the disaster are associated with similar behavior in the general population.

HUMOR

The phenomena of humor will be discussed according to the part it plays in the individual's coping process. Numerous stories, evidence of the people's continued sense of humor, are related by disaster workers. Some of these are as follows.

After the earthquake at Bakersfield, California, people used the pun "Quakersfield." Bumper stickers could be seen with the term and it has been rumored that letters which were addressed to residents in Quakersfield were correctly delivered.

In one residential area, a sign was posted that announced "open house." Behind the sign stood a badly damaged house with the entire second floor missing.

One disaster worker reported the following story of how a woman responded to the plea for evacuation from her apartment house in Anchorage, Alaska, during their major earthquake. The lady was taking a bath in her second floor apartment when she felt the movement of the earth and house. Immediately she heard men going through the complex shouting for the residents to get out. She quickly got up, ran out of the bathroom, and down the stairs. When coming down the stairs she met one of the men who was spreading the alert. He looked up at her and said "Say lady, haven't you forgotten something?" She looked down at herself (she was naked) and said, in effect, "Oh, thanks" and hurried back up the stairs to her apartment. But in a very short while, she came down the stairs again, this time seemingly much more in control of herself. However, as the man later said, she had her purse on her arm, but she still had not one stitch of clothes on!

A woman recounted this tale regarding her son-in-law in a recent tornado. She said that the warnings had come, one tornado had swept through the area and that they were having warnings about another tornado coming through. People were urged to leave their unsafe places and take shelter. The man rushed home to get his wife and child and found that they had already gone. Assuming that they had gone on to his mother-in-law's house that had a basement, he decided to grab what was important in the house and then join them. Because the electricity was off, he elected to empty the frozen food out of the freezer and take that with him. He hurriedly got a suitcase and filled it with the food. Now, a suitcase full of frozen food weighs a lot but the man left the house with the heavy suitcase full of food. He had only six blocks to go but the suitcase just kept getting heavier and heavier. His thoughts went something to the effect that this was ridiculous, he didn't have to take this food now, so he turned around and went back to the house. He emptied his suitcase and put the meat back in the freezer (all of this taking considerable time). He then took his suitcase to the bathroom and got out his wife's container of birth control pills. He put this in the suitcase, closed the suitcase and proceeded out again down the street to his mother-in-law's house. He reached the house safely and very proudly opened up the large suitcase to show what he had. In the large suitcase was his wife's birth control pills and nothing else! His only response later to the inevitable teasing was, "Well, I knew that if I ever saw my wife again she'd surely need those birth control pills!"

In conclusion, humor with accompanying laughter is a rather complicated human response. Laughing and being afraid or angry are closely connected. The unexpected event can frighten a person, but it also produces laughter. Laughing at the unexpected sometimes lessens the fear and serves as a release of tension. On a community level, humor serves to redirect the focus. It can turn the hardships of disaster into causes of involvement.

REFERENCES

American Psychiatric Association. First Aid for Psychological Reactions in Disaster. Washington, D.C.: American Psychiatric Association, 1966.

Fogelman, C.W., Parenton, V. Individual and group behavior in critical situations. Social Forces, 1959, *38*, 129.

Hocking, F. Psychiatric aspects of extreme environment stress. Diseases of the Nervous System, 1969, *31*, 120–121.

Howard, S.J. Treatment of children's reactions to the 1971 earthquake. Report presented to the American Association of Psychiatric Services. Beverly Hills, Calif.: 1971.

Janis, L.L. Psychological Stress. New York: Wiley, 1958.

Lachman, R., Tatsuoka, M., Bonk, W.S. Human behavior during the tsunami of May 1960. Science 1960, *133*, 1405–1409.

Laube, J. Response of the health care workers family-community role conflict in disaster and the psychological consequences of resolution. Unpublished doctoral dissertation, Texas Woman's University, 1974.

Lifton, R.J. Death in Life—Survivors in Hiroshima. New York: Random House, 1967.

Lifton, R.J., Olson, E. The human meaning of disaster. Psychiatry, 1976, *39*, 1–17.

Menninger, W.C. Psychological reactions in an emergency (flood). American Journal of Psychiatry, 1952, *109*, 128–130.

Moore, H.E. Tornadoes over Texas. Austin: University of Texas Press, 1958.

Quarantelli, E.L. The nature and conditions of panic. American Journal of Sociology, 1954, *60*, 267–275.

Quarantelli, E.L., Dynes, R.R. When disaster strikes. Psychology Today, 1971, *5*, 67.

Whalen, E.M. Observations of the June 1972 flood in the Wyoming Valley area of Pennsylvania. Paper presented to ad hoc consultant group, Office of Emergency Preparedness, October 26, 1972.

8

The Health of Postdisaster Populations: A Review of Literature and Case Study

Mary Evans Melick

Until relatively recently there has been little systematic study of the long-term health effects of disaster. Much of the disaster relief effort, including health services, has been concentrated in the immediate post-impact and remedy periods, lasting until several weeks following the disaster. After this time, disaster-related health services are withdrawn from the community and victims of the disaster are left to seek services from the functioning components of the local health care system. There may be several reasons for the lack of systematic follow-up. Among these reasons are the crisis orientation of the health service providers, the nondisaster responsibilities of volunteer health care providers, the lack of funding for follow-up studies, and possible geographic distribution of the disaster population, making follow-up technically difficult.

Probably the first systematic study of the long-term consequences of disaster was Cobb and Lindemann's (1943) study of the survivors of the Cocoanut Grove fire in Boston. Numerous studies since then have investigated the postdisaster community and survivor populations. Table 8.1 briefly reviews the studies of major disasters which have focused on health outcomes or consequences.

For several reasons it is difficult to draw firm conclusions regarding the long-term health consequences of disaster based on these studies. First, disaster, by its very nature is a unique occurrence. Few studies have compared several types of disasters to determine the importance of the characteristics of the disaster agent and the community in which the disaster occurs as these are related to the health and well-being of the postdisaster population. It seems likely, for example, that populations would respond differently to natural and man-made

TABLE 8.1. A SUMMARY OF THE HEALTH OUTCOMES OF MAJOR DISASTERS

Authors/ Publication Year	Event	Study Groups and Methods	Selected Findings
Cobb and Lindemann, 1943	Cocoanut Grove Fire, Boston, MA, November, 1942	Psychiatric interviews with 32 survivors. Emphasis on reaction (duration and characteristics).	14 of 32 survivors had neuro-psychiatric problems, half of which were reactions to bereavement.
Lorraine, 1954	Canvey Island floods, January 31 and February 1, 1953	Mortality study of Canvey Island population 1–2 months after flood.	Increased mortality rate during February and March 1953, compared to same period in 1952. The aged and those inclined to have respiratory conditions appeared to be especially at risk.
Moore and Friedsam, 1959	Tornado in Dallas, TX, 1957	142 survivors (72% female) studied for emotional problems through household interviews 4 months after event. No control group.	72% of respondents reported emotional distress among family members as a result of event. Those suffering—female respondents, children, adolescents, husbands, adult relatives, respectively.
Ciocco and Thompson, 1961; Schrenk et al., 1949	Smog episode, Donora, PA, October, 1948	Community survey (4092 Donora residents) of morbidity and mortality by household interviews. Emphasis on heart disease, asthma, and arthritis or rheumatism.	Those who had become ill at the time of event showed higher mortality and morbidity rates over the subsequent 9 years than other persons in the same area.
Archibald et al., 1962	World War II	57 combat veterans who had experienced combat syndrome, and 48 noncombat veterans from mental hygiene clinic were checked by	Validated presence of combat veteran syndrome 15 years after World War II involving startle reactions, sleep difficulties, diz-

Study	Methodology	Findings
	64-item questionnaire for symptoms indicative of combat veteran syndrome.	ziness, blackouts, avoidance of activities similar to combat experience, and internalization of feelings.
Bates et al., 1963	61 families (disaster victims) were studied 4 years after the event for behavior problems (children) and mental health problems (adults) through interview with victims and expert informants.	Generally negative health findings. Increase in cases of depression in adults. Physical/nervous exhaustion in leaders experiencing role conflict.
Hurricane Audrey, Cameron Parish, LA, 1959		
Leopold and Dillon, 1963	36 survivors studied for psychiatric disturbances 4 years after event.	Symptoms became worse over 4 years. Most victims required psychiatric treatment.
Marine explosion on the Delaware River, 1957		
Popovic and Petrovic, 1964	Psychiatric observations by mobile teams 1–5 days after disaster of persons in 27 evacuation camps and a psychiatric hospital.	Much of population was in mild stupor. Severe psychiatric disturbance was rare. Depression prevalent on days 2 and 3. Children evacuated to institutions were transiently disturbed.
Skoplje (Macedonia) earthquake, July 26, 1963		
Lifton, 1967	33 randomly selected survivors and 42 survivors especially articulate/prominent were studied 17 years after the event for mental and physical health by structured interview. No control group.	Apathy and despair in postimpact phase. Few psychiatric disorders. Radiation-related problems of leukemia, cataracts, cancer, and impaired growth and development of children. Psychosomatic bind (fear that any illness is related to radioactivity). Psychic numbing with fatigue and restricted vitality lasting into present. A-bomb neurosis.
Atomic bombing of Hiroshima, Japan, 1945		

(continued)

TABLE 8.1. (continued)

Authors/ Publication Year	Event	Study Groups and Methods	Selected Findings
Bennet, 1970	Floods, Bristol England, 1968	316 flood respondents and 454 non-flood controls studied for morbidity and mortality over 1-year period after flood.	Health status during 12-month period worse in flood group. Higher mortality in residents of flooded sections, especially among the elderly. More new psychiatric symptoms and more hospital admissions in males and females. Higher surgery rates in flood males who continued to live in own homes.
Eitinger, 1971	Concentration camp imprisonment, World War II	214 male and 13 female Norwegian former prisoners (most arrested at ages 20–30 years) examined approximately 30 years later, for health status, rate of aging, and mental health. No control group.	81% had cardiovascular, respiratory, gastrointestinal, neurologic, or mental diseases. Organic cerebral damage, impotence, and premature aging common.
Hall and Landreth, 1975	Flood, Rapid City, SD, June 9–10, 1972	Use of public records for changes in social indicators. Specific study of 35 families housed in public trailer sites.	For the community—number of nonterminated conceptions increased in 9 months postflood. Increase in arrests for public intoxication. For family sample—Indian families spent more days in the Public Health Hospital during the year postflood and made more outpatient visits. Much of the negative changes in social

Study	Sample	Findings
Abrahams et al., 1976	Brisbane floods, Australia, 1974	234 flood families (695 persons) and 163 nonflood families (507 persons) in same community studied by interview survey 3–12 months postdisaster; visits to physicians, psychological status, physical health.	indicators believed due to lower socioeconomic groups, especially transients, seeking work. Number of visits to physicians and hospitals increased in flood group during year following flood. Psychological problems more common in female victims. Persistent psychological problems, increased use of psychotropic drugs, sedatives, and hypnotics in flood respondents. No increase in mortality.
Melick, 1976	Flood, Tropical Storm Agnes, Wyoming Valley, PA, 1972	43 male flood, 48 male nonflood respondents (selected by multistage probability sampling from same working class community) studied 3 years after flood for physical and mental health problems by interview schedule and symptom checklists.	More victims indicated they were worse off then before flood; perceived that flood affected their health. Flood respondents did not have a greater number of illnesses or different kinds of illnesses but reported longer duration of illness. Emotional disturbance occurred in both groups, but its duration was longer in flood group respondents and their families.
Newman, 1976	Flood, Buffalo Creek, WV, 1972	224 children survivors studied by psychiatric interviews and analysis of pictures drawn 2 years after the flood.	Most were significantly or severely emotionally impaired by their experiences during and after the flood.

(continued)

TABLE 8.1. (continued)

Authors/ Publication Year	Event	Study Groups and Methods	Selected Findings
Penick et al., 1976	Tornado, Joplin, MO, 1973	Convenience sample of 26 victims interviewed 5 months after the tornado; physical and mental health. No control group.	75% of sample suffered psychological discomfort (anxiety, nervousness, or mild somatic complaints); 25% experienced interpersonal strain with family members.
Titchener and Kapp, 1976	Flood, Buffalo Creek, WV, 1972	654 survivors (224 children) taking legal action against company owning dam assessed for duration and severity of psychological disturbance by psychiatric examination 2 years after the flood. No control group.	80% had disabling psychiatric symptoms, maladjustments, and developmental problems (children).
Brownstone et al., 1977	Flood, St. Louis, MO, 1973; Tornado, Joplin, MO, 1973	136 flood and 26 tornado victims studied for psychological disability by survey 3–6 months after flood and 5 months after tornado. No control group.	No serious mental breakdown. Half felt more strained or nervous.
Janney et al., 1977	Earthquake, Peru, 1970	60 students from disaster city and 60 students from another city checked for number of life events by Peruvian Social Readjustment Rating Scales 1 year postdisaster.	Compared with controls, disaster victims reported a significant adverse change in health status in quake year and following year.
Parker, 1977	Cyclone Tracy, Darwin, Australia, 1974	Sample of 67 victims checked for psychological impairment and physical health by 30-item General Health Questionnaire at 1 week, 10 weeks (32 respondents),	39 victims characterized as "probable" psychiatric cases at 1 week (13 at 10 weeks, 4 at 14 months) postdisaster; 25% at 10 weeks, and 11% at 14 months

Reference / Disaster	Method	Findings
	and 14 months (18 respondents) postdisaster. Compared to the health survey of Sydney, Australia households.	indicated deterioration in physical health. Psychological morbidity higher at 1 and 10 weeks but not at 14 months.
Taylor, 1977 Tornado, Xenia, OH, April, 1974	350 interviews with workers in mental health and community agencies and interview survey with victims 6 months post-disaster and mail survey 1 year later.	Low rates of mental health problems including: only 3% thought they might have a nervous breakdown, 1% considered suicide; increase in tranquilizer and decrease in alcohol use; 27% reported trouble sleeping and 25% reported headaches. Number of emergency room visits and juvenile delinquency increased.
Logue, 1978 Flood, Tropical Storm Agnes, Wyoming Valley, PA, 1972	407 female flood respondents and 155 female nonflood respondents (systematic household samples) studied for mental and physical health status by mailed questionnaire approximately 5 years after flood: Zung scale, Langner scale, and modified SCL-90 for psychological status; 50-symptom checklist for physical symptoms; 23 life events.	Flood respondents showed more symptoms on Langner and SCL-90 (obsessive-compulsive). Physical health effects significant for immediate family (e.g., gastritis, constipation, severe headaches, bladder trouble), husband (hypertension), respondent (severe headaches, bladder trouble). Perceived health problems more frequent in flood respondents and immediate family members. Flood respondents stated flood had more deleterious effects on their health. Duration of psychological distress longer for flood group. Flood respondents experienced more "stress for major life events since flood.

(continued)

TABLE 8.1. (continued)

Authors/Publication Year	Event	Study Groups and Methods	Selected Findings
Nailor et al., 1978	Love Canal chemical dumpsite, Niagara Falls, NY, 1978	97 families in homes near Canal (230 adults, 134 children) studied for miscarriages, birth defects, liver functions, and blood mercury levels through medical records, blood tests, and medical histories.	More miscarriages and birth defects occurring in Love Canal females than before moving there and than expected based on general population. Especially frequent in southern Canal section. Women who lived on Canal longer had more miscarriages.
Price, 1978	Brisbane floods, Australia, 1974	246 flood families (695 persons) and 194 nonflood families (507 persons) living close to floods area were compared to psychological and physical health status at 3 and 12 months postdisaster by interview survey.	This extension of the study by Abrahams et al. focused on age-related health effects. Women less than 65 years of age experienced significantly more psychiatric symptoms than men. This sex difference did not appear in those aged 65 and over.
Takuma, 1978	Earthquake, Ebino, Japan, February 21, 1968	Interview (50 victims) and questionnaire survey (455 victims) of health status 7 weeks after event.	Majority of respondents complained of ill health after quake, but symptoms decreased over the 7-week period.
Dohrenwend et al., 1979	Nuclear accident at Three Mile Island, Harrisburg, PA, March 28–April 10, 1979	Several interview surveys during 5 months after event, including household probability samples within 32-km radius of plant, mothers of preschool children, school children, mental health center clients, Three Mile Island	Those upset: women, those under age 65, those with preschool children. 52% within 32-km radius evacuated, influenced by distance from Three Mile Island and having preschool children. Demoralization and perceived

Reference	Event / Method	Results
	plant workers, and control groups. Focus on mental health effects (perceptions and attitudes).	threat to health higher in April than later. Women, young people, and those with preschool children more unfavorable toward continued stay in area.
Faich and Rose, 1979	Blizzard, RI, February, 1978 State-wide record review of emergency rooms for storm period and 7 days prior to storm. Review of medical examiners' log and vital statistics for February 1978 and for previous 5 days.	Emergency room visits declined 64% and emergency admissions decreased 35% immediately after storm but returned to normal levels 3 days later. Admissions for myocardial infarction increased. Total mortality and ischemic heart disease deaths increased for 5 days after storm.
Glass et al., 1979	Blizzard, ME, 1978 Survey of records for morbidity (especially infectious disease) and mortality in population of eastern Maine during week after storm.	No outbreaks of infectious disease and no significant increase in mortality during week after blizzard compared to week before.
Wert, 1979	Three Mile Island nuclear accident, Harrisburg, PA, 1979 Questionnaire survey of 1435 Blue Shield employees (80% women) during early April for symptoms of distress and other health problems.	Most common symptom: trouble concentrating (increasing with distance from Three Mile Island). Other problems commonly cited: trouble going to sleep and staying asleep, earlier waking and headaches. Evacuees averaged more symptoms than stayers.

(continued)

TABLE 8.1. (continued)

Authors/ Publication Year	Event	Study Groups and Methods	Selected Findings
Bromet et al., 1980	Three Mile Island nuclear accident, Harrisburg, PA, 1979	Interview surveys of mothers of preschool children within 16-km radius of plant, unionized employees, mental health system clients, and respective control groups 1 year after event.	Survey demonstrated increase in mental health problems over the study period.
Keehn, 1980	World War II, Korean Conflict	Mortality study of 11,246 survivors of World War II and 7912 Korean Conflict survivors.	Increased risk of dying among former prisoners of war which diminishes over time. Excess of deaths due to cirrhosis appeared about the 10th follow-up year. No increased aging among POWs seen in mortality from chronic or degenerative diseases.
Paigen (reported to Holden), 1980	Love Canal chemical dumpsite, Niagara Falls, NY, 1978	Informal surveys of physical and mental health.	Residents perceived that effects such as miscarriages, stillbirths and birth defects, cancer, respiratory, urinary, liver, and kidney problems were due to environmental exposure.
Smith, et al., 1980	Richmond River Flood, Lismore, Australia, March 1974	Examination of hospital records for 1 year before and 1 year after flood.	Flood did not result in increase in hospital admissions or deaths. Pattern of admissions changed with doubling of admission rate for severely flooded males and halving of female rate. Deaths from heart disease increased

Reference	Disaster	Method	Findings
Ahearn, 1981	Earthquake, Managua, Nicaragua, December 1972	Longitudinal study of admissions to the Nicaraguan National Psychiatric Hospital.	significantly in year following flood for all of Lismore. Rates of admissions increased for the disaster area and immediately adjacent areas after the first postdisaster year. The diagnostic category showing the strongest (and significant) increase was neurosis which increased for both victims and nonvictims. Persons with a predisaster history of mental illness were at greater risk of hospital admission beginning about 1 year postdisaster and continuing for several years. Emotional problems persisted for about 3 years.
Gleser et al., 1981	Flood, Buffalo Creek, WV, 1972	Study of litigants (see Titchener and Kapp, 1976) 2–5 years postdisaster. Comparison with nonlitigants. Multiple measures were used including a symptom checklist, checklist of family disruption indicators, sleep disruption questionnaire, and Psychiatric Evaluation Form (Spitzer et al., 1968).	Over 30% continued to suffer debilitating symptoms 4–5 years postdisaster. 30% of families reported increased alcohol consumption, 44% increased cigarette smoking, and 52% increased use of prescription drugs. More than three quarters reported sleep disturbances 2 years postdisaster. Comparison with nonlitigants indicated that the nonlitigants were suffering more symptomatology than litigants.

(continued)

TABLE 8.1. (continued)

Authors/ Publication Year	Event	Study Groups and Methods	Selected Findings
Janerich et al., 1981	Flood, Tropical Storm Agnes, area around Almond, NY, 1972	Population study of leukemia/lymphoma incidence and spontaneous abortions in river valley during 5 years after event.	35% rise in spontaneous abortion rate starting 6 months after flood. Rate of leukemia and lymphoma increased in towns bordering streams approximately 2 years after flood, compared to nonriver valley and New York State.
Lindy et al, 1981	Fire, Beverly Hills Supper Club, Southgate KY, May 1977	125 of approximately 2500 survivors recruited through four outreach methods. Structured interview and Psychiatric Evaluation Form rating were completed 1 year postdisaster.	Survivors reported loss and subjective stress. Those located through the media tended to be a high-risk group.
Patrick and Patrick, 1981	Cyclone, November 23, 1978, Sri Lanka	Study of 100 contiguous households in one severely affected and one unaffected village. Data collected 2, 6, and 12 months following the disaster.	More than three quarters of the affected and 4% of the unaffected populations had psychiatric symptoms. Half of the affected population and all of the unaffected population began having symptoms within 1 month; the rest developed symptoms later. In three quarters of the affected population, symptoms persisted for 6 months. Most common were anxiety, depression, and phobia. Women were more likely to develop symptoms after 1 month postdisaster.

190

Bromet et al., 1982	Three Mile Island nuclear accident Harrisburg, PA, 1979	Comparison of 151 community mental health center patients from Three Mile Island area and 64 patients from a comparison site with a nuclear reactor. Interviews held immediately, 9–10 months and 12–13 months after the incident. Instruments included Schedule for Affective Disorders and Schizophrenia—Lifetime Version, social support interview schedule, and SCL-90.	No difference between two groups. Comparison of most and least distressed Three Mile Island patients showed that quality of support network and viewing Three Mile Island as dangerous were significantly associated with mental health.
Burke et al., 1982	Blizzard and subsequent flood, Revere, MA, February 6 and 7, 1978	64 preschool children in a Head Start program. Use of Connors Parent Questionnaire plus a storm questionnaire given 5 months postdisaster.	Increased behavior problems persisted for at least 5 months postdisaster. At particular risk were boys and children accepted for Head Start because their parents said they had special needs. School behavior improved and parents tended to deny behavior problems.
Goldsteen and Schorr, 1982	Three Mile Island nuclear accident, Harrisburg, PA, 1979	Telephone survey of random sample of Newberry Township and Goldboro (N = 409) in 1979 and interview of randomly selected subsample (N = 100) in March 1980.	Identified increasing levels of distress over time.
Ollendick and Hoffman, 1982	Flood, Rochester, MN, July 5, 1978	107 households selected from list of 2000 with which relief group had contact in 8 months postflood (124 adults and 54 children). Warheit, Holzer, and	68% sample reported being at least somewhat more depressed after the flood than before. About one third of adults noted improved functioning postdisaster. *(continued)*

TABLE 8.1. (continued)

Authors/ Publication Year	Event	Study Groups and Methods	Selected Findings
		Schwab depressive symptomatology scale and Milne's Before and Now Disaster Checklist used.	43% of children had continued problems.
Taylor and Frazer, 1982	Mount Erebus aircrash, Antarctica, November 28, 1979	Clinical interviews, structured questionnaires, and written and photographic materials were used to assess the distress experienced by 180 persons who handled or identified the bodies. Data were collected by researchers immediately after completing their work and 3 and 20 months later.	35% were in high-stress groups (Hopkins Symptom Checklist); 21% after 3 months and 23% 20 months. Membership in the high-stress groups varied over time.
Murphy, 1983	Volcanic eruption, Mount St. Helens, WA, May 18, 1980	39 bereaved of presumed dead persons, 30 bereaved of known dead, 21 experiencing loss of permanent residence, and 15 experiencing loss of leisure residence. Matched control group (N = 50). Instruments included: Life Experiences Survey, Hassles Scale, HSC-90, and items written by author.	Respondents reported they were only somewhat recovered 11 months following disaster. Bereaved of presumed dead reported higher scores than controls in life events and depression. Bereaved of confirmed dead reported higher scores than controls on negative life events, hassles, depression, and somatization. Permanent property loss group indicated higher score on negative life events than controls. Self-efficacy and social support buffered the effects of stress on depression.

disasters. Studies of man-made disasters, such as wars and prison camp internment, indicate that malnutrition and other physical deprivations may result in long-term sequelae seldom seen following natural disasters other than such situations as prolonged drought. It is uncertain what effects on health may result from identification with the oppressor, the attachment of blame to an individual or group, and the prolonged coping techniques necessary for survival (see Chapter 5). Likewise, we lack systematic studies comparing the health of populations prone to recurrent disasters with those of a once-in-a-lifetime disaster. Other factors related to the disaster that may influence health outcomes are the social supports of the victim population, the soundness of the economic base of the community, the proportion of the population which is fatally or seriously injured, and the duration and scope of the disaster. Also, little work has been done comparing the stress of disaster with other stressful life experiences to determine if the health outcomes are the same. It is also noteworthy that there are few studies comparing the pre- and postdisaster health and well-being of disaster populations. Recently several studies have used social indicators such as divorce (Aguirre, 1980), admission to mental hospitals (Ahearn, 1981), and admission to general hospitals (Glass et al., 1979; Smith et al., 1980) as indicators of change in the postdisaster community.

Although the picture is not perfectly clear, existing evidence indicates the following:

1. Not all studies of postdisaster populations have found long-term health consequences of disaster (e.g., see Taylor, 1977).
2. The preponderance of the evidence seems to indicate that disaster is associated with recovery period mental health problems. These problems include depression, anxiety, phobias, sleep disturbances, irritability and, in some cases, an increase in psychiatric illnesses and admission to mental hospitals. Such problems may last for several years.
3. Studies which use clinical assessment techniques (e.g., Titchener and Kapp, 1976) have often found higher rates of mental health problems than those which used self-report and/or mental health scales such as the Symptom Checklist-90 (SCL-90) (Derogatis, 1977) or Gurin Symptom Checklist (Gurin et al., 1960), (e.g., see Bromet, 1980; Logue, 1978; Melick, 1976).
4. A postdisaster increase in physical health problems has been reported by several investigators. These conditions have included, for example, a self-report of headache and bladder problems and hypertension in husbands (Logue, 1978) as well as an increase in spontaneous abortions and increased rates of leukemia and lymphoma (Janerich et al., 1981).

5. There is also a suggestion that the duration of illness is longer in disaster victims than in nonvictim controls (Melick, 1976).
6. Some positive effects of disaster have also been reported for a proportion of the victim population. This includes self-report of improved functioning (Ollendick and Hoffman, 1982).
7. Nonvictim control groups have sometimes been found to experience stress as a result of disaster. Such persons may be in need of mental health services (Shippee et al., 1982). This finding raises questions about identifying the victims of a disaster. Because of kin and friendship ties, a broader group of persons than the survivors of a disaster could be considered victims.
8. Although infrequently studied, it appears that rescue workers, body handlers and other "nonvictims" working at the disaster site may experience long-term mental health problems (Dunning and Silva, 1980; Taylor and Frazer, 1982).
9. Research to date has indicated that diverse groups of individuals have developed long-term health changes following disasters while little attention has been paid to high-risk groups. Bromet and co-workers' (1982) study of psychiatric patients' responses to disaster indicated no particular risk regarding the development or exacerbation of mental health problems following disaster. Logue (1978) indicates that the group at highest risk for health changes were women less than 65 years old with lower levels of education and incomes.
10. Although the postdisaster period is often identified by survivors as being stressful, the majority of victims are reluctant to take advantage of mental health services, including outreach services (e.g., see Lindy et al., 1981).

ASSESSMENT OF PHYSICAL HEALTH STATUS

An important aspect of studies focusing on postdisaster health and well-being is the selection of instruments and techniques used to assess health status. The use of standardized instruments and scientific methods of sample selection is critical in building a literature base which can be used for theory construction and as a basis for the development of practice guidelines. In evaluating the data available on postdisaster health status, it is important to recognize that various aspects of health are of central concern depending on the postdisaster period of study. Immediately following a disaster, for example, emphasis is placed on identifying the number of dead and injured persons and on classifying and treating those with injuries. During the remedy period the focus shifts to monitoring and controlling outbreaks or potential outbreaks of infectious diseases. During the recovery period, in contrast, the focus is on identification and treatment of secondary or stress-related illnesses which are in some way the result of the disaster, but which are not directly due to injury or to contact with a contaminated environment.

To date a variety of aspects of physical health have been assessed in the recovery period. These have included minor symptoms, diagnosed diseases or syndromes, and death. Several studies have focused on measurement of illness behavior or what the individuals who perceive some disease do about their health problem. Studies measuring illness behavior have included Abrahams et al. (1976) who studied office visits to a physician; Wert (1979) who recorded visits to an occupational health nurse; Faich and Rose (1979) who studied emergency hospital visits and admissions; and Bennet (1970) and Smith et al. (1980) who analyzed hospital admission rates and surgical rates.

Some studies have relied on objective measures of physical health while others have examined subjective perceptions of disaster victims. Objective measures have included the number of deaths recorded (Bennet, 1970; Glass et al., 1979. Lorraine, 1954), and the presence of disease as determined by physical examination (Eitinger, 1971) or through hospital or physicians' records (Faich and Rose, 1979). Examples of the types of illnesses which have been studied include: myocardial infarction (Faich and Rose, 1979); numbers of spontaneous abortions (Janerich et al., 1981; Nailor et al., 1978); the incidence of liver dysfunction or blood mercury levels (Nailor et al., 1978); and rates of leukemia or lymphoma (Janerich et al., 1981). Although these measures of postdisaster health are objective, there are several problems in relying on them to provide a detailed picture of the health status of victim populations. These problems include possible destruction of predisaster comparison records, the questionable validity and reliability of diagnoses, and a focus on disease rather than on illness behavior. Individuals may be ill, but may choose to ignore illness because other concerns such as shelter and providing for a family may be priority issues. Also, treatment facilities may not be conveniently located or individuals may be reluctant to seek care from providers they do not know personally.

In an attempt to obtain information which more accurately reflects the individual's health–illness experience, some researchers have used subjective measures of health, that is, self-report. A number of studies (e.g., Parker, 1977) have used health questionnaires or symptom and condition checklists (Logue, 1978) or have asked respondents about symptoms of disease and episodes of illness (Abrahams et al., 1976; Ciocco and Thompson, 1961; Lifton, 1967; Melick, 1976; Penick et al., 1976;

Takuma, 1978). In several cases, victims have been asked to compare their pre- and postdisaster health (Logue, 1978; Melick, 1976). Uniformly victims have indicated poorer postdisaster health even when they were unable to provide a history of a greater number of postdisaster illnesses as compared to predisaster illnesses.

To date there has been no ideal study of the physical health of a postdisaster population during the recovery period. Such a study would employ a control group, use a longitudinal design with follow-up over perhaps a 2-year period, and most likely employ both objective and subjective measures to assess a broad range of health outcomes. It would be necessary to determine the incidence and prevalence of types of illnesses, severity and length of illnesses, and the types of treatment sought and provided.

ASSESSMENT OF MENTAL HEALTH STATUS

There have been three major methods of obtaining data about postdisaster mental health. The first is the examination of admission and attendance records in which the researcher compares the pre- and postdisaster use of mental health services within a given locality (e.g., see Ahearn, 1981). In some community disasters, these records have been destroyed by the disaster agent. In addition, these records provide a limited view of the mental health status of individuals in the community since they provide information only on those who have received care.

Alternative approaches have been to obtain data directly from individuals either through clinical interviews and/or through the use of standardized psychological scales or instruments. Following the Buffalo Creek Dam disaster, for example, Titchener and Kapp (1976) used intensive clinical interviewing as well as projective psychological testing. Other researchers have relied primarily upon written standardized instruments. Bromet and associates (1980), for example, used the Schedule of Affective Disorders and Schizophrenia Lifetime Scale (SADS-L) developed by Endicott and Spitzer (1978) to assess the presence of severe mental disorder. They also used the 90-item Self-Report Symptom Inventory (Derogatis, 1977) to assess psychological symptoms such as anxiety, phobias, anger, and psychophysiological disturbances. Kasl et al. (1981) used several methods and instruments to collect data on workers at the Three Mile Island and Peach Bottom nuclear plants. One-hour telephone interviews were followed by mailed questionnaires and face-to-face interviews. The instruments used included the Demoralization Scale (Link and Dohrenwend, 1980) to evaluate self-esteem and a modification of the Langner 22-item screening score of psychiatric impairment (Langner, 1962) to assess psychophysiological problems.

In assessing the mental health of a postdisaster population, it may be beneficial to use several techniques and/or multiple measures to obtain a comprehensive picture of mental health problems, well-being, and mental health treatment. The use of standardized instruments has the advantage of permitting comparison of results across studies.

One of the important aspects of disaster research which has not yet been resolved is the identification of victims and their differentiation from nonvictims. Many times a victim is defined as someone whose home has been destroyed in the disaster (e.g., see Logue, 1978; Melick, 1976) or someone who has lost a loved one in the disaster. Those who live in the community, but who have not experienced loss are then assumed to be nonvictims. Research has shown what a popular song has told us, that one victim experiences the tragedy while another stops to observe it.* Because of kin and friendship ties, because those experiencing loss are often taken into the homes of those not experiencing loss, and because of the economic and political ties which bind a community, it is important that health providers and researchers not assume that persons who do not seem to have suffered a loss are defined as nonvictims without evaluation of life changes which they have experienced. Melick (1976), in her investigation of a postflood community, found that many nonvictims had an increase in their life events score and in episodes of illness following the flood. Although these increases tended to be somewhat more modest than those of persons who experienced loss of housing, they might nevertheless be associated with a decreased sense of well-being and possibly with illness. It is also possible that the near-miss phenomenon may produce stress with consequences for mental and physical health. Recently Murphy (1983) has reported a research study indicating that differential health effects result from different conditions of loss. Further research is needed to clarify the definition of victim so that providers of mental health care can make their services available to persons and groups who may benefit from their services.

A CASE STUDY OF POSTDISASTER HEALTH AND WELL-BEING: THE AGNES FLOOD, WILKES-BARRE, PENNSYLVANIA

Located in the northeastern part of Pennsylvania, Wilkes-Barre at the time of the flooding produced by Tropical Storm Agnes was a city of 58,865 (Department of Commerce, 1972). Across the river is a small

---

*Bob Seger, "No Man's Land," Bob Seger and the Silver Bullet Band. Capitol Records, 1980.

bedroom community, Kingston, which had a population of approximately 18,325 persons. These two cities are located in the Wyoming Valley which contains the Susquehanna River, the longest river draining into the Atlantic Ocean. The Susquehanna has its origin in Otsego Lake in Central New York State and flows in a generally southeastern direction toward the Chesapeake Bay.

At the turn of the century Wilkes-Barre was an important anthracite coal mining center. Anthracite production in the Wyoming Valley peaked in 1918 when 37.7 million tons were mined (Franke, 1974). The Valley still contains several reminders of this golden age of mining. These include the large homes of the wealthy former mine owners and industrialists which line the river common, the scars of strip mining borne by the surrounding mountains, and the ethnic diversity of the population. Many new immigrants came to the Wyoming Valley seeking employment in the mines. At the time of the flood persons of foreign birth or parentage constituted just over 29 percent of the population while less than 2 percent of the population was black (Franke, 1974). The largest ethnic groups were Polish and Italian. Many of these persons are now elderly, speak broken English, and maintain ties with ethnically homogeneous institutions such as churches and clubs. A significant number of the older men previously employed in the mines have anthracosilicosis or other mining-related disabilities.

Many of the largely working class towns and cities in the Wyoming Valley were just beginning to recover from the effects of the coal mining decline when the disaster occurred. The 1970 census showed an area that was economically depressed with a median income of $8047, a median real estate value of $9300, and a population with a median age well above the national average (Department of Commerce, 1972). About one-third of all workers, largely women in low-paying jobs, were employed in apparel manufacturing (Franke, 1974). Other important industries included electrical machinery, fabricated metals, tobacco, food processing, printing and publishing, and trucking.

The disaster reported here is widespread flooding resulting from Tropical Storm Agnes. This storm developed in Yucatan during the evening of June 14, 1972, and hit the Florida coast on June 18. It began moving up the eastern coast of the United States causing wind and water damage until it began to move out to sea the evening of June 21. Instead of continuing out to sea, like similar storms, Agnes's course shifted inland establishing a double center over the Wyoming Valley of Pennsylvania and the Corning-Elmira area of the southern tier of New York State. The storm then continued to move westward until it disintegrated over western Pennsylvania on June 24. By the time the storm was over, Agnes had dumped more than 28 trillion gallons of water on the eastern seaboard, mostly on the middle Atlantic states. The final statistics showed that an estimated 116,000 homes, 2400 farm buildings, and 5800 businesses were damaged or destroyed (Department of the Army, 1972). The loss of life was relatively low with 118 deaths attributed to the storm (Metropolitan Life Insurance, 1977). The greatest property damage occurred in the Wyoming Valley where about 25,000 homes were destroyed, although only three flood-related deaths were reported in this area.

Flooding has occurred before in this community. During this century, major floods occurred in 1902, 1904, 1936, 1940, 1946, and 1964 (Mussari, 1974; Romanelli and Griffith, 1972). In response to the 1936 flood, when the river crested at 33.7 feet, a 15-mile system of dikes was built to contain flood waters up to 33 feet. In addition, six reservoirs were built on tributaries of the Susquehanna upstream from the Wyoming Valley in an effort to prevent flooding. The Agnes storm, however, caused the Susquehanna to crest at 40.9 feet, 7.9 feet above the level of the dikes.

Approximately 80,000 people were evacuated. Many went to live with friends or relatives elsewhere in the Valley. The remainder were housed in public shelters established in local schools. The evacuation period lasted 3 days for most people. When allowed to return home, most residents found greater destruction than they had anticipated and many were forced to seek housing from others or to use mobile homes provided by the Federal government.

In Kingston all but 20 of the buildings were damaged. Approximately 150 industrial firms employing 11,335 workers were affected (Franke, 1974; Krantz, 1973), and it was estimated that the unemployment rate rose to nearly 20 percent in the Wyoming Valley (Department of the Army, 1972).

A number of researchers were active in this postdisaster community studying the effects of the flood. Two researchers in particular (Logue, 1978; Melick, 1976) were interested in studying the health and well-being of the population during the recovery period. Melick's study was conducted nearly 3 years after the flood. She was primarily interested in investigating the relationship between stress and physical illness and emotional disorder in a sample of working class men, ages 25–65 during the recovery period. The study focused on three time periods: 6 months before the flood (January to June 1972); the period from the impact of the flood to $2\frac{1}{2}$ years later (June 1972 to January 1975), and the most recent 6 months (January to June 1975).

This study was designed to compare the life change and illness experiences of two groups of men who were residents of the same community and who were similar except for their disaster experience. The study was limited to working class men for several reasons, including (1) the fact that they were probably employed at the time of the flood (2) a smaller sample can be used if one need not take account of differential rates of illness and reporting of illnesses if both sexes and other age groups were used, and (3) previous research had indicated that the lower classes are especially susceptible to the effects of disaster (Wilson, 1962). A sample of 120 working class men was selected using a multistage probability sampling technique (Melick, 1976). Each of the 60 flood and 60 nonflood group respondents was sent a letter requesting their participation in the study and advising them that an interviewer would be contacting them soon.

Testing of the study hypotheses required the collection of five types of data. These were demographic information, flood experience, life events (assessed by the Schedule of Recent Experience, Holmes and Rahe, 1967), social integration, and health–illness experience (assessed by the Checklist of Twenty Symptom Items, Gurin et al., 1960) as well as by other self-report items (e.g., number and length of illness episodes) developed by the researcher. The instrument was pretested on 10 subjects similar to the anticipated respondents, and revisions were made as necessary.

Data were collected by personal interviews conducted in the homes of the respondents. Despite the flood-related destruction and urban renewal taking place, the majority of the intended subjects were located. Data analysis was based on 91 cases, 43 flood and 48 nonflood respondents. A follow-up reliability study indicated 0.83 reliability.

Logue's study (1978) was conducted in the spring of 1977, 5 years postdisaster. The primary purpose of the study was to determine the long-term effects of disaster for two time periods, the recovery and postrecovery periods. This study was designed in part to complement Melick's study to present a more comprehensive picture of the health of this postflood community. The respondents, therefore, were women 21 years of age or older who lived in Kingston and surrounding towns. Women were also selected since they are at greater risk of mental disorders than men (Weissman and Klerman, 1977). This was an epidemiology study and large sample sizes were required in order to permit flexibility in stratifying the data base. The sample was selected using a multistage probability sampling technique. Following sample selection, a questionnaire was mailed to the targeted group, and 407 flood respondents (52 percent) and 155 nonflood respondents (21 percent) returned questionnaires. Follow-up analysis indicated that many flood nonrespondents gave poor health as a reason for not responding to the questionnaire. The overall result of this modest return, therefore, may have been a minimizing of the health effects of the flood.

Logue's instruments included several designed to assess mental health. These included Zung's 20-item Self-Rating Depression Scale (Zung, 1965); Langner's 22-item Screening Instrument (Langner, 1962); and a modified version of the 90-item Self-Report Symptom Inventory (SCL-90) (Derogatis et al., 1977). In addition there were demographic questions and a researcher-developed 50-item scale designed to measure the 5-year incidence of various health effects of disaster.

The outcomes of both studies provided support for the hypothesis that there are long-term health consequences of disaster. Both Melick and Logue hypothesized that the mere flooding of a dwelling unit would be a stressor of sufficient intensity to have long-term effects on mental health. Comparison of flood and nonflood respondents indicated that the former did have higher, although not statistically higher, levels of self-reported mental health symptoms, particularly anxiety and obsessive-compulsive behavior. The obsessive-compulsive symptom seems to correspond to the state of psychic numbing described by Lifton and Olson (1976) in their study of the victims of the Buffalo Creek flood. Two factors may have accounted for the failure to attain statistical significance in the Wilkes-Barre sample when Lifton and Olson had found sustained mental health problems. The first is that Melick and Logue used standardized self-report instruments to determine mental health status. Those studies that have used this technique have generally found lower levels of impairment than studies that have used clinical assessment techniques such as psychiatric interviews. The second reason was that the Agnes disaster produced minimal loss of life in the communities under study. Lifton (1967) indicates that immersion in a culture of death may have consequences for prolonged mental health problems. Disasters which produce property loss, but little loss of life may be associated with fewer mental health problems, in part because social support networks are less disrupted.

In Melick's study, respondents were asked if anyone in their family had experienced emotional distress as a result of the flood. If the respondent answered affirmatively, the interviewer asked about the person experiencing distress, the treatment and length of the episode. Flood respondents were significantly more likely to report emotional distress. They indicated that they, rather than another family member, were the person who experienced the distress. Emotional distress lasted significantly longer in flood than in non-flood respondents (mean of 190 days versus 120 days). The nature of the distress or emotional upset was often reported as anger or irritability with several respondents noting they had gotten into fights. Professional help was rarely sought to remedy the reported emotional distress.

Regarding physical health, Logue's respondents were asked to rate their health as well as the health of each family member. Reported health at the time of the survey was poorer for the flood respondents and their families than for nonflood respondents and families. Flood respondents indicated a greater association between the flood and ill health than did the nonflood group. Melick noted that flood respondents did not report a significantly greater number of illnesses, although the trend was in that direction. Nonflood group respondents reported a greater number of illnesses in the predisaster period while flood respondents reported greater numbers of illnesses in both postdisaster periods. Reported illnesses did not differ in type for the two flood conditions. It was interesting to note, however, that the duration of each illness was longer for flood than nonflood respondents (19.4 days versus 3.5 days). In addition, flood respondents were more likely to state that their present health status was poorer than a year ago. They also more frequently cited specific effects which the flood had had on their health while nonflood respondents overwhelmingly (94 percent) stated that the flood had no influence on their general health. Specific effects on health cited by flood group respondents included fatigue or loss of pep, anxiety or tension, and production of a specific, often chronic, disease condition.

Making use of a 50-item symptom checklist, Logue's flood group respondents were more likely to report severe headaches, bladder trouble, and the occurrence of at least one symptom than were his nonflood group respondents. Flood group husbands were more likely to have developed hypertension. The occurrence of gastritis, frequent constipation, bone or cartilage disease, cardiovascular and digestive illnesses, and bladder troubles were all more commonly reported for flood group than nonflood-group families.

It is interesting to note that the female respondents in Logue's study indicated that the average duration of emotional distress suffered by a family member was 2 years. The duration of physical distress for the family member suffering the greatest distress was $2\frac{1}{2}$ years. For married respondents, both studies found that husbands were mentioned most often as the family member suffering the greatest physical and emotional distress. This result, although no surprise to the researchers working in the community, is unlike that previously noted by Moore and Friedsam (1959) who found that their female respondents were more likely to report personal emotional upset. In general, husbands demonstrated longer duration of emotional upset than wives while wives experienced a significantly longer duration of physical distress than their husbands (3 years versus $2\frac{1}{2}$ years).

Many respondents in Logue's flood group believed that the flood hindered them from obtaining regular medical checkups (44 percent) or obtaining attention for specific medical problems (35 percent). Failure to attend to medical problems or engage in preventive care may have been an important factor associated with the longer duration of illness experienced by flood as compared to nonflood-group respondents. With additional demands on their finances and time, postdisaster victims may be less likely to seek preventive care or treatment early in the course of an illness. When they come for treatment, therefore, they are sicker than nonvictims and take longer to regain their health and strength. Additional research is needed in this area.

Melick and Logue were both interested in measuring the stress experienced by respondents. Melick used the Schedule of Recent Experience (Holmes and Rahe, 1967) while Logue used 22 major life events extracted from Bazeley and Viney's (1974) research plus an open-ended question regarding major events not found on the checklist. For the preflood period Melick's respondents received approximately the same life change unit score while flood group respondents had higher scores for the period from June 1972 to January 1975. Although the flood group respondents maintained a higher score for January 1975 to June 1975, this was not significantly different than nonflood-group scores. The number of illness was correlated with life change unit score with those scoring highest on life change, regardless of flood condition, experiencing the greatest number of illnesses. Logue's flood group demonstrated significantly more perceived stress than the nonflood group for life events experienced between 1972 and 1977.

Both investigators were interested in the role of stress buffering factors in shielding the person under stress from the development of illness. Melick's measure emphasized social support and included information on marital status, relationship with family and friends, and church attendance while Logue selected 10 psychosocial asset items from Nuckolls and co-workers' study (1972). Melick's measure failed to indicate a significant buffering effect of social support while Logue's analysis found that flood respondents who experienced high stress regarding the perception of life events and low psychosocial assets were at particular risk for physical health symptoms.

The final analysis with implications for postdisaster health and well-being relates to respondents' perceptions of the recovery period. This period has been reported to be a second disaster (Erikson, 1976) because of the changed conditions of life associated with it.

Unemployment is one of the changes which may occur postdisaster. Although both groups experienced similar rates of unemployment during the recovery period (about 20 percent for husbands and 30 percent for respondents), the flood group demonstrated significantly longer rates of unemployment than the nonflood group (9 months versus 6

months for husbands and 7 months versus 4 months on the average
for respondents). Much of this unemployment in the flood group seemed
to be the respondent's choice since considerable time and effort were
required to reestablish a family dwelling unit. Respondents who continued to work and to repair or replace their housing unit often reported
exhaustion. Despite long periods of unemployment, it is noteworthy
that 19 percent of Logue's flood respondents felt that work in the recovery period was so hard that some immediate family member became
ill as a result.

Because the recovery period seems to be a time of particular stress,
it may be important to determine the length of time that this period
continues. This information may be particularly helpful for health care
providers to have in order to plan for delivery of care, particularly outreach programs to high-risk groups. The research reported here asked
respondents for their perception of the length of the recovery period,
or the period it took them to get back on their feet. Respondents in
both studies indicated that the perceived mean and median length of
the recovery period was 18 months.

CONCLUSIONS

Community disasters, such as the Agnes flood reported here, are often
associated with long term health consequences for community residents.
Such consequences include physical health problems, emotional distress,
and impaired sense of well-being. Health professionals should be aware
of the prolonged effects of the disaster and of the recovery period, or
second disaster which follows, in order to identify persons at risk of
sequelae and to design intervention programs to treat and/or to prevent the development of secondary health problems. Recognition must
be given to the fact that disaster victims are often reluctant to seek
out health care services, particularly mental health services, following
disaster.

It is not entirely clear who should be designated as the victim of
a disaster since a number of persons who seem not to have been affected by the disaster agent suffer deleterious effects as a result of the
disaster. Some of these groups of "nonvictims" include persons experiencing the near-miss phenomenon, those whose economic, political, or
social status is affected by the disaster, those not living in the community who suffer loss of a loved one, evacuees, body handlers, health
care providers, and persons who give significant personal aid, such as
shelter, to victims. Although additional research is needed in clarifying the definition of victim, health care providers should be aware that

these and other groups of nonvictims may experience health problems postdisaster.

Future research should attempt to determine the relative risk of incurring health problems and to identify groups at particular risk. Specific intervention programs could then be developed and implemented for the group at greatest risk. This would have the advantage of conserving scarce resources in the recovery period.

Considerable research is still needed in identifying the health effects, both positive and negative, of disaster and the length of time over which disaster-related stressors exert their effects. Research designs should be as rigorous as possible, including the use of control groups, standardized instruments and data collection techniques, and the use of scientific sample selection, in order to permit cross-study comparisons, replications and generalizations of findings. Various types of disasters—community and individual, natural and man-made, disasters caused by different agents—should be compared in order to determine the similarity of health outcomes. Finally, it is important to carefully document and evaluate intervention programs to determine the transportability and effectiveness of such programs for the identification and relief of postdisaster health sequelae.

ACKNOWLEDGMENTS

This research was supported in part by a Special Nurse Fellowship, Public Health Service, Department of Health, Education and Welfare. The author acknowledges the secretarial assistance of Leslie Long and Theresa Flansburg in the preparation of the manuscript. Special thanks is extended to Dr. James N. Logue whose research is discussed in the case study.

REFERENCES

Abrahams, M.J., Price, J., Whitlock, F.A., et al. The Brisbane floods, January 1974: Their impact on health. Medical Journal of Australia, 1976, 2, 936–939.

Aguirre, B.E. The long term effects of major natural disasters on marriage and divorce: An ecological study. Victimology: An International Journal, 1980, 5, 298–307.

Ahearn, F.L., Jr. Disaster mental health: A pre- and post-earthquake comparison of psychiatric admission rates. Urban and Social Change Review, 1981, 14, 22–28.

Archibald, H.C., Long, D.M., Miller, C., et al. Gross stress reactions in combat—A 15 year follow-up. American Journal of Psychiatry, 1962, 119, 317-322.

Bates, F.L., Fogelman, C.W., Partenton, V.J., et al. The social and psychological consequences of a natural disaster: A longitudinal study of Hurricane Audrey. Disaster Study No. 18. Washington, D.C.: National Academy of Sciences, National Research Council, 1963.

Bazeley, P., Viney, L.L. Women coping with crisis: A preliminary community study. Journal of Community Psychology, 1974, 2, 321-329.

Bennet, G. Bristol floods 1968. Controlled survey of effects on health of local community disaster. British Journal of Medicine, 1970, 3, 454-458.

Bromet, E., Parkinson, D., Schulberg, H.C. et al. Three Mile Island: Mental health findings. Washington, D.C.: National Institute of Mental Health, 1980.

Bromet, E., Schulberg, H.C., Dunn, L. Reactions of psychiatric patients to the Three Mile Island nuclear accident. Archives of General Psychiatry, 1982, 39, 725-730.

Brownstone, J., Penick, E.C., Larcen, S.W., et al. Disaster-relief training and mental health. Hospital and Community Psychiatry, 1977, 23, 30-32.

Burke, J.D., Jr., Borus, J.F., Burns B.J., et al. Changes in children's behavior after a natural disaster. American Journal of Psychiatry, 1982, 139, 1010-1014.

Ciocco, A., Thompson, D.J. A follow-up of Donora ten years after: Methodology and findings. American Journal of Public Health, 1961, 51, 155-164.

Cobb, S., Lindemann, E. Neuropsychiatric observations during the Cocoanut Grove fire. Annals of Surgery, 1943, 117, 814.

Department of the Army, Corps of Engineers (Baltimore District). Wyoming Valley flood control, Susquehanna River, Pennsylvania. Baltimore, Md., 1972.

Derogatis, L.R. The SCL-90 Manual 1: Scoring, Administration and Procedures for the SCL-90. Baltimore: Johns Hopkins University School of Medicine, Clinical Psychometrics Unit, 1977.

Dohrenwend, B.P., Dohrenwend, B.S., Kasl, S.V., et al. Technical staff analysis report on behavioral effects. Presented to the President's Commission on the accident at Three Mile Island, October 31, 1979.

Dunning, C., Silva, M., Disaster-induced trauma in rescue workers. Victimology: An International Journal, 1980, 5, 287-297.

Eitinger, L. Organic and psychosomatic aftereffects of concentration camp imprisonment. International Psychiatry Clinics, 1971, 8, 205-215.

Endicott, J., Spitzer, R.L. A diagnostic interview: The schedule for affective disorders and schizophrenia. Archives of General Psychiatry, 1978, 35, 837-844.

Erikson, K.T. Everything in Its Path: Destruction of Community in the Buffalo Creek Flood. New York: Simon and Schuster, 1976.

Faich, G., Rose, R. Blizzard morbidity and mortality: Rhode Island, 1978. American Journal of Public Health, 1979, 69, 1050-1052.

Franke, D. America's Fifty Safest Cities. New Rochelle, N.Y.: Arlington House Publishers, 1974.

Glass, R.I., O'Hare, P., Conrad, J.L. Health consequences of the snow disaster in Massachusetts, February 6, 1978. American Journal of Public Health, 1979, 69, 1047–1049.

Gleser, G.C., Green, B.L., Winget, C. Prolonged Psychosocial Effects of Disaster: A Study of Buffalo Creek. New York: Academic Press, 1981.

Goldsteen, R., Schorr, J.K. The long-term impact of a man-made disaster: An examination of a small town in the aftermath of the Three Mile Island nuclear reactor accident. Disasters, 1982, 50, 59.

Gurin, G., Veroff, J., Feld, S. Americans View Their Mental Health. New York: Basic Books, 1960.

Hall, S., Landreth, P.W. Assessing some long-term consequences of a natural disaster. Mass Emergencies, 1975, 1, 55–61.

Holmes, T.H., Rahe, R.H. Schedule of Recent Experience. Seattle, University of Washington, School of Medicine, Department of Psychiatry, 1967.

Janerich, D.T., Stark, A.D., Greenwald, P., et al. Increased leukemia, lymphoma and spontaneous abortion in western New York following a flood disaster. Public Health Reports, 1981, 96, 350–356.

Janney, J.G., Masuda, M., Holmes, T.H. Impact of a natural catastrophe on life events. Journal of Human Stress, 1977, 3, 22–34.

Kasl, S.V., Chisholm, R.F., Eskenazi, B. The impact of the accident at the Three Mile Island on the behavior and well-being of nuclear workers (Parts I & II). American Journal of Public Health, 1981, 71, 472–495.

Keehn, R.J. Follow-up studies of World War II and Korean conflict prisoners: Mortality to January 1, 1976. American Journal of Epidemiology, 1980, 111, 194–211.

Krantz, D. Trouble with Agnes. Wilkes-Barre, Penn.: D.L.K. Associates, 1973.

Langner, T.S. A 22-item screening score of psychiatric symptoms indicating impairment. Journal of Health and Human Behavior, 1962, 3, 269–276.

Leopold, R.L., Dillon, H. Psychoanatomy of a disaster. American Journal of Psychiatry, 1963, 119, 913.

Lifton, R.J. Death in Life: Survivors of Hiroshima. New York: Random House, 1967.

Lifton, R.J., Olson, E. The human meaning of total disaster: The Buffalo Creek experience. Psychiatry, 1976, 39, 1.

Lindy, J.D., Grace, M.C., Green, B.L. Survivors: Outreach to a reluctant population. American Journal of Orthopsychiatry, 1981, 51, 468–475.

Link, B., Dohrenwend, B.P. Formulation of hypotheses about the true prevalence of demoralization in the United States. In B.P. Dohrenwend et al. (Eds.), Mental Illness in the United States: Epidemiological Estimates. New York: Praeger, 1980.

Logue, J.N. Long-term effects of a major natural disaster: The Hurricane Agnes flood in the Wyoming Valley of Pennsylvania, June 1972. Ph.D. dissertation. Division of Epidemiology, Columbia University School of Public Health, 1978.

Lorraine, N.S.R. Canvey Island flood disaster, February, 1953. Medical Officer, 1954, *91*, 59–62.

Melick, M.E. Social, psychological and medical aspects of stress-related illness in the recovery period of a natural disaster. Ph.D. dissertation. State University of New York at Albany, 1976.

Melick, M.E. Life change and illness behavior of males in the recovery period of a natural disaster. Journal of Health and Social Behavior, 1978, *19*, 335–342.

Metropolitan Life Insurance Company. Catastrophic accidents—A 35 year review. Statistical Bulletin, March 1977, *58*, 2–4.

Moore, H.E., Friedsam, H.J. Reported emotional distress following a disaster. Social Forces, 1959, *38*, 135–139.

Murphy, S.A. Advanced practice implications of disaster stress research. Journal of Psychosocial Nursing and Mental Health Services, 1984, *22*.

Mussari, A.J. Appointment with Disaster: The Swelling of the Flood. Wilkes-Barre, Penn.: Northeast Publishers, 1974.

Nailor, M.G., Tarlton, F., Cassidy, J.J. Love Canal: Public health time bomb—A special report to the Governor and Legislature. Albany: New York State Department of Health, September 1978.

Newman, C.J. Children of disaster: Clinical observations at Buffalo Creek. American Journal of Psychiatry, 1976, *133*, 306–412.

1970 Census of population and housing: Census tracts. Wilkes-Barre and Hazelton, Pennsylvania. Department of Commerce, Bureau of Census, 1972.

Nuckolls, C., Cassel, J., Kaplan, B. Psychosocial assets, life crises and the prognosis of pregnancy. American Journal of Epidemiology, 1972, *95*, 431–441.

Ollendick, G., Hoffman, M. Assessment of psychological reactions in disaster victims. Journal of Community Psychology, 1982, *10*, 157–167.

Paigen, B., Holden, C. Love Canal residents under stress: Psychological effects may be greater than physical harm. Science, 1980, *208*, 1242–1244.

Parker, G. Cyclone Tracy and Darwin evacuees: On the restoration of the species. British Journal of Psychiatry, 1977, *130*, 548–555.

Patrick, V., Patrick, W.K. Cyclone '78 in Sri Lanka—The mental health trail. British Journal of Psychiatry, 1981, *138*, 210–216.

Penick, E.C., Powell, B.J., Sieck, W.A. Mental health problems and natural disaster: Tornado victims. Journal of Community Psychology, 1976, *4*, 64–67.

Popovic, J., Petrovic, D. After the earthquake. Lancet, 1964, *2*, 1169.

Price, J. Some age-related effects of the 1977 Brisbane floods. Australia New Zealand Journal of Psychiatry, 1978, *12*, 55–58.

Romanelli, C.J., Griffith, W.M. The Wrath of Agnes. Wilkes-Barre, Penn.: Media Affiliates, 1972.

Schrenk, H.H., Heimann, H., Clayton, G.D., Gafafer, W.M. Air pollution in Denora, Pennsylvania. Public Health Bulletin, No. 306, 1949.

Shippee, G.E., Bradford, R., Gregory, W.L. Community perceptions of natural disasters and post-disaster mental health services. Journal of Community Psychology, 1982, *10*, 23–28.

Smith, D.I., Handmer, J.W., Martin, W.C. The effects of floods on health: Hospital admissions for Lismore. Canberra, Australia, Center for Resource and Environmental Studies, 1980.

Spitzer, R.L., Endicott, J., Mesnikoff, A.M., Cohen, M.S. The Psychiatric Evaluation Form. New York: Biometrics Research, 1968.

Takuma, T. Human behavior in the event of earthquakes. In E.L. Quarantelli (Ed.) Disaster: Theory and Research. Beverly Hills, Calif.: Sage Publications, 1978, 159–172.

Taylor, A. J. W., Frazer, A. G. The stress of post-disaster body handling and victim identification work. Journal of Human Stress, 1982, 8, 4–12.

Taylor, V. Good news about disaster. Psychology Today, 1977, 93, 94, 124, 126.

Titchener, J.L., Kapp, F.T. Disaster at Buffalo Creek: Family and character change at Buffalo Creek. American Journal of Psychiatry, 1976, 133, 295–299.

Weissman, M.M., Klerman, G.L. Sex differences and the epidemiology of depression. Archives of Genral Psychiatry, 1977, 34, 98–111.

Wert, B.J. Stress due to nuclear accident: A survey of an employee population. Occupational Health Nursing, 1979, 27, 16–24.

Wilson, R.N. Disaster and mental health. In G.W. Baker, D.W. Chapman (Eds.), Man and Society in Disaster. New York: Basic Books, 1962.

Wyoming Valley flood control, Susquehanna River, Pennsylvania. Baltimore, Md.: Department of the Army, Corps of Engineers (Baltimore District), 1972.

Zung, W.W.K. A self-rating depression scale. Archives of General Psychiatry, 1965, 12, 63–70.

Health Care Providers as Disaster Victims

Jerri Laube

Health care providers, by virtue of their training and occupation, are looked upon by the community as having responsible roles in disaster. They are perceived by laity and medical personnel alike as the most competent group to deal with crises. Although subject to the same emotional trauma as the general population, health care providers must continue to function in their roles yet maintain psychological stability (Fig. 9.1).

Considering the community expectations of the health care provider, what happens to the provider's family responsibility? Should the health care provider assume the community role over the family role? If the health care workers do not first determine their families' safety, would not this added stress result in increased psychological reactions? To answer these questions, a research study was conducted by the author. This chapter briefly reports how the study was conducted and reports pertinent findings.

ROLE CONFLICTS

Event
The event was a tornado that swept through Xenia, Ohio, a midwestern town in the United States, leaving a path of destruction one fourth mile wide by 15 miles long. Winds had been clocked up to 212 miles per hour (Figs. 9.2, 9.3, 9.4).

Thirty-four people were left dead. Seven hundred and eighty-five people were sent to hospitals for treatment, with 155 admitted. Total number of homes damaged was 2757, with 41 percent destroyed, 25 percent having major damage, and 31 percent having minor damage. One hundred fifty businesses were destroyed and 200 businesses re-

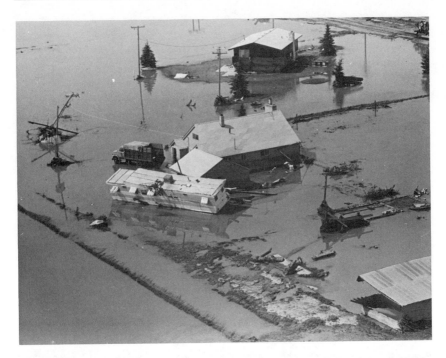

Figure 9.1. Teton dam disaster, June 1976. *(Photo courtesy of the American Red Cross)*

ceived some sort of damage. Nine schools were severely damaged, and one college was 80 percent destroyed. Three thousand families suffered some type of loss (American Red Cross, 1974).

Purposes of the Study
The purposes of this study were: (1) to determine the response of the health care provider to family/community role conflict in disaster; (2) to validate the need for outside agencies, such as American Red Cross, to provide immediate emergency action for service to disaster victims and providers; and (3) to determine the long-term effects of disaster in the health care provider.

Hypotheses
The following hypotheses were tested:

H_1: During time of disaster, an equal number of health care providers choose their family roles as do those who choose their community roles.

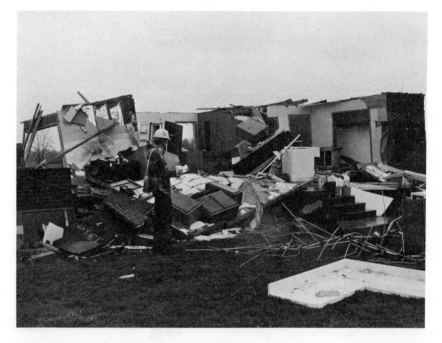

Figure 9.2. Decatur County, Indiana. Damage caused by April 3, 1974 tornadoes. *(Photo by Max Galloway courtesy of the American Red Cross)*

H_2: During time of disaster, the psychological stress level is proportionally the same in health care providers who choose the family role and in those who choose the community role.

Definition of Terms

For the purpose of this study, the following definitions were used:

TIME OF DISASTER: refers to the data-collecting period of this study which was from 1 to 12 days after the tornado.

PSYCHOLOGICAL STRESS: as evaluated with the Psychiatric Status Schedule (PSS), is determined by the summary symptom and role impairment scores. The higher the score, the greater is the level of stress.

HEALTH CARE PROVIDER: an individual who, in his or her occupational role, provides direct or indirect health care services.

REGISTERED NURSE (RN): a person who holds a valid license to practice the profession of nursing.

FAMILY/COMMUNITY ROLE CONFLICT: refers to the forced choice that must be made by individual family members who have well-de-

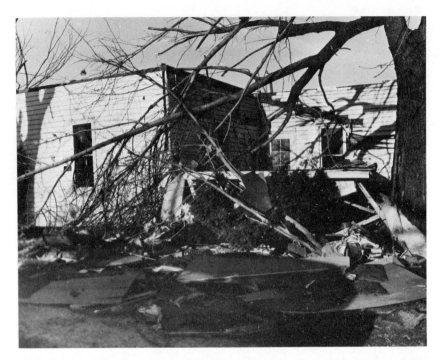

Figure 9.3.   Grant City, Indiana. Destruction caused by April 3, 1974 tornadoes. *(Photo by Florine Rogers courtesy of the American Red Cross)*

fined and important disaster roles in the community, such as health care work.

Limitations
One limitation of the study concerned sample selection. Since the disaster was not predictable for either time or place, the subjects could not be obtained before the disaster occurred. Therefore, conclusions were drawn without the benefit of comparison to preimpact data. A convenience sample of all of the health care providers the researcher could locate and interview in a 12-day period was used.

Another study limitation regards perception of past events. However, the difficult problem of recall for victims was diminished in this study because details of the disaster were not the data needed to fulfill the study purposes. The researcher did not experience difficulty in establishing rapport with the workers, even though they may have been victims themselves.

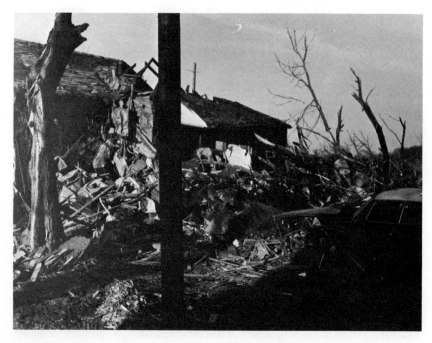

Figure 9.4.   Grant City, Indiana. Destruction caused by April 3, 1974 tornadoes. *(Photo by Florine Rogers courtesy of the American Red Cross)*

BACKGROUND

Effect of Disaster on the Provider

Medical personnel are expected to maintain composure in any type of stress situation although they may be exposed to suffering, pain, and death. According to Coombs and Goldman (1973), they develop "detached concern," which is the ability to care for the critically ill, yet maintain an acceptable emotional detachment.

Not all reports about disaster relief workers are positive. Lifton (1965) found, in his study of the survivors of Hiroshima, many strong negative feelings in the relief provider, such as fear, anger, hatred, and resentment. These feelings resulted in disruption of team functioning, thus hindering the necessary relief work.

Rayner (1958) found that nurses continued to function effectively in disaster, even though they experienced strong emotional responses. She identified two types of role conflict, nurse–mother and nurse–doctor, as responsible for the emotional difficulties experienced by the nurse.

In Laube's (1973) study of the Hurricane Celia disaster, the majority of the nurses coped with their anxiety without impairment of the professional role. However, there were nurses who left work or did not report for duty during the disaster period. Major stresses identified by the nurses were excessive physical demands, concern for own or patient's safety, inadequate supplies, seeing the poor suffer, hurt children, the disorganization, and concern for own family's welfare.

Shader and Schwartz (1966) believe professional people, such as doctors and nurses, begin to function in a disaster sooner than the untrained. However, they agreed that family roles are intensified in the inventory phase of disaster, with family loyalty a strong force in human behavior. This is also borne out in Feld's (1973) reflections on the Agnes flood. In his words, he was a "flood victim who happens to be a social worker" (p. 46). Apparently Feld directed all of his energy to his family role as he made no remarks about assuming any type of community role.

Although Hill and Hansen (1962) have a theoretical framework for viewing families in crisis, this has not been applied to crisis in disaster. There is much work yet to be done before it is known how disaster affects families and how families and individual family members react in disaster. A suggested proposition for study, as identified by Hill and Hansen, is: "Individual family members who have well-defined disaster roles in the community will experience role conflict between family roles and community roles" (p. 211).

Kin relations are very important in disaster. It is believed that if individuals have any doubt concerning their family's safety, they will choose the family role instead of the community role. Furthermore, even if the individual's family is safe, choosing in favor of the community role may endanger the family's adjustive capacity (Hill and Hansen, 1962).

In summary, this brief review of literature suggests that although medical and nursing personnel may be expected to function effectively in a period of disaster, this cannot be assured. Individuals differ in their reactions, depending more on type and duration of stress than on education, experience, or predisaster personality. Typical reactions to disaster include shock and disbelief, apathy, sleep disturbances, irritability, somatic distress, and overdependency. Long-term psychological effects have not been substantially documented.

Family roles are important, particularly during times of crisis such as in disaster. Health care workers, who are also from the disaster area, have an exceptional amount of stress, for they must not only work through their own reactions to the disaster, they must resolve the family/community role conflict.

METHOD

The Research Design

A mixed design was used incorporating a survey approach and an ex post facto quasi-experimental approach. Ex post facto research is defined as: "research in which the independent variable or variables have already occurred and in which the researcher starts with the observation of a dependent variable or variables. The investigator then studies the independent variables in retrospect for their possible relations to, and effects on, the dependent variable or variables" (Kerlinger, 1967, p. 306).

Determination of the health care provider's family/community role conflict and subsequent resolution was obtained in a survey. These data were then incorporated into a three-group, quasi-experimental design. The explanatory variables were the independent variable, family/community role conflict, and the dependent variable, psychological stress. (See Figure 9.5.)

Research Tool

After careful deliberation, the Psychiatric Status Schedule (PSS) was chosen as the research tool for this study. The PSS is a standardized interview schedule to evaluate a subject's social functioning, role functioning, and mental status. Two levels of scores are obtained. The first level consists of 17 symptom and 6 role scales. The second level summarizes the first level scales into four symptom scales and one role scale (Spitzer et al., 1970). (See Table 9.1.)

The second-level scales—subjective distress, behavioral disturbance, impulse control disturbance, reality testing disturbance, and summary role—were used in the analysis of data. In addition, a total score was computed.

Validity and reliability studies of the PSS indicate acceptable coefficient levels. The internal consistencies of the four summary scales range from 0.80 to 0.89. Interjudge reliability coefficients range from 0.90 to 0.98 for the four summary symptom scales and 0.94 for the summary role scale.

Validity studies were based on: (1) correlations between the PSS scales and similar items from other instruments, (2) data from population expected to differ on various dimensions, and (3) demonstration of expected changes in psychopathology in the same subjects at different points in time. The findings of these studies support the use of the PSS in research (Spitzer, et al., 1970).

Demographic information, obtained at the beginning of each interview, included: gender, marital status, education, occupation, religious

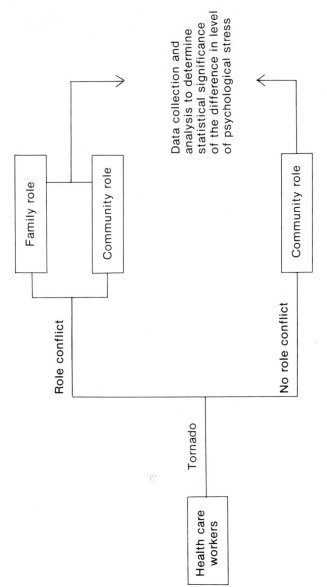

Figure 9.5. The Research Design Employed to Compare Health Care Workers.

**TABLE 9.1. BASIC SCORING SYSTEM OF THE PSYCHIATRIC STATUS
SCHEDULE**

	First Level	Second Level (Summary Symptom and Role Scales)
Symptom scales	Depression–anxiety Daily routine–leisure time impairment Social isolation Suicide–self-mutilation Somatic concern	Subjective distress
	Speech disorganization Inappropriate affect, appearance, behavior Agitation–excitement Interview belligerence–negativism Disorientation–memory Retardation–lack of emotion	Behavioral disturbance
	Antisocial impulses or acts Drug abuse Reported over anger	Impulse control disturbance
	Grandiosity Suspicion–persecution–hallucinations Alcohol abuse	Reality testing disturbance
Role scales	Denial of illness Wage earner role Housekeeper role Student or trainee role Main role Parent role	Summary role

(From Spitzer, R.L., et al. The Psychiatric Status Schedule. Archives of General Psychiatry, July 1970, 23, p. 45. Courtesy of the American Medical Association.)

preference, race, and the head of the household's occupation and education. Such information was used in checking the adequacy of samples.

Additional questions were asked about: (1) family characteristics, for example, family constellation, family responsibility, health of family members; (2) subjects' behavior in the disaster, for example, where subjects were at impact, when subjects determined the welfare of their family and condition of their home, when subjects first reported for duty or began rescue operations, number of continuous hours worked without rest; and (3) subjects' attitude toward their experience with disaster, for example, was their loss greater than those of their neighbors, how they saw their community role, major stress experienced, and how they coped with their stress.

As in Laube's (1973) interview schedule, the interviews were closed with the question, "What is the funniest thing that has happened during this disaster?" in order to lessen any anxiety that may have been aroused in the course of the interview.

Subjects

The sample was comprised of 101 health care providers, 49 RN, and 52 others—MDs, aids, orderlies, and x-ray and laboratory technicians. The disaster-struck community was in the midwestern part of the United States and had a population of 22,700.

The subjects selected themselves into groups by virtue of their family/community role conflict. Health care workers from the disaster area, but without family responsibility and thus no role conflict, served as controls.

Collection of Data

The researcher was on site within 24 hours of the disaster and remained 11 consecutive days, eight to ten hours each, conducting personal interviews on all available, consenting health care providers and Red Cross workers. Providers from each duty shift were contacted as the researcher arranged her hours to coincide with the various schedules. Subjects were assured anonymity and confidentially.

A letter of introduction was first secured from the American Red Cross chapter disaster headquarters. This letter served as a pass into the disaster area and insured cooperation in the Red Cross centers and shelters. To interview subjects in the community hospital, permission was obtained from the administrator and director of nursing service. Permission was granted from the medical director and director of nursing service in the County Health Department to interview their staff. In addition, the researcher received permission to interview from each worker who participated in the study.

ANALYSIS AND INTERPRETATION OF DATA

Test of the Hypotheses

H_1: During time of disaster, an equal number of health care providers choose their family roles first as do those who choose their community roles first.

TABLE 9.2. HEALTH CARE WORKERS BY CHOICE OF ROLE AND FAMILY RESPONSIBILITY[a]

Family Responsibility	Family Role	Community Role
No	3 (3%)	14 (14%)
Yes	52 (53%)	27 (30%)

[a]χ^2 = 10.54640; degrees of freedom (DF) = 1; p = 0.0012.

The hypothesis was rejected at the 0.05 level of significance (see Table 9.2). Of the total health care providers, 3 percent of the providers lived alone and chose to stay home, 14 percent of the providers lived alone and chose the community role, 53 percent of the providers had family responsibilities and chose the family role, and 30 percent of the providers had family responsibilities but chose the community role. Altogether, 56 percent of the providers chose the family role and 45 percent of the providers chose the community role.

Regrouping the sample population data by gender, analysis of the female health care providers revealed that 4 percent lived alone and chose to stay home, 15 percent lived alone and chose the community role, 50 percent had family responsibilities and chose the family role, and 26 percent had family responsibilities but chose the community role. For the total group, 59 percent chose the family role and 41 percent chose the community role. (See Table 9.3.)

Of the male health care workers, none who lived alone chose to stay home, 12 percent who lived alone chose the community role, 41 percent had family responsibilities and chose the family role, 47 percent had family responsibilities but chose the community role. Inferential statistics were not run because of the small numbers of subjects per "cell." (See Table 9.4.)

H₂: During time of disaster, there is no difference in level of psychological stress among health care providers with family/community role conflict according to whether they choose the family or community role first.

TABLE 9.3. FEMALE HEALTH CARE WORKERS BY CHOICE OF ROLE AND FAMILY RESPONSIBILITY

Family Responsibility	Family Role	Community Role
No	3 (4%)	12 (15%)
Yes	45 (55%)	21 (26%)

TABLE 9.4. MALE HEALTH CARE WORKERS BY CHOICE OF ROLE AND FAMILY RESPONSIBILITY

Family Responsibility	Family Role	Community Role
No	0	2 (12%)
Yes	7 (41%)	8 (47%)

The hypothesis was rejected at the 0.05 level of significance for subjective distress. The mean "subjective distress" scores on the PSS of health care providers with family/community role conflict were higher for those who chose the community role than for those who chose the family role first. However, all of the groups had lower mean scores than the standardized mean scores, indicating that there were no extreme responses. (See Table 9.5.)

Comparison of Characteristics of Subject Groups

The groups were compared by age, gender, education, continuous hours worked without rest, and damage incurred in the disaster.

- Group I—Health care providers with family/community role conflict, chose family role.
- Group II—Health care providers with family/community role conflict, chose community role.

TABLE 9.5. MEAN SCORES OF THE PSYCHIATRIC STATUS SCHEDULE SUMMARY SCALES FOR HEALTH CARE WORKERS FROM THE DISASTER AREA

Summary Scale	Groups			Standard Score
	Role Conflicts		No Conflict	
	Family Role	Community Role		
Subjective distress	32.39	34.25	33.35	35.74
Behavioral disturbance	41.21	41.59	41.24	42.11
Impulse control disturbance	45.00	45.00	45.00	45.56
Reality testing disturbance	44.04	44.06	44.00	44.47
Summary role impairment	41.38	41.31	40.53	42.11
Total	31.13	32.03	31.52	Not available

• Group III—Health care providers without role conflict (live alone).

Groups I, II, and III (see Table 9.6) were similar in average of subjects and number of years in school, although groups I and II had subjects who did not finish high school. The average number of continuous hours worked without rest was about the same for groups II and III, 15.59 hours and 14.25 hours, respectively; but the average number of continuous hours worked for group I was 9.79. The maximum number of continuous hours worked by anyone in group I and group II was 36, and the maximum number of continuous hours worked in group III was 49. Group I had 13.5 percent men, group II had 28.1 percent men, and group III had 11.8 percent men. Twenty-five percent of group I had tornado damage, 56 percent of group II had tornado damage, and 47 percent of group III had tornado damage. The major differences in the groups was by design; subjects in group I and II had family responsibility and subjects in group III lived alone.

TABLE 9.6. COMPARISON OF CHARACTERISTICS OF HEALTH CARE WORKERS IN THE EXPERIMENTAL AND CONTROL GROUPS

	Experimental		Control
	Role Conflict		
	Family Role (1)	Community Role (2)	No Role Conflict (3)
Characteristics	(N = 52)	(N = 32)	(N = 17)
Age			
Mean	39.13 years	36.59 years	36.94 years
Range	18–61	19–65	20–63
Education			
Mean	14.69 years	15.41 years	14.65 years
Range	9–22	9–23	12–20
Continuous hours worked			
Mean	9.79 hours	15.59 hours	14.25 hours
Range	0–36	4–36	0–49
Sex			
Men	7 (13.5%)	9 (28.19%)	2 (11.8%)
Women	45 (86.5%)	23 (71.90%)	15 (88.2%)
Damage incurred			
Yes	13 (25%)	18 (56%)	8 (47%)
No	39 (75%)	14 (44%)	9 (53%)

Discussion

As in previous disaster field studies, interpretations must be made cautiously.

H_1:   During time of disaster an equal number of health care providers choose their family roles as do those who choose their community roles first.

The hypothesis was rejected. More health care workers chose their family roles over their community roles. This finding supports the assumptions of Hill and Hansen (1962) that if the provider has any doubt concerning his or her family's welfare, the health care provider will choose the family role and neglect the community role. The study results also support observations made by Fogelman and Parenton (1959) that disaster victim's behavior is primarily family oriented. Studies by Lynch (1970), Moore and Friedsam (1959), and Drabek (1970), in which the importance of family relationships were identified, were clearly supported also.

Considering the American culture today, one might expect that the majority of female health care providers would choose the family role over the community role, whereas the male health care provider would choose the community role. Men probably feel greater internal and external pressure to assume community roles and women may feel the pressure to stay with families at home because of the gender division of labor in households which was prevalent when data were collected. With the trend toward women's rights and responsibilities, one's sexual identity is expected to have less influence on role choice in the future.

H_2:   During time of disaster, there is no difference in level of psychological stress among health care providers with family/community role conflict according to whether they chose the family or community role first.

The hypothesis was rejected for subjective distress. As the summary subjective distress scale includes the following symptom scales—depression, anxiety, and somatic concern—it was not surprising to find some elevation. Tyhurst (1957), Howard (1971), McHugh (1972), and Whalen (1972) all identified depression, anxiety, and somatic concern as psychological reactions that occur in disaster.

It was not unexpected that health care providers who chose the community role would manifest the most psychological stress, but it was unexpected that the health care providers who chose the family role would manifest the least psychological stress, with control groups ranked in between. This finding suggests that all providers would have a lower level of psychological stress if they could first ascertain the well-being of their families and/or the condition of their personal and real property.

In interpreting the results, one must also consider the possible impact of such extraneous variables as family constellation and continuous hours worked without rest. The control group was made up of health care workers who lived alone as compared with the experimental groups who lived in some type of family relationship.

In reviewing the continuous hours worked without rest, there appears to be a relationship with the level of psychological stress. The experimental group that chose the family role first had a variance of none to 36 continuous hours worked with an average of 9.79 h, the control group had a variance of none to 49 h with an average of 14.25 h, and the experimental group that chose the community role first had a variance of 4 to 36 h and an average of 15.59 straight hours of work.

It is fairly well documented that psychological reaction to disaster occurs in sequential phases, without well-defined beginnings and endings, and that these phases may differ in length according to the individual. Therefore, individuals may have been in different phases of the reaction process when interviewed, even though the data collection was completed in a short 12-day period. The research would have been strengthened if all subjects could have been interviewed at the same point in their reaction process.

The researcher was aware of distinct changes in the emotional climate of the disaster-struck community. Shock and disbelief were prevalent when the researcher arrived 24 h postdisaster, and this continued for a period approaching 7 days. There was a profound quiet in the shelters, hospitals, and throughout the disaster-struck community.

As the shock began to dissipate, there were open expressions of emotions, generally sadness with crying, and thankfulness for life of self, family, and friends. In the last few days of the study, physical tiredness was evident, people became impatient, and anger was expressed in various ways.

Rescue agencies took their share as scapegoat, as described by Whalen (1972) and Drabek and Quarantelli (1967), although the most obvious target of anger was insurance companies. As illustration, when providers were asked what had affected them the most, in the first week the responses generally dealt with the destruction. In the last interviews, the respondents often angrily lashed out at the inconveniences "caused" by insurance agencies.

The researcher was well received wherever she went. Individuals openly responded in the interview and were most generous with their time. Only two individuals refused to be interviewed. One subject, 2 hours after the interview, requested that he be deleted from the study.

Although the majority of health care workers checked first on their family before reporting for work in the community, it must be noted that generally there was only a short time spent with their family. Those that stayed to comfort their children or just be with family for a while admitted to guilt feelings. Providers expressed guilt because their home or families were safe, with destruction all around them.

There was a spirit of community altruisim with a high value on disaster relief work of any kind. People came from far and near, saying they had to do "something." Nurses reported for duty who had not worked for years. Hospitals were generously staffed, and could have well afforded for the providers with family responsibilities to stay at home for a while. In fact, personnel were encouraged to see about their family. When subjects recounted this to the interviewer, they appeared grateful for the hospital management's concern, but nevertheless felt a strong need to stay on duty.

TWO YEARS POSTDISASTER

In 1976, the same subjects were contacted by mail with the request to complete the PSS adapted for self-administration. Letters and 101 PSS questionnaires were sent out. Of those, 42 were returned "nondeliverable," 30 subjects returned their completed questionnaires, and the remaining 54 subjects did not respond. Of the 30 returns, 19 were from group I—had family responsibility and chose the family role first; 6 were from group II—had family responsibility and chose the community work first; 5 were from group III—lived alone. For analysis of the longitudinal data, the responses of the population returning the questionnaire in 1976 were compared with that same population's responses in 1974.

Three hypotheses were formulated for testing. Data were analyzed by the t test for related measures.

H_1: There is no significant differences in psychological functioning during disaster and 2 years postdisaster in health care providers with role conflict who choose the family role over the community role.

Rejected at the 0.01 level of significance for subjective distress. There were no significant differences in the remainder of the scales.

Symptoms of subjective distress increased over the 2-year period.

H₂: During the time of disaster and 2 years postdisaster there is no significant difference in psychological functioning in health care providers with role conflict who choose the community role over the family role.

Rejected at the 0.01 level of significance for subjective distress. There were no significant differences in the remainder of the scales.

H₃: There is no significant difference in psychological functioning during disaster and 2 years postdisaster in health care providers who had no family responsibilities.

Rejected at the 0.2 level of significance for subjective distress. There were no significant differences in the remainder of the scales. Symptoms of subjective distress increased over the 2-year period postdisaster for health care providers who had no family responsibilities.

Group responses by role choice were not analyzed because of the very small number.

CONCLUSIONS

The following conclusions were made on the basis of the findings in this study:

1. During time of disaster, a significantly greater number of health care providers with family/community role conflict chose the family role over the community role. Therefore, there is a need for outside assistance until the local health care providers can put their homes in order.

2. During time of disaster, health care providers who resolved their family/community role conflict by choosing the family role had significantly less psychological stress, as evaluated on the "subjective distress" scale of the PSS, than did health care providers who resolved their family/community role conflict by choosing the community role.

3. Health care providers manifest more subjective distress, which is yet still within normal range, 2 years postdisaster than they do during the disaster period.

4. Health care providers, in a disaster-struck community, maintain normal psychological functioning.

Caution must be taken in generalizing the findings of this study. As in all longitudinal research requiring data from the same individual at more than one point in time, limitations were posed. An important limitation was that of distinguishing between effect of maturation and effect that resulted from historical events or the time of year at which measurements were taken. The major limitation, however, was that of sample diminishment.

ACKNOWLEDGMENTS

This research was partially funded by the American National Red Cross.

REFERENCES

American Red Cross. Survey Statistics. Dayton, Ohio, April 5, 1974 (typewritten).

Coombs, R.H., Goldman, L.J. Maintenance and discontinuity of coping mechanisms in an intensive care unit. Social Problems, 1973, 20, 342-355.

Drabek, T.E. Methodology of studying disasters: Past patterns and future possibilities. American Behavioral Scientist, 1970, 13, 331-343.

Drabek, T.E., Quarantelli, E. Scapegoats, villains, and disasters. Trans-action, 1964, 4, 12-17.

Drabek, T.E., Stephenson, J.S. III. When disaster strikes. Journal of Applied Social Psychology, 1971, 1, 187-203.

Feld, A. Reflections on the Agnes flood. Social Work, 1973, 18, 46-51.

Fogelman, C.W., Parenton, V. Individual and group behavior in critical situations. Social Forces, 1959, 38, 129-135.

Hill, R., Hansen, D. Families in disaster. In G.W. Baker, D.W. Chapman (Eds.), Man and Society in Disaster. New York: Basic Books, 1962.

Howard, S.J. Treatment of children's reactions to the 1971 earthquake. Paper presented to the American Association of Psychiatric Services, Beverly Hills, Calif., 1971.

Kerlinger, F.N. Foundations of Behavioral Research. New York: Holt, Rinehart & Winston, 1967.

Laube, J. Psychological reactions in disaster. Nursing Research, 1973, 22, 343-347.

Lifton, R.J. Psychological effects of the atomic bomb in Hiroshima. In R. Fulton (Ed.), Death and Identity. New York: Wiley 1965.

Lifton, R.J. Death in Life—Survivors of Hiroshima. New York: Random House, 1967.

Lynch, D. Tornado, Texas Demon in the Wind. Waco, Tex.: Texian Press, 1970.

McHugh, R. Observations related to hurricane Camille. Paper presented at the Office of Emergency Preparedness Conference on the Psychological Effects of Disaster. Washington, D.C., October 26, 1972.

Moore, H.E., Friedsam, H.J. Reported emotional stress following a disaster. Social Forces, 1959, 38, 135-139.

Rayner, J. How do nurses behave in disaster? Nursing Outlook, 1958, 6, 572.

Shader, R., Schwartz, A.J. Management of reactions to disaster. Social Work, 1966, 11, 99-104.

Spitzer, R.L., Endicott, J., Fleiss, J., Cohen, J. The Psychiatric Status Schedule. Archives of General Psychiatry, 1970, 23, 41-51.

Tyhurst, J.S. Individual reactions to community disaster. American Journal of Psychiatry, 1957, 107, 764-769.

Whalen, E.M. Observations of the June 1972 flood in the Wyoming Valley area of Pennsylvania. Paper presented at the Office of Emergency Preparedness Conference on the Psychological Effects of Disaster, Washington, D.C., October 26, 1972.

PART THREE

The Interface Between Victims, Health Professionals, and Community Systems

10

The Planning and Administration of a Mental Health Response to Disaster

Frederick L. Ahearn, Jr.

This chapter addresses the issue and problems of planning and implementing a human service program in response to an unanticipated situation, such as a community disaster. Although the administrative elements and principles which guide a response are equally applicable to expected as well as unexpected events, there are several notable differences. Disastrous occurrences cause individual and collective trauma resulting in crisis. There is an urgency to act in an environment that may be unfamiliar or unknown as the system of relief care varies from the usual context of human services. Time limitations impose pressures upon the administrator to fully understand the nature of the problem and to consider appropriate alternatives for action.

The response process encompasses two phases, design and implementation, which require that the administrator possess sociopolitical and analytical skills (Bolan, 1974). These abilities, although interrelated and complementary, contribute dimensions that are unique and necessary to the problem-solving endeavor.

First, the administrator must demonstrate a range of sociopolitical skills in order to gain participation and acceptance by others. The principal assumption to this dimension is that problem-solving tasks take place within a specific social and political context, compelling the administrator to be proficient in inter- and intrasystem relationships and exchanges. Thus, this phase fosters participation, seeks sanction and support, marshalls resources, and facilitates decision-making.

Second, the design and implementation of a response strategy emphasizes analytical elements, such as thinking, imagining, reasoning, and deliberating. For the administrator, these skills are employed in gathering and analyzing data, assessing need, identifying and weighing alternatives, setting priorities, and planning the detailed design of a program.

This chapter reviews the elements in the design and implementation of a response to an unanticipated occurrence, using the 1978 Massachusetts Blizzard as a case example. During both phases of design and implementation, sociopolitical and analytical roles are discussed for a range of response activities which include sanction and support, assessment of need, resource development, program design, program implementation, and intersystem strategies. Finally, the author presents some implications of this case study for administrative practice and theory which are relevant for all types of social programs.

CASE BACKGROUND

The most severe blizzard in 109 years struck eastern Massachusetts Monday and Tuesday, February 6 and 7, 1978. Before the storm ended, it had dumped 27 inches, a record for the most snow in any one storm. The blizzard raged for almost 33 hours as winds roared to 90 miles per hour—hurricane force. High tides reached 15 feet above the mean low water level. The combination of the violent winds coming from the northeast (off the ocean), high tides, and a full moon produced serious flooding along the coast. The disaster caused tremendous personal and community loss.

Eighty-four persons died and over 4400 were injured as a direct result of the storm. Two thousand one hundred and thirty-three homes were destroyed and another 9360 damaged. More than 30,000 inhabitants were evacuated to nearby schools, churches, and shelters. Some 10 miles from the coast along Boston's circumferential highway (Route 128), 3000 motorists were trapped in their cars, some for as long as 36 hours. Financially, the cost of the storm exceeded 463 million dollars.

From the beginning, a representative of the Massachusetts Department of Mental Health (DMH) was assigned first to the Governor's Disaster Control Center and, once the storm became a Presidentially declared disaster, with the relief efforts of the federal government. As the initial concern of DMH was the emergency needs of its inpatient and outpatient populations, area directors went into action to meet these emergencies which were usually emotional crises brought about by the lack of medication, and by fear of the storm and its consequences.

A major administrative problem from the beginning was the staffing of ongoing and new service programs. Department of Mental Health employees and volunteers were organized into relief teams to staff existing mental health programs and provide crisis counseling services to aid victims and their families at the shelters. Disaster Assistance Centers, and in their own homes. Training and orientation concerning behavioral reactions to disaster and intervention techniques to provide psychological aid were given to volunteers, DMH employees, and other relief workers. Another key activity included a public information program designed to enlighten the community about the emotional feelings that they may be experiencing.

During these first postcatastrophe days, DMH decided to apply for Federal disaster funds to conduct an ongoing crisis counseling program for storm survivors. The proposal was approved March 8, 1978 and $380,000 was granted to implement a program for a 6-month period; another $100,000 was received to extend services for an additional 3 months. When the grant terminated in November 1978, a total of 3824 clients had received crisis counseling services.

ADMINISTRATIVE RESPONSE TO AN UNANTICIPATED EVENT

When confronted with a crisis situation, the administrator must decide whether or not to act and, if action is required, what the most appropriate strategy would be given the situation. The administrator may be perplexed and unsure how to respond in the face of chaos and uncertainty. To arrive at a decision, an administrator ascertains the needs created by the event and assesses the nature of the crisis, calculating how his or her organization will fit within the total context of the response system.

Through a thorough and clear understanding of the implications of what has happened, the administrator must assume responsibility for making the call to action, mobilizing required resources, and initiating a program of services to assist those impacted by the crisis. To do this, the administrator must recognize how the event affects people, what services they may need, how best to deliver that service, and ways in which to coordinate one's actions with others in the response system.

Administrative decision-making in an environment of crisis requires patience, knowledge, and flexibility. Accurate data about what has occurred and who is affected are essential, but these data are generally lacking, inadequate, or difficult to collect. In the aftermath of an unanticipated event, the administrator must work long hours to decide what to do and how to do it. The administrator's actions will vary depending upon the crisis, the community, and the agency and its resources. The following guide has been devised to assist the social service administrator in his/her efforts. Specifically, this guide considers the requirements for:

1. Sanction and support
2. Assessment of need
3. Resource development
4. Program design
5. Program implementation
6. Intersystem strategies

As these steps in taking administrative action are interrelated and often overlapping, the administrator may work on several elements at the same time.

Sanction and Support

Before proceeding very far, the administrator will need legitimation and sanction for action. In some instances, administrators may possess authority to act by virtue of position or legal status, but in other instances, they may have to seek approval of a superior or a board of directors. Lack of early legitimation may lead to misunderstanding, conflict, or competition, thus reducing the chances for success.

> The idea of a mental health response to the blizzard arose from a number of sources, all independent of the other. The Commissioner assigned a deputy to serve on the Governor's Disaster Control Center where emergency needs of mental health programs and agencies were coordinated. This deputy lived closest and could walk to the Control Center, a definite advantage since no automobile travel was permitted for 8 days. In addition, the directors of several catchment areas immediately responded by providing service to shelters, hotels, and Disaster Assistance Centers. From the first days of the storm, the Commissioner of Mental Health had approved Departmental action and those involved received approval from others in the relief system.*

The administrator may take several immediate steps to secure sanction. First, the administrator's superior or Board President should be contacted by telephone and briefed as to the current assessment of need

---

*Case material has been drawn from several sources. These include: (1) the author's personal experience working during the Massachusetts Blizzard; (2) interviews with mental health professionals who staffed Project Concern, the crisis counseling program for disaster victims; and (3) the final report of Project Concern, Project Concern: Crisis Counseling After The Blizzard Of '78. (Boston: Massachusetts Department of Mental Health and Research for Social Change, 1979.)

and the potential for organizational action. Of course, this assumes that the telephone system is operational. Any informal contact should be followed-up with meetings to clarify issues of responsibility and sanction. All lines of authority and delineation of activities must be clear to all. Finally, approval to act should be put into writing to avoid confusion or conflict later.

To strengthen the organization's legitimacy to act, there is a need to develop informal and formal systems of support in the shortest possible time span. The activities of human service agencies in response to an unanticipated event usually cannot operate in a vacuum, but must be interrelated with a variety of services that spring up after the event. How does the administrator collaborate with these other programs and how does the agency gain access to an arena of relief care? And, who has the responsibility and perhaps the authority to direct and coordinate relief services.?

A human service response may require the approval and support of authorities. For example, Civil Defense is in charge of all who respond to a local emergency. In seeking the support of relevant community agencies, the administrator attempts to gain cooperation, formally and informally, for anticipated activities. It is hoped that these administrative initiatives result in interagency agreements for cooperation and mutual support.

One of the mental health workers who volunteered was a psychiatrist, a person with previous experience with disaster victims. As she entered a refugee shelter, she observed representatives of the Red Cross and various governmental agencies discussing procedures and attempting to clarify their roles. The scene was one of confusion. She invited a small group of these relief workers to gather in an adjoining room and took several minutes to explain who she was and what resources she could bring to the shelter. Producing a copy of the Federal regulations on disasters which indicated that crisis counseling is part of the relief effort, she was able to orient the workers to her role which resulted in acceptance and support of the mental health person as a team member.

The psychiatrist continued her work at the shelter for several weeks receiving positive collaboration from the other relief workers. Without their legitimation of her role and their subsequent referrals, the psychiatrist would have been an isolated member of the relief team.

Another way to maintain support and legitimacy for a special response to a crisis is the establishment of a task force to assist in aspects of planning and managing a program. This could be a subcommittee of the existing board of directors or it could be an ad hoc group created solely for this project. In putting together such a group, the administrator should attempt to recruit participants who represent a wide

range of interests and although the group may vary in size, a committee of 10 to 15 members is usually suggested. These participants should
reflect four distinct elements of the community (Burke, 1979):

- *Experts:* These are professionals in human services who have
  knowledge of the client population, service needs, delivery models,
  and program evaluation
- *Power group:* Individuals who, by virtue of their social status or
  position, exert influence on decisions made in the community and
  have access to resources. Examples include politicians, clergy, industry or banking executives, or businesspeople.
- *Sentiment group:* Frequently there are associations which reflect,
  in a broad sense, the values, the norms, and sentiment of a community. Such groups may be the League of Women Voters,
  unions, or other civic or social entities
- *Needs group:* Individuals who know the problem first hand, that
  is, victims, clients.

Such a task force can legitimize and support efforts to determine
need, shape program goals, access financial resources, and interpret services to the community at large.

When the decision was made to fund a crisis intervention program for victims of the storm, the Department of Mental Health set up a Steering Committee composed of 12 members. Included were the Project Director, seven
directors of mental health areas impacted by the blizzard, a representative from the Red Cross and Catholic Charities, and two university profes-
sors, experts in disaster work. Meetings were held monthly, focusing on
program assessment, modification of policies, and interagency collaboration.

Assessment of Need

Before making any decision in response to an unanticipated event, the
administrator should:

- Understand the consequences of the crisis and the various definitions of the problem/need
- Survey groups affected by the aftermath
- Ascertain the availability of community resources to combat the
  effects of the crisis
- Utilize these data to set program goals and service delivery
  strategies

In assessing need created by crisis, the administrator has to be
sensitive to how groups within the community define the problem. As

these definitions depend upon the interaction of norms and values and on culture and tradition, communities delineate problems differently. A case in point is what constitutes mental health since there are many views as to what is health and what is illness. Deviant behavior in one place may be perfectly acceptable in another. Therefore, administrators must be consciously aware of these distinctions when determining need.

Methods for collection of data concerning the impacts of an unanticipated event usually include a combination of primary and secondary sources of information. In the latter instance, one may review the literature concerning reactions to similar hazards, noting their impacts and service solutions. Reports or studies of similar situations may be available through the Health and Welfare Council, local library, or neighboring university. Such information hopefully will detail the types and degree of problems/needs usual in situations like these, how individuals and families manage the aftereffects, and ways that human service agencies may intervene to assist victims. Also, the examination of case records in the agency or neighboring agencies in the first days after an event may enable the administrator to judge the types of resulting problems. Naturally, these information gathering activities require time which may not be available to administrators and their staffs.

Another approach relies more on primary or first-hand data. Selecting a sample of individuals suffering from the crisis and interviewing key informants, such as police, human service workers, local physicians, clergy, or pharmacists are two methods of determining the types of problems people are presenting. These approaches are time consuming and expensive. In addition it is difficult, in the immediate aftermath, to attend to the requirements of random sampling and sound questionnaire construction. On the other hand, data from primary sources almost always have a richness and relevance difficult to obtain from secondary sources.

When Project Concern began, there was concerted effort to determine the types of emotional problems that individuals and families were experiencing and to estimate how widespread these problems were. In the first weeks after the blizzard, mental health professionals completed a brief form on every victim that they had seen in a shelter, motel, school, or Disaster Assistance Center. At the end of each day, the forms were sent into the central office where the information was aggregated. Forms were simple and easily completed. They contained the following information:

- Background data, for example, age, marital status, number in family, address, and so forth
- Presenting symptoms, classified in broad catagories, to focus on problems in functioning, and avoiding psychiatric labeling
- Degree of loss from storm, including death of a loved one, unemployment, financial hardship, and destruction of home and property

- Mental health status prior to storm
- Nature of victim's support system.

Analysis of this information revealed a certain percentage of those seen who were suffering psychological effects of the blizzard. To determine total need, administrators applied this percentage to the overall number of victims.

The major purpose of an assessment of need is to understand the problems that people have so that relevant services may be planned and implemented for them. Once the effects of the event are known, the administrator extrapolates the findings of a needs study to the population in question. This is a difficult task and estimates such as the one used in the above example are quite common. Perhaps the crucial question for the administrator at this point is whether or not there is sufficient need that requires the agency to respond.

For example, the needs assessment cited above documented that mental health volunteers had seen 2189 disaster victims who were presenting a number of signs of distress such as anxiety, depression, passivity, somatic complaints, phobias, and the like. Also within 30 days of the storm, the Department of Mental Health received 733 referrals from other agencies. Thousands of victims were still residing in temporary housing and evidence from other disasters showed that dislocation often led to emotional consequences. Based upon these data, the Department of Mental Health decided to apply for a grant from the National Institute of Mental Health (NIMH) to provide crisis counseling services to disaster victims and their families. Thus a response was decided upon because of the increase in referrals and victims seeking psychological aid.

Resource Development

Resources provide the organizational means for achieving its goals and objectives. The administrator must be acutely aware of the organization's need for and control over resources and, if there are not sufficient internal resources, then a sociopolitical strategy to gain these from the environment will be necessary. In the analysis to develop a strategy for resource development, the social administrator considers the following:

- Type of resource
- Source
- Amount available
- Process for resource distribution
- Short- and long-term cost to the organization for accepting resources (quid pro quo)

- Transferability of resources—can they be used for anything or only for a specific use?
- Control over resources

An activity related to the process of documenting need is a careful inventory of community resources. Gaps in service become apparent by comparing need with available resources. Therefore, the administrator must be knowledgeable about what services are already or may be available for those suffering the consequences of an unanticipated event, and also how to mobilize these resources on behalf of clients. Resources consist of community services such as nutrition programs, food stamps, and temporary housing or health services. In analyzing these resources, the administrator is aware of services offered (health, food, income, shelter, or information) and organizational auspices (voluntary or governmental at the local, regional, state, or Federal level).

During the needs assessment and program design phases, the administrator has calculated program costs and the availability of resources, estimating the amount of additional resources required to mount a new program. Oftentimes some form of fundraising activity may be essential as the administrator plans special events or benefits, puts together a campaign, approaches benefactors, or prepares a formal proposal which seeks assistance from public or private sources. Financing will depend upon the administrator's ability to demonstrate need, rationalize the soundness of the program approach, and document capacity to mobilize additional community resources.

Mental health leaders were aware that in the case of a Presidentially declared disaster, they could request funds for their program to provide psychological assistance to disaster victims. Under Section 413 of the Disaster Relief Act of 1974 (Public Law 93–288) monies were available for this purpose. The law reads as follows:

Sec. 413. The President is authorized (through the National Institute of Mental Health) to provide professional counseling services, including financial assistance to states and local agencies or private mental health organizations to provide such services or training of disaster workers, to victims of major disasters in order to alleviate mental health problems caused or aggravated by major disasters or their aftermath.

Administrators at the Massachusetts Department of Mental Health prepared a formal proposal citing the need for the service and describing a program of crisis counseling services. As this was being prepared, staff requested technical assistance from NIMH, asked for input and support from the Federal Coordinating Officer (the President's appointed manager), and approached Rep. Thomas P. O'Neill, speaker of the House of Repre-

sentatives, and Democrat from Massachusetts, for his support. After a week
of negotiations and a review by NIMH, the proposal was funded for
$380,000.

Once resources have been attained, the question of who gets what
is decided by a process of resource allocation. Some view this process
as rational, citing specific criteria for ensuring fairness and others perceive the process as a means for ensuring system homeostasis and enhancement. In either case, resource allocation is a basis for power that
defines what an administrator and the organization can do (Gummer,
1980). This approach stresses the political nature of resource allocation decisions which, in turn, influence the social interactions among
all organizational actors.

Program Design

The result of the analysis of need and development of resources is a
clarification and identification of problem areas and the examination
of strategies to resolve them. Program goals are formulated which specify priorities and groups targeted for assistance. In a word, the administrator, usually in concert with the agency's board or planning task
force, sets a course for agency action by proposing a generalized approach to problems caused by the unanticipated event.

Goals are broad statements of value, indicating choice and priority which are translated into action through a variety of program strategies. There are frequently a number of possible approaches and solutions
to a given problem and each is to be examined by use of certain agreed
upon criteria. Type of intervention or combination of intervention may
distinguish approaches. For example, an administrator may be forced
to decide whether a short-term crisis intervention approach is preferred
over long-term therapy. Another criteria of importance is cost. This,
of course, will be considered within the context of the agency's resources
and the potential outcome or benefit of a given strategy. And approaches vary by administrative structure as the following example
shows:

> When the Department of Mental Health made a commitment to serve the
> emotional needs of the blizzard's victims, much discussion ensued about
> relevant treatment modalities. It was pointed out that victims were not
> mental health patients, but rather ordinary people who have had an extra-
> ordinary experience. Their problems for the most part were the stresses
> of disaster, expressed in a variety of physical and emotional symptoms.
> Mental health practitioners advised that a concrete, reality-oriented ap-
> proach which emphasized information and hopefulness would be the most
> effective method of returning victims to prior functioning.
> In the first weeks after the snowstorm, victims were scattered through-

out the area. Some were living with relatives, others in hotels, motels, or shelters. Given their goal to provide crisis counseling services to those victims, mental health administrators opted for a decentralized administrative structure, employing a strong outreach component to identify survivors, define levels of psychological assistance required, and spell out specific treatment plans.

Program alternatives, therefore, are weighed in relation to potential beneficial outcomes, preferred treatment modalities, differential service delivery strategies, and the requirements of program structure. Decisions are made which maximize the agency's potential for achieving stated program goals and objectives. Three issues clearly needed attention during this process. First, the administrator carefully and creatively imagines alternative schemes to resolve the need at hand. Second, the administrator reviews the pros and cons of each approach, given clearly articulated and understood criteria. And, finally, the administrator involves relevant others, for example, boards, staff, and advisory committees, in this process which is essentially participatory in nature.

It is clear that each decision the administrator makes during this process influences and shapes the subsequent steps. There is a logical and integral relationship among the phases of sanction and support, need assessment, resource development, plan design, program implementation, and intersystem strategies. But as the administrator enters the plan design phase, there are still many choices to be made.

As goals are general statements concerning the direction in which the agency desires to go, they are descriptions of the agency's mission, a guide to future action. Objectives spell out in clear and specific fashion how goals are reached. These are targets that together enable the organization to achieve its purpose and are key elements which direct the administrator in program design.

A number of techniques may be employed by the administrator to plan a program. Some are rather simple benchmarks for program construction while others tend to be more complex criteria which guide the design process. Management by objectives (MBO), cost benefit analysis, cost efficiency criteria, and program planning budgeting systems (PPBS) are a few of the tools available to the administrator during this phase. One approach for understanding the elements in the design process has been introduced by Perrow (1967) where four key factors are emphasized. These are the functional, technological, efficiency, and systemic requirements necessary to design a project. In understanding these factors, the following definitions are offered.

Functional requisites consist of the identification and listing of anticipated program activities and/or services, including which groups are the target of service, and specific approaches and interventions to be employed. Activities such as daycare services, counseling, case management, screening and diagnosis, referral, and follow-up services are some examples.

> In deciding to mount a program of psychological assistance, mental health administrators assumed that victims were adversely affected by the blizzard and the resulting tidal flooding. It was known that these individuals regardless of need would not seek mental health aid as they did not consider themselves "patients." In order to avoid the stigma attached to mental health care, the program was detached from the mental health system and referred to as Project Concern.
>
> Key functions in providing psychological assistance to survivors were outreach, provision of information, counseling services, and, if needed, referral to other programs. Outreach was particularly needed for the reasons stated above. Victims are generally quiet and undemanding and usually will not seek out help. When they do come, they are experiencing the stresses of loss. Some need counseling; others need information concerning loans, rebuilding their homes, and so forth. If the victim has had serious problems prior to the event or demonstrates serious impairment of functioning, referral to a mental health clinic may be required.

To carry out these program activities, certain *technological requirements* are necessary. These consist of the need for resources—personnel, financial, and material—to perform program functions. Managers consider the need for type and number of staff, space, and facilities, and equipment, supplies, and furniture.

A third consideration in program design is the imperative of *efficiency*. The human service manager formulates a plan for type of administration and for the system of accounting, information collection, and evaluation. A key question is how each of the subunits of the program interrelate and how the project as a whole can operate efficiently. Some of the issues that administrators face are:

- Length of project
- Program sponsorship auspice and administration
- Centralization versus decentralization
- Costs and budget
- Nature of information systems
- Forms of internal and external accountability
- Types of program supervision

No program operates in a vacuum as there is always a need to understand the environment in which the program will function and to develop the necessary linkages to meet program goals. By tying the proposed plan to existing services in the community through formal and informal agreements, board representation, and contracts, the administrator addresses the last factor in program design, *systemic requisites*. The main ingredient of this element is a collaborative arrangement for the purposes of support, survival, avoiding competition and conflict, and offering clients the range of quality services that they need. By linking the agency's program with existing resources in the community, the administrator creates a vehicle for making referrals, educating the public, and seeking financial, material and political support.

> The Department of Mental Health designed a decentralized program with eight different sites operating out of storefronts or churches. Each site had a mental health team with a professional administrator answerable to the director of the regional mental health clinic. Other members of the team were nonprofessionals trained in interviewing, information giving, referral, and supportive counseling.
>
> Although service delivery was decentralized, the budget and accountability activities were maintained by the central office. An incorporated private firm was contracted as a conduit of grant funds received from the Federal Emergency Management Agency and the National Institute of Mental Health and served as the mechanism to hire the staff, thus avoiding the restraints of civil service.

In designing a program to meet needs created by an unanticipated event, the administrator employs a variety of tools and techniques. One such approach emphasizes the requirements of program functions, technology, efficiency, and system linkage. Once developed, the plan is reviewed and approved by the agency's planning committee, task force or board of directors.

Program Implementation
Program implementation is the process of translating ideas, notions, mission statements, goals and objectives into action. In linking knowledge to action, the administrator takes into account the context of the problems, trying to understand the complexity of forces which influence, positively or negatively, the process of implementation. Slavin (1980) wrote, "The administrator of a social agency always functions in a dynamic field of forces in which conflicting constituency interests contest for attention and response." With this in mind, the administrator sets into motion administrative activities which result in the performance of new services. To this end, the elements of control, service delivery, approach, information system, and evaluation structure become important.

How does the new program fit within the overall organizational structure and what is the pattern for organizational control? The administrator is ultimately accountable to the board of directors, but may also be answerable to an advisory group set up especially for the project. The board of directors or the advisory committee usually will approve policies regarding the program's mission and monitor activities to see that policies are implemented.

Also, administrators generally receive their sanction and authority from the board of directors, but in larger agencies this may actually emanate from an executive director. Authority and responsibility to carry out the programs and policies enacted to meet its goals and objectives are distributed to various levels of staff which have been defined as executive management, program management, supervisory, and front line staff (Patti, 1982). Questions of authority, control, obligation, and responsibility must be clarified for each level of staff involved in the new program.

The identification of the various service activities help to specify major program components which are then packaged into administrative structures. These groupings may be formally organized, such as departments or sections, or they may be, as is the case in small agencies, rather informally grouped under some form of central administration. Examples include such agency services as intake, information and referral, consultation, and treatment (i.e., crisis intervention, long-term care).

Service delivery models require varying administrative structures which address the following:

- The conceptualization of the helping process
- Identification of specific helping activities
- Division of labor and assignment of roles
- Delegation of authority

Some approaches emphasize a decentralized structure, focusing on service accessibility or specialized target groups. Other strategies may stress a comprehensive model of service delivery, requiring all services under one roof using a centralized or federated administrative structure. Obviously, there are many variations of the decentralized-centralized theme given the service delivery model, program organization and delegation of authority.

Once the structure for service delivery is set and there is clarity of program activities, the organization initiates a process to recruit the staff necessary to carry out the functions of the program. Professional, nonprofessional, clerical, and maintenance personnel may be necessary to operate the project. Their number and duties should be clearly specified in job descriptions.

When Project Concern began, ads were placed in the Boston Globe, the Bay State Banner, and El Mundo, searching for area coordinators, clinical team leaders, community service workers and secretaries. The advisory committee had decided to staff seven teams assigned to specific geographic areas. In hiring area coordinators, the task force looked for:

- Administrative experience and ability to make decisions, handle budgets, write reports, and analyze data
- Expertise in offering clinical orientation, training, and consultation
- Intimate knowledge of the community and its resources
- Skill in mobilizing community groups and resources for action
- Ability to communicate and get along with a variety of people.

Characteristics required for clinical team leaders were essentially clinical skills in diagnosis, crisis intervention, and supervision of the community service workers. In all instances, these individuals were Master's level social workers or psychologists.

The search for community service workers stressed the following personal attributes:

- Maturity, motivation, and emotional stability
- Ability to relate well with others
- Skill or potential skill in offering counseling assistance to victims
- Intimate knowledge of the community and its resources

Administrators tried to recruit people from the affected area to fill the community service worker positions. A Bachelor's degree plus 2 years of experience was required.

Each program requires a structure to gather information and keep records and accounts. As the administrator may be responsible for the management of program funds, it is important to set up accounting and bookkeeping procedures to have accurate records of expenditures for space, equipment, materials, supplies, and salaries. Records which collect service information, noting client progress, are also an essential part of an information system. In the design of these systems, care must be given by the administrator to the issues of confidentiality. Finally, the training of the staff in the use of the forms and documents of the information system is an often-overlooked activity. To avoid resistance and to insure accurate record keeping, one should hold regular training sessions concerning the various procedures and requirements of the information system and the rationale for collecting these data.

Evaluation and accountability are the major reasons for establishing a sound information system. As the program progresses, there exist requirements to evaluate individual and collective performances as well as to report to authorities on program activities. By reviewing individual and program data, the administrator is able to alter program activities and make individual reassignments of work tasks. From time to time, it is helpful or necessary to aggregate program information for the purpose of providing a board of directors, task force, community leaders, or the funding source with a report on program activities.

In review, the process of implementation addresses the design of administrative structures, coinciding with authority and control, service delivery, information systems, and the need for evaluation and accountability.

Intersystem Strategies

Intersystem strategies also depend heavily on analytical and sociopolitical skill. In the first instance, the administrator must possess abilities in performing technical tasks which facilitate a better understanding of one's environment and ways in which to link resources and to intervene. Knowledge of the external environment, the relationship of the various subelements, and a sense of what is possible given these relationships is crucial to the agency's administrator. To act on one's analytical appraisal of the external system, the administrator must also be proficient in sociopolitical processes.

Administrators and their agency may be viewed as part of a social interactional network as suggested by Talcott Parsons. This network has four principal aspects: (1) a set of units which interact; (2) rules by which the interaction takes place; (3) a patterned and organized system for the interaction; and, (4) the environment of systemic interactions (Parsons, 1968). Bolan's analysis (1971) of the basic social network in the planning process is helpful in conceptualizing the administrator's sociopolitical interactions. These take place at two distinct levels: with clients, and with the environment. For our purposes, therefore, we will analyze strategies based on interactions with:

- Client groups
- Institutional network
- Community decision network

Intersystem strategies have a number of purposes, including the search for sanction, resource development, gaining participation and support, giving and exchanging information, providing service, advocating policies, and resolving conflict. Each of these involve clients, organizations, and community decision makers. Thus, there is an interactional skill for the social administrator which can be translated into a number of roles at each of these levels.

In dealings with the *client group*, the administrator usually focuses upon:

- Defining client need and required services
- Gaining participation and support for program services

- Providing information concerning services available as well as for the purpose of referral
- Advocating for client groups, particularly those which do not have power

It is not usual that administrator and the agency seek sanction from the client group, but program support and participation are more important tasks. Important roles for the administrator with this unit are those of facilitator, interpreter, enabler, and advocate.

The *institutional network* is the aggregate of human service agencies that make up the service system. To operate within this system, any new program would primarily require support and, if required, sanction. "Turf issues" are not uncommon and the development of a new service without the participation of relevant organizations can be the cause of serious conflict. The exchange of information is crucial to this process, stressing the roles of enabler and facilitator.

Oftentimes the purpose of the intersystem strategy is to emphasize service intergration through interorganizational collaboration, resource sharing, and the avoidance of duplication. To accomplish this, the administrator concentrates on, in addition to those roles stated above, bargaining and negotiation. These roles are also employed in resolving organizational conflicts, frequently the effects of differing interests and values.

The mental health team in Revere, Massachusetts actively sought affiliations and agreements with other agencies. The first level of agreement was developed at the refugee center with various private and public agencies for the purpose of securing reciprocal referrals and providing case consultation. Later as victims dispersed to temporary housing or the homes of relatives, the team collaborated with the local interagency council, resulting in procedures to share information, making referrals and exchanging resources and technical assistance.

The interactional process may also actually be the vehicle to advocate for other organizations to change their policies and procedures. If advocacy results in conflict, then bargaining and negotiation are the methods of resolution

When interacting with the *community decision network*, the administrator is usually attempting to influence the nature of a decision. Representing the client group or speaking on behalf of the agency, the administrator actively seeks (1) sanction to act, (2) support (moral and financial) for a program strategy, and (3) changes in or adoption of policy.

This *community decision network* consists of key organizations in the political, economic, religious, and social spheres. Examples are legislative bodies, judicial or regulatory agencies, banks, manufacturing or industrial units, churches and synagogues, and groups such as the League of Women Voters or taxpayers' groups. Obviously, the composition of the decision network differs from community to community and from issue to issue.

The types of roles played by the administrator within the community decision network include:

- Interpreter and analyst of need
- Advocate for policies and services
- Resource developer—fundraiser
- Catalyst for new services initiatives
- Spokesperson for program accomplishments
- Defender from attacks on programs

An integral element of program implementation is the development and execution of intersystem strategies. To accomplish these, the administrator has to be particularly skilled in sociopolitical strategies. The translation of these skills into professional behaviors guides social administrators in their interaction with the client group, institutional network, and community decision network.

FURTHER IMPLICATIONS FOR ADMINISTRATIVE PRACTICES

This case highlights administrative responses to unanticipated events which may be of major proportions such as a tornado, toxic waste spill, or even the closing of an industrial plant. Such events have a serious impact on individuals as well as communities, human service systems, and individual agencies. Or, these events may be relatively minor, such as a fire affecting individuals and families who then turn to the human service network for help. In either case, the event places pressure on the administrator to understand the nature of the problem and consider modes of organizational action within a time frame which is usually very limited.

With the exception of the pressures cited above, the administrative principles reviewed in this chapter are applicable to all administrators. In other words, the administrator needs the sociopolitical and analytical tools to seek sanction and support, assess need, develop resources, plan and implement programs, and deal throughout this process with a dynamic set of forces within his or her environment.

Perhaps the single most important lesson from this case example is the necessity to be prepared, not only for the expected but also the unexpected. One should occasionally ask, "What would happen to this community, agency, or our clients if the unthinkable happens? How would my organization respond?" One form of preparedness is the design and review of an annual plan which details required administrative responses to expected and unexpected events.

The process of preparing a preplan considers and answers, where possible, a number of questions. These include:

1. What are the major risks faced by this community and by this agency?
2. If any of these occur, what would be the population at risk? What methods can we use to assess need?
3. In what ways can the agency respond to the event and what specific services can be delivered to those in need?
4. What kind of sanction and support are necessary for an agency response and how can these be attained?
5. What resources, financial, material, and human will be needed to implement a planned response?
6. Who in the agency will be responsible for carrying out the initial response effort?
7. What is the nature of the environment in which action is proposed and who are the relevant actors? Prior to an anticipated or unanticipated event, can our agency establish formal and/or informal linkages with key organizations and individuals?

An administrator may be able to prepare a plan that answers all of these questions, but the process of attempting to respond will be a very beneficial exercise. When a problem-solving process is then called for, the administrator will follow steps similar to those listed above.

This case example has illustrated the importance of both the sociopolitical and analytical dimensions in carrying out the various administrative responses to expected and unexpected events, but oftentimes the importance of the former dimension is overlooked. The training of human service administrators must include the principles of analysis, planning, and management, as well as content and practice in politics, decision-making processes, communication, and community organization. Thus, it is crucial for the administrator to be equally knowledgeable and skilled in the sociopolitical processes as well as the analytical techniques of these administrative responses.

Finally, in response to either an unanticipated or anticipated event, the administrator must demonstrate knowledge and skill during both the planning and implementation of programs and services. As we have seen, administrative expertise is required for gaining sanction and support, documenting need, developing resources, designing plans, implementing programs, and interacting with the organization's environment. Thus, sociopolitical as well as analytical abilities are crucial requirements for carrying out these planning and implementation activities.

REFERENCES

Bolan, R.S. The social relations of the planner. Journal of the American Institute of Planners, 1971, *37*, 6, 386–396.
Bolan, R.S. Mapping the planning terrain. In Planning in America: Learning from Turbulence. Washington, D.C.: American Institute of Planners, 1974.
Burke, E.M. A Participatory Approach to Urban Planning. New York: Human Sciences Press, 1979.
Gummer, B. Organizational theory for social administration. In F.D. Perlmutter, and S. Slavin (Eds.), Leadership in Social Administration. Philadelphia: Temple University Press, 1980.
Parsons, T. Social interaction. In International Encyclopedia of the Social Sciences, Vol. 7. New York: Macmillan and the Free Press, 1968.
Patti, R. Analysing agency structures. In M. Austin, Jr., and W.E. Hershey (Eds.), Handbook on Mental Health Administration, San Francisco: Jossey-Bass, 1982.
Perrow, C. A framework for the comparative analysis of organization. American Sociological Review, 1967, *32*, 3, 194.
Slavin, S. A theoretical framework for social administration. In F.D. Perlmutter, S. Slavin (Eds.), Leadership in Social Administration. Philadelphia: Temple University Press, 1980.

11

Working Side by Side: Collaboration of Mental Health Professionals and Clergy at a Temporary Morgue

Jacob D. Lindy
Thomas Eisentrout

> Dr. Rieux (the physician) speaking with Father Paneloux (the priest) as the plague rages: "We're working side by side for something that unites us—beyond blasphemy and prayers. And that's the only thing that matters."
>
> Albert Camus, *The Plague*

One hundred sixty-five people died in the fire which destroyed the Beverly Hills Supper Club, Southgate, Kentucky, May 29, 1977. The deaths resulted from smoke inhalation as people struggled behind two blocked doorways in the Club's Cabaret Room. News of the fire and its growing toll shocked the region. As part of the disaster rescue operation, volunteer firemen retrieved the dead from the smoldering fire. Police and Red Cross volunteers transported the bodies to a nearby gymnasium which was hastily being converted to a temporary morgue.

During the next hours and days, hundreds of families and friends of those stricken in the fire came to the morgue to claim their dead. Some were among those who escaped the fire themselves; others first learned of the blaze on the 11 P.M. news; still others traveled hundreds of miles in search of a missing relative.

The circumstances of those traumatically bereaved families, amidst the harsh grayness of dread and death in the temporary morgue is difficult to imagine and more difficult to convey.

Those who came to assist became painfully aware of the dread of the grotesque; of the helplessness, grief, outrage, and powerful defenses of denial, disavowal, disbelief, and heroism which permeated that experience (Titchener and Lindy, in press).

Families were suddenly being confronted with news of unexpected deaths, the awesome task of viewing burned bodies of loved ones, informing relatives including children, preparing funeral arrangements. The fire had turned their world literally into a "dis-astrous" place (derivation: "ill-starred").

For the many professional and volunteer agencies responsible for rescue operations (Red Cross, police, and so forth) the challenge was to make available the best possible support for these families in the most efficient way. But who was best qualified to meet this task?

Traditionally, clergy have played the major role in comforting suddenly bereaved families in tragedy. Chaplains carry out this task in hospitals every day. Further, studies of the delivery of mental health services to survivors following recent tornadoes in Xenia, Ohio (Taylor, 1976), and Wichita Falls, Texas, point out the central role of clergy in delivering human services. In each of these instances an interfaith council took major responsibility for follow-up to survivors.

An accepted role for mental health professionals (MHPs) with bereaved families in disaster is less established.

Grief and mourning are untoward but expected psychological stresses in the course of a life cycle. It is generally assumed that the internal work of such mourning occurs spontaneously. Freud (1917) suggested that mourning was a normal process that does not require medical attention.

Further, one group of sociologists has argued in recent years that severe mental illness to survivors following disasters is a myth. Further, this group argues that goals of mental health intervention are imprecise, and that traditional mental health resources are often poorly prepared to offer relevant and immediate services (Taylor, 1976).

On the other hand, psychiatrists working with bereaved survivors, beginning with the work following the Cocoanut Grove fire (Adler, 1943; Lindemann, 1944) delineated the symptoms of "morbid" or pathologic grief reactions and reported significant long-term impairment on follow-ups.

These symptoms are characterized by impaired concentration, loss of energy, psychosomatic disorders, preoccupations with images of the deceased, nightmares, guilt, episodes of rage, and appearances of traits of the deceased in the behavior of the bereaved.

In addition to pathological grief, clinical studies demonstrate that many survivors experience a short-term stress response syndrome (Horowitz, 1974), while some go on to experience significant long-term chronic impairment as in the survivor syndromes (Neiderland and Krystal, 1968). Following certain disasters, such as the Buffalo Creek Dam break, the incidence of long-term impairment was of epidemic proportions (Titchener and Kapp, 1976). Of special interest in that disaster was the finding of a significant relationship between bereavement and extent of long-term psychological impairment (Gleser et al., 1981).

Within recent years then, the traumatically bereaved have been increasingly viewed by MHPs as constituting a population at-risk for short and long-term psychological impairment. They would be, therefore, a legitimate concern for immediate psychological support and potentially preventive services.

In keeping with these ideas, mental health teams have visited survivors still living in flooded houses (Heffron, 1977), set up quarters in temporary camps outside a town destroyed by earthquake (Cohen, 1976), and worked side by side with other relief agencies in postdisaster one-stop centers (Algona, Iowa; Xenia, Ohio).

The traumatically bereaved constitute, then, both a legitimate concern of the clergy and of MHPs. At Beverly Hills, both groups of professionals were asked to help; both responded.

To date there have been no reports of clergy and MHPs working together in the impact phase of disaster and, of course, no assessment of its effectiveness.

Over a 4-day period, 60 psychiatrists, psychologists, and social workers from the University of Cincinnati, working in 4-hour shifts, joined 40 clergy from the greater Cincinnati area in providing front line mental health support for traumatically bereaved at a temporary morgue. The remainder of this report is a description and assessment of what these two groups did, and how they worked together.

PREDISASTER PLANNING

As in disasters of comparable size with heavy death toll, a variety of formal and informal rescue organizations mobilized in order to put a temporary morgue into place: In this instance, such groupings included Red Cross, Southgate city administration, Campbell County coroner's office, local and regional police, pathologists, embalmers, nurses, dental technicians, a Federal Bureau of Investigation (FBI) disaster squad, fire departments (including volunteers), life squads, high school volunteer stretcher bearers, and the Salvation Army.

Three organizational links preceding the fire gave clergy access to the overall rescue structure: (1) a well-functioning police-crisis clergy team was already attached to the Cincinnati Police Department, (2) a disaster planning team of the developing Cincinnati Regional Clergy Association had recently met, and (3) FBI regulation called for clergy to assist in body identification.

One organizational link preceding the fire gave MHPs access to the morgue operation. The University of Cincinnati Department of Psychiatry disaster preparedness plan called for close liaison between the University and Red Cross, in case of disaster.

CLERGY RESPONSE

Shortly after midnight the first clergy arrived at the temporary morgue in response to police and citizen band radio communications calling for help. Two chaplains negotiated with the coroner primary responsibility for two activities: (1) setting up and managing a family holding area, and (2) guiding families through the morgue in order to view bodies and make identification.

Soon, more help arrived. First was the police-crisis clergy; then there were other hospital chaplains, parish priests, seminarians, and local and regional pastors. Clergy arrived as individuals and as groups such as members of the developing Cincinnati Regional Clergy Association. They provided continuous manpower for these two activities for 96 hours—until the last charred body had been identified and the temporary morgue closed. Leadership was provided by two chaplains (also pastoral counselors by training) and by police crisis-clergy.

PSYCHIATRY RESPONSE

Shortly after 1 A.M. the first MHP arrived at the morgue. Their route and charge were different. As per disaster plan, MHPs gathered at the emergency room of the University Hospital. From there an advance team was sent to Red Cross Headquarters. As the morgue neared completion Red Cross sent the advance team to evaluate the need for psychiatric assistance to the coroner and his staff as families came in to identify the dead.

Phase I
The advanced psychiatric team negotiated with the coroner and the clergy already on the scene a consultative role, in the following plan. Families and friends of people missing in the fire were to gather in the ambulatory wing of the Veterans Administration facility 150 yards from

the gymnasium (morgue). This was to be the family holding area. Each family was to be met by a clergyman who would stay with the family throughout the identification procedure. The family would check at the main desk (manned by Salvation Army personnel) to see if the missing person(s) were on the list of the already identified dead. If so, one or more members of the family would walk with the clergyman to the morgue. A designated relative or friend would then go with the clergyman through the rows of bodies and confirm the identification. On the way out of the morgue, forms were to be signed: death certificates, funeral arrangements, and so forth. The clergyman was to stay with the family during the period following the identification until they seemed ready to go home. A "roving" clergyman was to observe this process from a distance. If there seemed need of psychiatric assistance, the "rover" was to contact the mental health worker on the scene for consultation.

Phase II

By Sunday morning the scene at the morgue had shifted. Nearly 150 bodies were now in the gymnasium. A steady flow of families was arriving at the holding area. Many clergy were leaving the morgue to return to their churches for Sunday services. The psychiatrists were able to bring more help. The advance party arranged with those still back at the emergency room to activate a network of clinicians by telephone. Over the next day six teams, of eight MHPs each, worked in 4-hour shifts at the morgue. During this phase one MHP was to join one clergy at the initial meeting with a given family and proceed throughout the process side by side with the family. Each new team had a designated leader, was briefed prior to assignment and held a debriefing upon completion of a shift.

At times during this period there were breakdowns in the orderly flow of the families. Some families bypassed the holding area and entered the morgue directly. Other families had to wait long hours for word. Also, during this phase there were temporary breakdowns in the role definitions of the two groups. In all, 60 psychiatrists, psychologists, social workers, and psychiatric nurses participated in the plan.

Phase III

Finally, only the charred remains of a few bodies were left in the morgue. Families, some coming from hundreds of miles, waited endlessly for positive identification of those feared to be dead (matching of dental imprints on the remains with dental records). Here a single clergyman and a single psychiatrist shared the tedious hours with the few waiting families.

TABLE 11.1. QUESTIONNAIRE—REFLECTIONS OF THE EXPERIENCE OF
CLERGY AND UNIVERSITY OF CINCINNATI MENTAL HEALTH TEAMS WORKING
TOGETHER AT THE BEVERLY HILLS TEMPORARY MORGUE

1. Have you even worked with members of the other professional group (clergy or mental health professionals) before? If so, describe briefly.

2a. What were the qualities you most appreciated in members of the other group? Please give examples.

b. What qualities did you find most difficult about the other group? Please give examples.

3. Please describe your sense of "fit" of the two groups.

4. If there were times when you felt unhelpful or inadequate to the task, please describe these.

5. In what way were you and your professional group effective? Anecdotes of personal or observed experience would be helpful.

6. What were some of your experiences in working together with the same family?

Thus three models for collaboration evolved, each of which suited a different phase of the work. Phase I called for the MHPs as consultants only; phase II called for the clinician and clergyman to work side by side with the family in a team; and phase III called for a single collaborative pair.

This report is a critical assessment of the working relationship between clergy and psychiatry at the temporary morgue. It examines the differential and common functions of the two groups as well as the successes and failures of the collaborative effort. It is based largely on the questionnaire responses of clergy and MHPs working at the morgue (Table 11.1).

RESPONSE TO THE QUESTIONNAIRE

Forty-seven percent of clergy contacted (9 of 19) responded to the questionnaire. Forty percent of MHPs (20 of 50) responded to the questionnaire.

1. Previous Collaborative Experience Between Clergy and MHPs.

1. Seven of nine clergy responding to the questionnaire reported extensive previous work with MHPs.

2. Eleven of the MHPs reported extensive prior work with clergy, 3 brief work, and 6 no previous collaborative work with clergy.

2. Qualities Most Appreciated and Most Difficult About the Other Group

Clergy appreciated the depth of the MHPs' sensitivity to psychological reaction. Mental health professionals appreciated the clergys' comfort with this situation of sudden death and their capacity to support often simply and nonverbally (including physical contact).

There were several trigger issues for each group. When members of the other group "passed" the test on this issue, they would be praised; when certain members of the other group "failed the test" they were criticized. For the clergy, such trigger issues were: (1) not intruding on the time-honored role of clergy with the dead and their stricken families. For one respondent this meant that only the consultative model was acceptable. For the MHPs trigger issues included: (1) not interfering with normal grief responses by, for example, proselytizing, moralizing, excessive controlling, or excluding a mental health presence; or being insensitive to psychological trauma.

One general criticism of the clergy from the MHPs was that individuals stayed at the scene too long—often beyond the point of exhaustion.

3. Sense of "Fit" Between the Two Groups

1. Clergy (89 percent) reported that the fit between clergy and psychiatry was good.

2. Six MHPs were positive in their descriptions of the fit, two negative, and seven mixed.

4. Reported Feelings of Inadequacy at the Morgue

1. Many clergy understood this question to refer to the task of relieving pain, suffering, and helplessness at the morgue, and in the face of this task felt inadequate (67 percent).

2. Six of 20 (30 percent) MHPs described feeling inadequate initially as a result of role confusion. Three reported feeling technically inadequate as to the timing or appropriateness of grief facilitating or affect clarifying interventions.

5a. Reports of Effective Intervention (Mental Health Workers)

Mental health professionals reported verbal interventions directed at the following themes:

1. Management of psychic overload: for example, assessing and titrating the potentially traumatizing effect of making a body identification

2. Empathy and education regarding defenses which tended to wall off the experience of trauma and loss
3. Acceptance of outbursts of rage
4. Facilitating beginning grief work
5. Acceptance and understanding of survivor guilt.

Mental health professionals organized their accounts around clinical management skills: history, diagnosis, disposition, and follow-up. One social worker was struck at the impact of an earlier suicide by a parent which preceded the death by fire of the second parent. The surviving son was clearly distraught in making the identification. The social worker elected to pursue follow-up of this case in light of the *history* as well as the trauma. A psychiatrist *diagnosed* a manic psychosis in one of the waiting "relatives." Indeed, this was not a survivor, but a man drawn to the scene by the power of his mental disorder. Another psychiatrist concluded that immediate prolonged childlike tearfulness in a man who had lost both parents represented more a resistance to identifying the bodies than grief over acknowledged loss. He assisted in the *disposition* to take the next step and view the bodies directly.

Some clinicians broadened their perspective to the capacity of the surviving family to be a mutual support group for each other. A psychiatrist separated a quarrelsome stepfather from the father so that two separate support groups could form as they both anticipated word on the fate of a missing daughter. A psychologist chose to run after an angry son in an effort to provide wholeness to a family's support for each other. Mental health professionals were attentive to the traumatogenic potential of the environment. They looked for ways to monitor the climate of the morgue so as to reduce unnecessary overload on the family. A freshly arriving social worker noted that charred body remnants were now exposed in the gymnasium as dental imprints were being made. She thought such exposure unnecessarily traumatic to families identifying other bodies. Other workers in the gymnasium seemed to have become numbed to the traumatic impact. Clinicians hung sheets as curtains to minimize trauma.

5b. Reports of Effective Intervention (Clergy)

Clergy were clear with regard to their primary professional role at the morgue. They were performing a time-honored and religiously sanctioned ritual for the dead; they were providing traditional comfort for the families of the deceased. Within this spiritual context, clergy could and did offer prayer, spiritual strength, and the "silent symbolic presence of the Infinite in the midst of calamity." Clergy assisted in making funeral arrangements and in certain instances conducting them.

Clergy were less clear in verbalizing their psychological role. They reported familiarity in "dealing with people who have suffered great and sudden loss." There was, however, a wide spectrum of reported responses to that situation. One clergyman was clear that his role was to "keep appropriate distance, not in any way to interfere with the family's perferred reaction, be it silence, sobbing or indifference." By contrast, another clergy wrote, "my witness was to be there supporting, crying, touching, sharing," Most, however, took a middle ground of offering a "simple presence," to "sit with, stand with, care."

Broadly, clergy saw their activities in the identification process and funeral preparations as providing a focus through which families could actively structure their immediate experience to manage psychic overload by mastering details of specific behavior. In their report of their activities, clergy were largely inattentive to defenses against trauma and loss. They were largely inattentive to survivor guilt. They were variable in their response to rage and the value of activating grief work.

6a. Difficulties in Collaboration

At times role distinctions between MHPs and clergy broke down with mixed results. A young woman was walking hesitantly across the 150 yards to the morgue, a psychiatrist to her right, family and minister to her left. She was frightened of the physical condition in which she would find her brother's body; how much pain had he endured before he died, and asked, "How fast does a soul get to heaven? Does it wait here? Is it in pain?" The psychiatrist responded instinctively, "Souls get there right away." Nearby the family and the minister continued the conversation. "The Lord will be there to meet him when he arrives," the minister said more reassuringly.

A social worker became theological: a young man working as a stretcher bearer said, "If God is love, what is this?" She pointed out that he, in the very hard work he was doing, was loving the families of the dead through his help for them and that could be a way of restoring the meaning of a loving God.

A chaplain initiated treatment on the spot. A young man seemed overwhelmed at his helplessness and rage after identifying his father in the morgue. He was about to strike out at someone. The chaplain quickly ushered him to a large punching bag in the rear of the gymnasium and instructed him to release his fury on the punching bag.

Sometimes, the clergyman and MHPs disagreed. A pastor insisted on counseling a woman who was awaiting identification of her mother with the resigned phrase, "It's God's will." This "reassurance" did nothing to aid the woman's growing agitation. By insisting that a psychologist be given an opportunity to listen, she patiently permitted the woman to admit her fear that she expected to break down and lose control with the bad news. The woman then alluded to difficult memories and troubles between her and her mother. She also recalled sharing hobbies, tastes for needlework and other crafts. Candor and openness about troubles in mother-daughter relations were balanced by recalling the love in the relationship; grief work had begun.

6b. Successful Collaboration

CASE EXAMPLE 1

The 60-year-old mother and 32-year-old sister of a fire victim waited interminably for word that the charred remains behind the curtain were in fact D. A psychiatrist and minister waited with them. Mother had become agitated and pale during the waiting. She developed dyspnea and diaphoresis. The daughter seemed restless but better defended and in better physical health. Neither could accept the reality of D.'s death. Dental imprints now confirmed the identification, but it would be necessary for one family member to view the remains. Both mother and sister insisted on viewing the remains "to be sure." While all shared in the discussion which followed, the psychiatrist's view that exposing the mother to this scene would be severely and perhaps unnecessarily traumatizing, seemed to hold sway.

On viewing the charred remnants, alongside the clergyman, the sister responded quickly "That's him—I can recognize the jaw." She exited quickly, then said confidently to her mother, "It's definitely D.—he's been killed in the fire." Her mission accomplished, sister felt some relief. Mother now broke into deep sobs and began to grieve for her son. Sister's relief was, of course, only temporary. She had fended off traumatic overexposure by "recognizing" one of the few humanoid forms left amidst the charred remnants. She had transferred onto herself the family's disavowal that the son had died. She was puzzled by her own preoccupation with the traumatic sight, her own disbelief, and sense of weirdness, rather than what she viewed to be the more healthy grieving responses of the mother. At this point the mother asked the clergyman to pray for her son (he prayed); the daughter asked the psychiatrist what was wrong with her that she wasn't having any feelings. He explained that she was going through a horrible experience, that sometimes our minds protect us from the full impact of disaster until we're more ready to deal with it. The right time would come; hers was a normal first reaction to the kinds of fright and loss she was enduring.

CASE EXAMPLE 2

A young woman searched up and down rows of identifiable bodies failing to find her mother. She steadfastly held on to the belief that mother was alive, only to be informed later that imprints confirmed her mother's death. Now she was guided to the body that was her mother. Clearly she had walked past her mother 20 times without recognition. She attacked herself guiltily for failing to recognize her own mother. The psychiatrist pointed out that grief and disaster are overpowering; that the mind blocks what it wishes it did not see. Then she began sobbing, wanting to understand the meaning of her mother's death; she turned to the pastor. He comforted her, reminding her of her own deep convictions about God and the acceptance of death.

SUMMARY

Clergy and MHPs working together at a temporary morgue devised de novo three models for collaboration near the scene of the Beverly Hills fire.

One called on the psychiatrist as consultant only. This was employed during the first few hours when the number of families was small and the morgue relatively quiet and orderly. The second model called for one clergyman and one mental health clinician joining each family from start to finish. This was employed when the number of families became large and the overall climate in the morgue was of greater confusion. The third model called for a clergyman and a MHP to "stand by" with those few families who waited days to learn the news.

The primary function of each group was different. Mental health professionals attended to: management of psychic overload, empathy with affects of trauma and loss as well as defenses against them, acceptance of rage and survivor guilt and initiating grief work. These activities both complemented and were distinguishable from the primary function of the clergy: providing ritual for the dead, comfort for the bereaved, prayer, spiritual strength, and the presence of the Infinite in the midst of the calamity.

When collaboration worked best, clinicians responded to affects connected with trauma and loss and the understandable defenses against them, while clergy worked with the reality of death and the poignance of our human search for its meaning.

Together they formed a temporary psychological-spiritual buffer, trying to titrate trauma which by its very nature was overwhelming, and to support the forces of healing which for the moment were in danger of being overcome.

While competitive issues between the two groups were latently and at times overtly present, the overall fit was good. Indeed, collaboration may well have potentiated either's independent effectiveness.

We suggest that mental health preparedness in other communities may benefit from studying the Cincinnati clergy-mental health model and applying it to suit the needs and resources of a particular region.

ACKNOWLEDGMENTS

The authors wish to acknowledge the contributions of Jessica Murdaugh, M.S.W. and James Titchener, M.D. who designed and distributed the questionnaire in this study; and Joanne Lindy, Ph. D., the other half of the psychiatry "advance team."

REFERENCES

Adler, A. Neuropsychiatric complications in victims of Boston's Cocoanut Grove disaster. Journal of American Medical Association, 1943, *123*, 1098-1101.

Cohen, R.E. Post disaster mobilization of a crisis intervention team: The Managua experience. In H.J. Parad, H.L.P. Resnik, L.G. Parad (Eds.), Emergency and Disaster Management. Bowie, Md.: Charles Press, 1976.

Freud, S., Mourning and Melancholia, The Complete Psychological Works of Sigmund Freud, Vol. 14. London: Hogarth Press, 1917.

Gleser, G.C., Green, B. Winget, C. Prolonged Psychosocial Effects of a Disaster: A Study of Buffalo Creek. New York: Academic Press, 1981.

Heffron, E. Project outreach: Crisis intervention following natural disaster. Journal of Community Psychology, 1977, *5*, 103-111.

Horowitz, M. Stress response syndromes: Character style and dynamic psychotherapy. Archives of General Psychiatry, 1974, *31*, 768-781.

Lindemann, E. Symptomatology and management of acute grief. American Journal of Psychiatry, 1944, *101*, 141.

Niederland, W., Krystal, H. Clinical observations on the survivor syndrome. In H. Krystal (Ed.), Massive Psychic Trauma. New York: International University Press, 1968.

Taylor, V. Delivery of mental health services in disasters: The Xenia tornado and some implications. Columbus, Ohio: Ohio State University, Disaster Research Center, Monograph No. 11.

Titchener, J., Kapp, F.T. Family and character change at Buffalo Creek. American Journal of Psychiatry, 1976, *133*, 3.

Titchener, J., Lindy, J. Affect and Insight in the Clinician: A Psychoanalytic Study of the Beverly Hills Supper Club Fire. In press.

12

Social Upheaval and Recovery in Guatemala City after the 1976 Earthquake

JoAnn Glittenberg

Recovery and reconstruction following major social upheavals such as disasters and war have multiple health concerns. Besides loss of life and emotional trauma due to the direct efforts of the catastrophe, there are also long-term residuals of loss and change in the lives of survivors. Chiefly because of the financial expense, most research studies of disasters are limited to short-term follow-up studies of several weeks to a year or so after the traumatic event. Many scientists have urged the importance of longitudinal studies (Baker and Chapman, 1962; Marris, 1974).

Because of the magnitude of the 1976 Guatemalan earthquake, as well as the unprecedented outpouring of disaster relief and reconstruction aid, a longitudinal study funded by the National Science Foundation (NSF) was begun in 1977 (18 months after the event) and extended through 1982 (in selected areas). This study had as an overall goal the study of the process of recovery over a 5-year period postearthquake.* A quasi-experimental design was used to compare the recovery process in 19 experimental and 7 control sites. The overall guiding research question was: Does a catastrophe or social upheaval stimulate the recovery of the society so that the level of living postdisaster is higher than the predisaster state? The factor, level of living, was operationalized to include housing conditions and cost of living as well as measurements of the quality of life.

The results of a specific portion of the 1976 NSF study (as it is popularly called) the urban resettlements, are presented in this report. The

---

*Copies of the Final Report are in five volumes and may be obtained by writing to: Mr. Frederick L. Bates, Department of Sociology, University of Georgia, Athens, GA 30601.

goal of this presentation is to conceptualize the mediators needed for attaining an optimal level of functioning (health) on an aggregate (or settlement) level.

SOCIAL UPHEAVAL AND RECOVERY IN GUATEMALA CITY AFTER THE 1976 EARTHQUAKE

Social upheaval following a major disaster, natural or man-made, has profound effects upon individual lives as well as aggregate populations such as neighborhoods, cities, and towns. Losses include more than mere physical materials as we consider the magnitude of human suffering and disruption of political, religious, economic, and social systems. As the reverberations of a calamity shudder throughout a nation, as it did in Guatemala on February 4, 1976, individuals and groups experience the impact differently. The impact takes a variety of forms as the complexities of natural and social environments interplay.

How do we, as researchers, begin to deal with the magnitude of factors that affect humans? How do we determine the best way, the most effective manner of responding, in the longer term, to human suffering on a human scale? Do hasty emergency decisions have negative, long-lasting impairments—2, 3, or 5 years later? And, how do we as researchers measure the impact of relief measures in the complex, emotion-ridden arena of a disaster?

These are profound, difficult questions that cannot be answered simply or superficially. If we are to respond to catastrophic losses through relief agencies then we must do so with specific, targeted actions based upon sound research and not mere willy-nilly convulsive outpourings and an influx of eager helpers. Disasters, like human illnesses, are events that can be studied and lessons can be learned. The lessons to be learned, as described in this chapter, come from a complex, longitudinal study: The 1976 Guatemala Earthquake. The magnitude of the study need not discourage those readers engaged in smaller scale studies but rather the research design is applicable to various units of analysis. The lessons learned concern human adaptation, at the aggregate level, to stress and the coping mechanisms used. Such lessons should be meaningful for those involved in health care and social policy related to social upheaval.

BACKGROUND

Guatemala, the second largest of the Central American countries, with a population of 5.2 million people (1973 census) has suffered frequent natural disasters, for example, volcanic eruptions, flooding, and numerous devastating earthquakes. However, no previous disaster was of the magnitude of the 1976 earthquake. The fault line of the 1976 earthquake stretched across the center of the Republic and the magnitude, 7.5, on the Richter scale was sufficient to leave one million people homeless, 75,000 severely wounded, and 25,000 killed. Over 100 relief agencies came to the rescue of the victims; the outpouring of aid was unprecedented and was as surprising to some natives living in remote villages as was the disaster itself. The destruction to the tiny developing country was a significant blow to an economy that was, for the majority of the natives, only slightly above a subsistence level. The struggle against low economic production, high birth rates, and low literacy rates was now compounded with heavy economic and human losses. In some towns all the official leaders were killed; infrastructures such as water and sewage systems were completely destroyed. Some believed that Guatemala would never recover, but that was not the case. The findings show that there is variation in the recovery and reconstruction process and it is the study of this variation that is of interest to the discipline of nursing. Variation in the recovery process will point out that the coping process is strengthened or weakened, just as in crisis intervention, by numerous situational factors. By analyzing such situational factors, disaster relief agencies as well as social policy makers can intervene effectively for those who, at an individual or aggregate level, are victims of a catastrophe.

METHODOLOGY

Utilizing a quasi-experimental research design, 19 experimental sites (sustained heavy property damage and loss of life) and 7 control sites (sustained no or slight property damage and no loss of life) were chosen according to the following criteria:

1. Degree of loss of life
2. Degree of property damage
3. Geographical location (highland/lowland)
4 Ethnicity (Indian or Ladino)
5. Degree and type of relief and reconstruction aid
6. Degree of social organization.

A research team of eight Guatemalans who spoke both Spanish and Cakchiquel (a Mayan language) were the household interviewers using a pretested, inclusive 2-hour interview on a 1400 random sample households. The household interview was done twice, once in 1978 and again toward the end of 1980. Pre-earthquake data were used for many of the sites as well as from retrospective questions. In addition to the random household interview, community inventories, leader scheduled interviews, special project analysis, agency studies, ethnographies, and participant observation became the general data bank of findings.

The *urban settlements* were a part of the general study, but because the victims that were found in the urban sites were distinct, a special portion of the study was devoted to them.

The data were analyzed in the following ways: the household data were analyzed using recovery and reconstruction as the dependent variable, and the independent variable was the impact of the disaster. Intervening variables included type of social organization and access to aid. The statistical analysis included analysis of variances and multiple regressions; content analysis was used on the leader interviews. Descriptive analysis were made from the ethnographic data.

THE URBAN SAMPLE

Guatemala City, in 1982, had a population of over a million people. When founded in 1776, as the capital of the Republic, there were about 24,000 inhabitants. Growth was slow until after World War II when the influx of rural migrants began to increase. These migrants were poor and tended to live in squatter settlements and slums along the steep sides of deep ravines throughout the City. For over two decades these marginal settlements were inhabited by the poorest of the poor (most with family incomes of less then $50/month). These settlements were hardest hit by the 1976 earthquake. Over 60,000 of these houses were destroyed (Marroquin, 1978). Almost all of the former owners were squatters or renters whose landlords could not rebuild. Housing for over 200,000 people was desperately needed. Temporary shacks and shelters were set up by the people; over 120 such settlements, of about 10,000 people each, were established. Most of them were self-help settlements rebuilt with leftover scraps of cardboard and wood. Some victims were fortunate to have the help of a relief agency to plan and construct safe housing for them out of sturdy cement blocks reinforced with steel beams and tin roofs. For the NSF Study we chose to compare the recovery and reconstruction process in four different settlements that showed variation in the type and amount of aid given. The settlements were: Roosevelt, a forced refugee settlement; Carolingia, a planned settlement; 4th of February, an unplanned squatter settlement; and New Chinautla, a planned resettlement. Each of the settlements was inhabited by 10,000 to 15,000 people who had completely lost their houses and possessions in the disaster. Each will be described briefly.

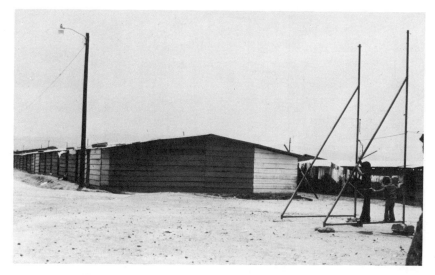

Figure 12.1. Roosevelt, forced settlement, 1977.

Roosevelt was a forced refugee settlement of 10,000 people who had lived predisaster in various sections in the City. It was a dismal setting with families living in long shed-like dwellings of 54 households each (Figs. 12.1, 12.2, 12.3). There were no curbs and the dirt roads became deeply eroded during the 6-month rainy season. Electricity was brought in 2 years after the disaster, but then only to the main street.

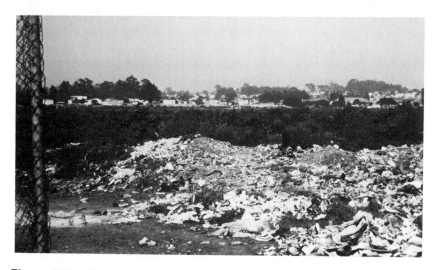

Figure 12.2. Site where Roosevelt, forced settlement, formerly existed, 1982.

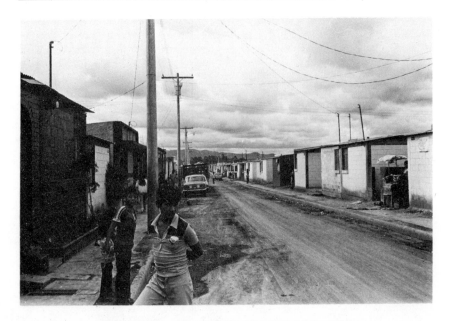

Figure 12.3. New Roosevelt (Qinta Mal), 1983.

Water was in very short supply at a few public faucets. Sixteen toilets and showers were shared by every 2000 inhabitants. The school was surrounded by a high fence; the crime rate was very high, although police patrolled the streets. The people were without hope for four years; the fifth year (1981) a total change occurred as the Guatemalan government built new homes for them to buy on a long-term loan basis. The quality of life changed from anomie to one of hope and expectation.

Carolingia, a planned settlement for 15,000 people was a model of what can be done with outside help and shared decision-making with the settlers. Sharing the same demise of their already poor predisaster existence, the Carolingians had consistent, quality help from a Norwegian agency, a Guatemalan church group sponsored by a church in the United States, and Church World Services, a nondenominational international religious group. Strong leaders evolved within the settlement; the land was developed with cement block houses assigned by lottery number. Schools and health clinics were soon in place. The psychological state within 1 year was of high expectation, and the community continued to grow and prosper (Figs. 12.4, 12.5).

Fourth of February, named for the date of the disaster, was an unplanned squatter settlement of about 15,000 people. The residents had lived prior to the earthquake in the deep ravines and with the loss of

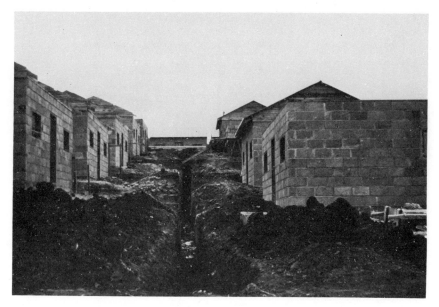

Figure 12.4. Carolingia, planned settlement, 1977.

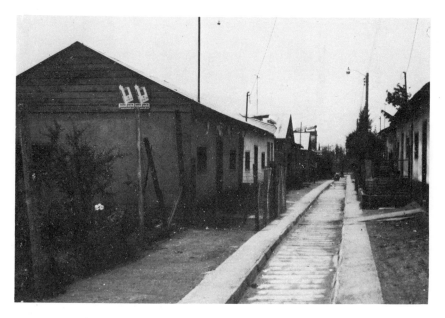

Figure 12.5. Carolingia, planned settlement, 1983.

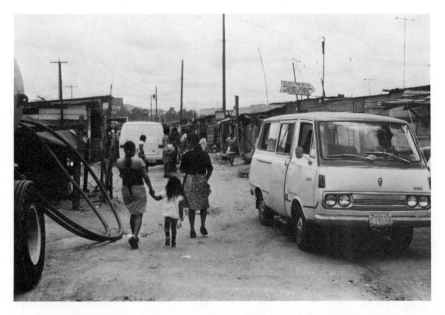

Figure 12.6. 4th of February, unplanned settlement, 1978.

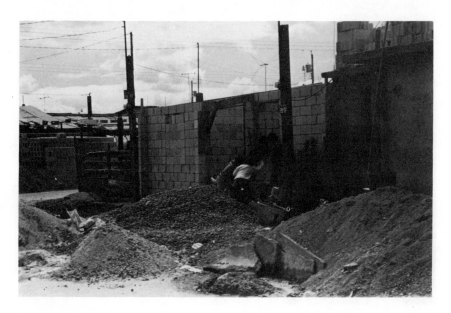

Figure 12.7. 4th of February, unplanned settlement, beginning planned reconstruction, 1982.

their houses they merely moved up to solid, flat ground and possessed the land by mere strength of numbers. Shacks of all types sheltered these energetic folk for 5 years as the settlement grew in formal organization with widening streets, a "community" center, illegal electricity tappings, a sanitary system, a school for 600 children, open markets, and water brought in by tank trucks. Without outside aid, however, the residents would have remained in their low level of living standards. In 1980 the Guatemalan government began a building program by which individuals could get long-term loans and help in buying and building permanent, cement block houses. Strongly organized, this settlement will become a positive influence on the City (Figs. 12.6, 12.7).

New Chinautla, a planned resettlement of ethnically mixed victims, in 1982 achieved the highest level of living of the four settlements (Figs. 12.8, 12.9). The settlement had deep roots in Guatemalan history with origins in the famous town of Chinautla. The old town was nearly destroyed by the earthquake and about half the residents (400 families) took shelter on flat land above their former town. Aided by Church World Services, Mennonites, and the Guatemalan government, the resettlement began by building cement block houses. The ethnic clash of Ladinos (mixed Spanish and Mayan Indian) and the Pokomam (Mayan) Indians created havoc for about 4 years in the new settlement.

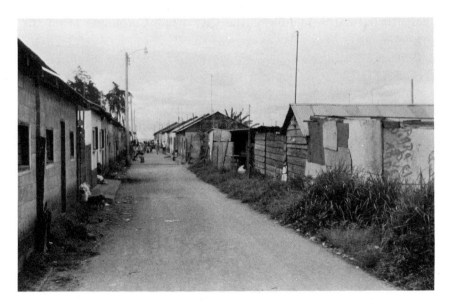

Figure 12.8. New Chinautla, planned settlement, 1978.

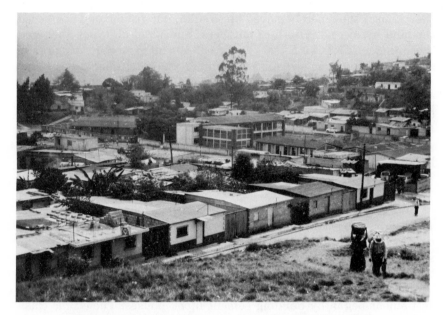

Figure 12.9.   New Chinautla, planned settlement, 1983.

During the fifth year (1981) the groups integrated and began to cooperate. The settlement in 1982 is similar to Carolingia, except New Chinautla is in the middle of the City while Carolingia is on the periphery.

THE SAMPLE

By studying the same household units over a period of 5 years, changes in level of living (the measurement of reconstruction) are important indicators of adjustment. The urban household sample consisted of the following:

Roosevelt: N = 53 in 1978,   N = 44 in 1980
Carolingia: N = 101 in 1978, N = 84 in 1980
4th of February: N = 117 in 1978, N = 95 in 1980
New Chinautla: N = 49 in 1978,   N = 45 in 1980

The total loss in the sample was 16 percent.

Food Shortages
Food shortages were severe for 67 to 79 percent of the people lasting from 2 weeks to 3 months (the longest period of shortage was for those in New Chinautla). The food items they found in shortest supply were

the staple foods of beans, corn, rice, bread, and sugar. Eighty-one to 94 percent received free, donated food. Few experienced receiving unfamiliar food and the majority believed the distribution was fair.

Housing
Temporary housing of cardboard, plastic sheeting was experienced in each settlement for a period of about 2 months to 1 year by 80 to 90 percent of the victims. Few could remember the agency's name that helped during the Emergency Period except for the Guatemalan Red Cross and the Army. Few listed medical care as a high priority need during the Emergency Period.

Social Relations
Changes in family relations and with authorities were seen as equal or better by 90 to 99 percent of the people in the Planned Settlements, but only 80 percent in the Unplanned Settlements (these data are prior to the 1982 changes in housing) viewed social relations as equal to predisaster conditions.

Reconstruction
Reconstruction, the dependent variable, was measured by multiple indicators; in this report one measurement will be used: level of living changes. This measurement is cost weighted according to functional items in the household. (Note: A report on how these figures were established has been prepared by the research team but will not be described further in this study.) Changes in Level of Living (Table 12.1) indicate a statistically significant ($p < 0.001$ level of probability) decrease in the means of each household from predisaster to 1976 postdisaster. This finding was expected, as housing was the chief item considered in the scale of 11 items. Figure 12.10 illustrates the changes over the 5-year period in the control sites as compared with the experimental sites. For both groups there was a gradual raising of levels of living but the experimental group was slightly higher at the beginning of 1975 and slightly lower in 1980, 5 years later. In the meantime, the disaster devastated the experimental group and drove its level of living down by around 60 percent. During the next 4 years the experimental group recovered to near its original level. Meanwhile the control group, which was only slightly affected by the disaster, gradually improved in level of living.

Figure 12.11 indicates that the mostly highly organized entity, Guatemala City, recovered more quickly and exceeded the predisaster level of living. The aldeas, small villages, and department capitals (similar to state capitals, but smaller) recovered more slowly and neither had in 1980 attained the predisaster level of living.

TABLE 12.1. DIFFERENCE IN LEVEL OF LIVING T_1-T_2[a]

Settlement	Inferential Statistics		Significance of Difference		
	Mean	S.D.	t	DF	Prob.
Roosevelt	(1) 1453.28	(1) 645.27	−5.40	104	<0.001
T_1-T_2	(2) 740.07	(2) 713.22			
Carolingia	(1) 1273.15	(1) 537.97	−9.24	200	<0.001
T_1-T_2	(2) 727.34	(2) 568.95			
4th of February	(1) 1143.49	(1) 447.70	−9.04	232	<0.001
T_1-T_2	(2) 597.30	(2) 475.99			
Chinautla	(1) 1135.76	(1) 484.37	−13.12	96	<0.001
T_1-T_2	(2) 414.95	(2) 522.72			

Abbreviations = DF, degrees of freedom.
[a]T_1, predisaster; T_2, postdisaster time 1976.

The urban settlements as depicted in Figure 12.12 indicate an even greater degree of variability in the process of reconstruction. Note the very sharp rise in Carolingia and New Chinaulta, the planned settlements as compared with the unplanned settlements. The changes in Carolingia and New Chinautla between 1980 (T_5) and (T_1) were an *increase* of $1259 and $1981, respectively, and for 4th of February and Roosevelt, a *decrease* of $433 and $596, respectively. The changes were due to the presence or absence of outside assistance. However, it would appear from the 1982 ethnographic data that both unplanned settlements are or soon will be equal to the planned settlements. In conclusion, outside assistance (the mitigating factor) was a critical factor in the reconstruction process whether the assistance was early (e.g., 1976) or late (e.g., 1981).

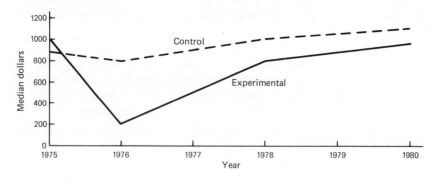

Figure 12.10. Level of living changes by control and experimental sites.

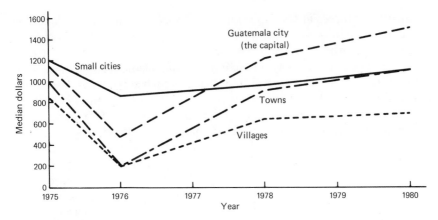

Figure 12.11. Level of living changes by level of social organization.

THE RECOVERY PROCESS FROM A STUDY
OF THE AGGREGATE UNIT

How individual households receive and utilize aid in the recovery process is essential information when planning for disaster relief. Another important aspect of maximizing on the aid given is understanding the

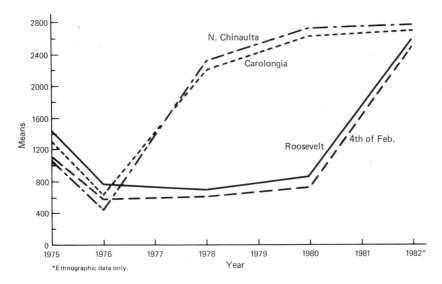

Figure 12.12. Level of living—urban settlements.

sociocultural forces at the aggregate level such as community or settlement that enhance, aid, or impede the recovery process. Given the opportunity to study the process for over 6 years, certain aggregate characteristics are clearly identifiable from ethnographic data and leader interviews. Certain characteristics of each settlement were summarized at the end of 1980 and again in 1982. Of the four characteristics studied (decision-making, leadership style, social matrix, and psychological state), it is evident that the communities that progressed socioeconomically most rapidly were those that were democratic and highly integrated with a high level of participation. The characteristic, psychological state, is dependent upon the other three characteristics. Events specific to each settlement were either stimulants or barriers to reconstruction. For instance, the conflict that arose between two leaders in 4th of February constrained active recovery for a period of about a year; yet, following resolution of the conflict both sets of followers were highly vitalized and established new settlements. Such conflict behavior is often seen in other settings of overcrowding and competition for territory or resources. Anticipation of such a normal process of conflict and resolution might alleviate undue pressure and stress.

Another aspect of the recovery process that impeded the reconstruction was the autocratic control of New Chinautla by one leader and his loyal family. Although he had some fine leadership qualities, not allowing for other leaders to emerge became a devisive force. Finally community members became a sufficiently strong force as to expel the autocratic leader. Instead of anarchy the community redefined its goals and reestablished priorities and community cooperation.

The example of Roosevelt as a forced settlement and the resultant loss of hope, anomie, and internal decay was a highly visible external process. Leaders had left, decision-making was abated, and hopelessness had become widespread within 3 to 4 years after the disaster. A startling change occurred in the four characteristics (decision-making, leadership style, social matrix, and psychological state), once the new settlement, named Qinta Mal, was opened. The resiliency and recovery of victims was a lesson in survival. Once opportunity for improvement was made possible, the residents advanced swiftly. Social scientists who challenge a culture of poverty would find evidence for their debate in the remarkable change in the lives at a household level of the former residents of Roosevelt

Similar comments could be made about the recovery process in 4th of February. Once an organized solution was formalized the residents seized the opportunity for improvement. The difference in the two groups is chiefly that settlers in Roosevelt had probably a higher standard of living prior to the earthquake; however, they did not have the survival strategies that the residents of 4th of February had had before the disaster. Strong leadership was a positive influence for the residents of 4th of February.

Table 12.2 depicts in a longitudinal time-ordering sequence the process that each settlement underwent from bereavement for each of them in 1976 to various states of recovery in 1982. Close evaluation of the years 1978, 1979, and 1980 shows the widest spread of differences. Notable are the high levels of recovery for Carolingia and New Chinautla in each subsequent year following the disaster. The essential element was the aid in reconstruction given by outside agencies. Only in 1982 are changes visible in 4th of February and Roosevelt when these settlements also received outside assistance for reconstruction.

FUTURE OF THE SETTLEMENTS AND LESSONS LEARNED FOR FUTURE DISASTERS

As documented by the 1982 ethnographic data, it appears all four settlements now are approximately equal in the recovery process. The characteristics of the communities as of 1982 are summarized in Table 12.3. This summary clearly illustrates the interplay between the factors of decision-making, leadership style, social matrix and psychological state. The final characteristics of each community as of 1982 are the same with decision-making: high-level participation; leadership style: democratic local control; social matrix: highly integrated. However, psychological state as a characteristic varies from settlement to settlement. The planned settlements, Carolingia and New Chinautla, are reintegrated; the unplanned or forced settlements, 4th of February and Roosevelt, are revitalized.

Residents have permanent, well-constructed housing with legal access to property tenure; also, the settlements each have electricity, water, sewage, and asphalted roads. We cannot be certain that the present-day residents are the same victims of the disaster, but from the 1980 Household Survey we found 84 percent of the 1978 urban household residents were still in the same location. It can be argued that the temporary, refugee-type housing of Roosevelt and 4th of February was *not* unlike their predisaster housing as depicted from the 1973 census study. What has changed for all residents, as of 1982, is that their housing is more valuable, safer from subsequent earthquakes, and privately owned. Each settlement should continue to improve as

TABLE 12.2. DYNAMIC PROCESS OF RECOVERY

	1976-1977	1978	1979	1980	1982
	State of	State of	State of	State of	State of
Planned settlement (Carolingia)	Bereavement	High activity reconstruction	Pride	Power and cooperation	Settled cooperation
Unplanned settlement (4th of Feb.)	Bereavement	Conflict	Cooperative competition	Fission and new beginnings	Power and achievement
Forced settlement (Roosevelt)	Bereavement	Waiting maintenance	Helplessness	Hopelessness and alienation	New beginning and high
Planned settlement (Chinautla)	Bereavement	Reconstruction	Competition	Conflict	Power and cooperation

TABLE 12.3. CHARACTERISTICS OF COMMUNITY ORGANIZATION

Settlements	Decision-making	Leadership Style	Social Matrix	Psychological State
Planned (Carolingia)	High-level participation	Democratic Local control	Highly integrated	Reintegrated
Unplanned (4th of Feb.)	High-level participation	Democratic Local control	Highly integrated	Revitalized
Forced (Roosevelt) (1976–1980)	Low-level participation	Autocratic Outside control	Shallow integration	Anomie Internal decay
1982	High-level participation	Democratic Outside input	Highly integrated	Revitalized
Planned (New Chinautla) (1976–1980)	Moderate-level participation	Autocratic Local control	Ethnic schisms	Competitive
1982	High-level participation	Democratic Local control	Integrated	Reintegrated

each has access to a market and employment environment as well as progressive social institutions such as education and health facilities. The future should be better in each settlement. What has been learned from the postdisaster recovery and reconstruction process are five major points. They are:

1. Economically poor people with limited income production need outside financial, organizational, and legal assistance in recovery to a predisaster level. Left without assistance, such persons remained at a much lower level of living than predisaster; however, a paternalistic attitude (as seen in Roosevelt) also was a destructive force postdisaster. The people lost hope and despaired.

2. Shared decision-making seems essential and most productive (as seen in Carolingia and New Chinautla). Roosevelt victims had little participation in making decisions and although predisaster they had a higher level of living than any of the other victims, they remained on a lower level. How the aid is delivered is as important as how much.

3. The motivation of the agency seems clearly reflected in the satisfaction of the aid given. The most praised agencies were those who were part of the community; that is, they lived and worked there.

4. It seems that all aid given is important, but over time permanent, safe housing was the most significant aid given. Also, planning the total settlement *before* beginning the actual reconstruction also led to a more productive resolution and best use of resources.

5. Continued control of the settlement by the residents makes for a long-term commitment (as seen in Carolingia and New Chinnautla). A usury clause was included, that is, recipients of a new house from a relief agency were prohibited from selling the house. The house could be used as inheritance property, however. This clause protected the agency's investment, and avoided dealing with opportunistic "victims."

CLINICAL IMPLICATIONS

Important strategies used by a therapist or a relief agency are similar in that the strengths of the victim (an individual or an aggregate unit) are mobilized and maximized and new options and resources are identified or provided. These new supports offer an individual, family, or community opportunities for change and growth. Another finding from the NSF Earthquake Study was that even after stagnating for over 4 years, when an opportunity for change was given to the settlers in the Forced and Unplanned Settlements, they were able to rejuvenate and to recover. Human resiliency does not seem to diminish or die, but hope seems to spring eternal. A critical, nonreversible condition does not appear to be pervasive, and change does appear to be a human potential.

REFERENCES

Baker, G., Chapman, R. Man and Society. New York: Basic Books, 1962.

Marris, P. Loss and Change. New York: Random House, 1974.

Marroquin, H. El problema de la vivienda popular. Guatemala City: CIVDU, 1978.

13

The Media in Disaster

Don M. Hartsough
Dennis S. Mileti

It is generally recognized that the mass media are the conduit by which society receives information and on which it forms images of any major disaster. But do the media contribute to disaster psychological effects—both positive and harmful? This chapter will address this general question and provide a brief overview of the influence of the mass media on the psychological effects of disaster. In addition, selected comments will be made specifically regarding the accident at Three Mile Island (TMI).

The TMI accident which began on March 28, 1979, was not under control for several days and remained an incident of international significance for even longer. During that time most of the information and impressions regarding TMI were conveyed to the public by the mass media. Thus, the media actually conveyed to the general public the major dimensions of the accident as it was unfolding. As in other technological incidents, it is only natural that those concerned with assessing the psychological impact of the TMI accident be highly conscious of the likely role played by the mass media as a major determinant of the impacts observed.

For the purposes of this report, media will be defined as television, radio, newspapers, news magazines, and the wire services. Other mass media of interest to researchers would include entertainment media, such as films, fiction and nonfiction books, and others; however, these seem beyond the scope of this report.

There is a great deal of opinion, usually in the form of "conventional wisdom," about the topic of psychological disaster impacts and the mass media, but very little systematic data are actually available. There have been, however, many studies of the effects of mass media on disaster populations regarding warnings. See, for example, Anderson (1969, 1970), Bates et al. (1963), Danzig et al. (1958), Drabek (1969), Leik et al. (1981), McLuckie (1973), Mileti (1974, 1975), Mileti et al. (1981),

Moore (1964), Quarantelli and Taylor (1978), and Turner et al. (1981). To our knowledge, the only study on the topic of postdisaster mass media-related psychological effects is reported by Murphy (Chapter 3). In fact, there seems to be a paucity of scientific studies on the effects of mass media (e.g., television news, newspaper stories) on behavior in general, including all the behavior that occurs in nondisaster situations. The area also seems to lack a comprehensive theoretical base, as noted by the participants at a 1979 workshop on mass media and disasters (Disasters and the Mass Media, 1980). Our aim in this chapter will be to summarize the relationships between the mass media and psychological impacts in reference to two research areas. These are: (1) postdisaster effects (however scarce the information is in this area) and (2) the effects of the media in emergency warning situations as they serve to alter psychological states—thoughts, perceptions, and so forth—and to mobilize people for warning response.

CONVENTIONAL WISDOM REGARDING MASS MEDIA EFFECTS ON DISASTERS

Observers of the mass media in disasters have two different positions. One sees the media as having a positive effect, while the other concludes that they have a net negative effect. The negative position was well stated by Gary A. Kreps, a participant in the National Research Council Workshop:

> There appears to be a long-standing assumption among disaster researchers that the media are deficient in disaster reporting. The media have been accused of inaccurately reporting disaster impacts, of giving undue emphasis to the sudden and dramatic, and of conveying false images about disaster behavior. Concern has been frequently expressed about these and other supposed deficiencies while, at the same time, there is the inevitable admission that very little is known about the effects (positive or negative) of disaster reporting on human behavior. (Kreps, 1980, pp. 40-41)

The media, in other words, are seen as caring less for accurate reporting than sensationalism or at least giving their readers or viewers a "newsworthy story." This position was supported by interview data obtained by Murphy (see Chapter 3).

Conventional wisdom among disaster researchers and observers also has a positive side. The media are seen as having the potential for informing the public of threatening situations, for giving precise warnings, for giving information about disaster impact, and for helping to prevent inappropriate and unwanted behavior, such as widespread convergence on the disaster scene. The media also help to bring aid to the disaster-struck populations. Kreps sees this role of the mass media as simply an extension of what we expect from the media under normal circumstances, that is, the rapid transfer of information to a widespread audience.

There is little doubt that the media occupy an ambivalent position with regard to disaster relief managers and others who have important responsibilities associated with any disaster. A disaster site is filled with emotional tensions, especially if there has been an unexpected, sudden catastrophe. Along with this tension, there is an urgent need to gather, transmit, and receive information. Disaster managers are dependent on the mass media, for example, to convey information to the public that will help the public come to behave in appropriate ways. Because of this extreme dependency, there may be a reluctance to recognize the limitations of the media. To quote Kreps (1980), "We expect a great deal from the media, and we are easily disappointed if expectations are not fulfilled." (p. 47) The media are also highly dependent on disaster managers. If the media are to report information, some reliable source must give this information. Someone must be willing to be quoted and take responsibility for what is said. Given these conditions, it is easy to see how major tensions develop between those with emergency manager roles in a particular disaster and the media that report it. It is not surprising that once the disaster is over, and discrepancies are found, mutual fingerpointing and even scapegoating may take place.

DISASTERS AND NEWSWORTHINESS

Nearly all disaster-type incidents start out as local events reported only by the local media. It is only after they reach a certain level of "newsworthiness" that disasters are reported widely and become national or international events or news. Precisely what is it that propels an incident to become a nationally reported disaster? In so many words, Kreps says that an incident must have significant *physical impact* in order to achieve this status. And how does one assess physical impact? To quote Kreps (1980), "With regard to measurement of impact the focus must necessarily be on relatively readily available measures of the scope (geographic) and the intensity (deaths, injury, property damage, rates of disease, and so forth) of physical impact." (p. 53) The *scope* and *intensity* of a situation are the criteria that determine newsworthiness;

a harmful situation must achieve widespread destruction and/or great geographic significance before it is reported. Kreps also notes in a footnote that, "Social impact is very imprecisely defined and there is little agreement on how it can be measured. Even measures of physical impact may not be finally determined until weeks or months after the disaster—if, in the end, they are ever unequivocally presented." (p. 53)

The point regarding newsworthiness is an extremely important one for understanding the dynamic relationships among disaster events, the general public, and the mass media. It may also be especially important for the long-term psychological effects of disaster. The long-term psychological effects of disaster include not only the immediate effects of the agent itself, but also, and perhaps more importantly, the meaning or significance that that disaster experience comes to have in the life of the individual.

As a case in point, why did TMI become so newsworthy? The TMI reactor accident did not fit the typical pattern of disasters that are widely reported by the mass media. It was limited in geographic *scope* to the Island (to be literal about where it was happening) or to an undefined area downwind of the Island up to about 10 miles. It was also quite limited in *intensity* because there were no deaths or injuries or property damage or diseases to be reported. Three Mile Island came to have great social impact by virtue of the mass evacuation of approximately 144,000 residents, but even before the evacuation was advised, it was newsworthy almost instantly. Why did TMI suddenly become a nationally reported incident, one that carried many of the characteristics of the reporting of more conventional major disasters?

An obvious hypothesis regarding the newsworthiness of TMI concerns the potential danger in the situation. That is, nuclear energy may be perceived to be highly potent and possess great destructive powers if it is not carefully controlled. Moreover, the fact that a nuclear power plant involves a highly complex technology which neither the media nor the public generally understands could fuel public interest in events at such facilities. So the newsworthiness of the TMI incident likely was generated by *potential danger* rather than by actual loss or destruction as was originally suggested by Kreps.

A different hypothesis would cast these perspectives into a somewhat more dynamic arrangement. One might hypothesize that reporters emphasized the potential dangers in the situation in order to *justify* reporting the incident nationally. That is, from an objective point of view, TMI was a serious problem with the machinery at a utility's plant. This was hardly the kind of story that usually achieves instant national notoriety. Perhaps it could not have been reported in an objective way and still have carried the justification for national attention. This alternative hypothesis supposes that to achieve national newsworthiness, the potential scope and intensity of the incident had to be elevated. That is, the focus of reporting came to be as much on what *could* happen as to what *was* happening in order to justify national coverage.

It is unlikely that media reporters consciously or deliberately went through this logical process (as described by the alternative hypothesis). Instead, it is likely that reporters covering the TMI accident unconsciously added their justification for national attention to their story, that is, the potential dangers that they perceived to the area around Middletown and eastern Pennsylvania.

After the TMI accident, it was very difficult to separate a media-induced psychological effect from an "actual" effect, since there were potentially very real dangers at TMI. From one viewpoint, one could call TMI a "media event." This argument would presume that psychological effects stemming from TMI could be laid on the doorstep of the mass media. This view would be just as much in error as one that ignores the very real influence that the media were likely to have had on people's reactions to the TMI incident.

SOME QUESTIONS TO AID IN THE ASSESSMENT OF THE MASS MEDIA IN DISASTERS

Participants in the National Academy of Sciences panel (Disasters and the Mass Media, 1980) posed some questions that helped to guide their assessment of the effects of the mass media on disasters. Five similar questions are proposed here:

1. How accurate are the mass media in reporting disasters and postdisaster situations?
2. How thorough are the mass media in reporting disasters?
3. Do the mass media contribute to the impressions and images of a disaster and its effects?
4. Regardless of the answers to the three questions above, how do the mass media actually affect the behavior of individuals, either positively or negatively, in disaster situations?
5. What are the specific psychological effects of concern, that is, what are the dependent variables and are they adaptive or dysfunctional for individuals and groups involved?

How Accurate Are the Mass Media in Reporting Disasters and Postdisaster Situations?

The mass media are often accused of being inaccurate in basic news reporting. However there seem to be relatively little hard data to demonstrate whether the source of inaccuracy lies more in the sources of information (e.g., disaster managers) or in the reporting of that information. One study, however, does document how the media inflated the status of a disaster prediction study from a scientific hypothesis about an impending earthquake to an actual earthquake "prediction-warning" with ensuing public alarm (cf. Mileti et al., 1981, pp. 39–44).

One repeated fault of media reporters seems to be that of demanding precise and certain information where none exists. They may press disaster managers, such as incident commanders and relief management personnel, for damage estimates, projected decisions, and descriptions of disaster populations which turn out to be pure conjecture. One might easily imagine that the media reporters are in turn responding to other pressures, that is, the needs of editors and ultimately the viewing or reading public, for precise information where none may exist. The result is that the need on the part of reporters can create situations which unfortunately result in inaccuracy in their work. First, they can pressure interviewees until they get information that is unreliable, but which is reported as reliable information. Second, they may get a "no comment" from a legitimate news source but then seek out someone else who is not a legitimate news source but who is willing to give a news story. Third, the media also seek to present both sides of an issue. In disaster situations or in emergency warning settings this practice can create confusion on the part of the public that receives that information (Mileti et al. 1981). These actions produce conflicting information which is inaccurate. At TMI, accurate reporting was particularly difficult because of the complex technology involved in the accident.

How Thorough Are the Mass Media in Reporting Disasters?
The issue of thoroughness is just as important as that of accuracy, because media may wittingly or unwittingly omit certain crucial aspects of a disaster situation from their report of it. The omission may produce a distorted understanding of the total disaster situation. Over the last several decades, media reporting has become more professional, and thus more attention has been given to confirming a news story before reporting it. Still, the pressure of deadlines in disaster situations forces incomplete reporting by the media. Incomplete reporting may be one means of developing or maintaining a "story line," and this pertains to the third question, that of images conveyed to the general public by the media.

Do the Mass Media Contribute to the Impressions and Images of a Disaster and Its Effects?
This question has to do not only with *what* is reported but *how* it is reported. Included here are all the nonverbal cues such as tone of voice

and gesture, and the communication techniques of word selection, scene selection (for television reporting), the use of context, and so on that are used to enliven and give depth to straight reporting. It is widely accepted that news teams select a "slant" or story line which will form the context for reporting of a news event (Frank, 1973). The slant of a news story gives interpretation and meaning to the factual information embodied in the story. For example, the hypothesis was proposed that the slant of the TMI incident was the potential danger of the situation, and it was this slant that allowed the TMI story to become a national event.

It is likely that the general public forms an impression or image of a disaster situation based in large part on the way in which it is conveyed. This is especially true with those who are not familiar with the situation, for example, those who are informed of it only through the mass media.

The general public seems particularly susceptible to image creation, because apparently many people are unaware of the practice of taking slants or story line approaches, and feel that they are getting "straight news." This is especially true for TV news reporting, the medium which is under the greatest constraints to condense its information and thus produces the least amount of factual information. An Opinion Research Corporation poll in 1972 showed that television news reporting was considered as most objective (53 percent) and most complete (63 percent) of all the news media (Frank, 1973). (In contrast to the "most complete" rating given television reporting, newspapers achieved only 19 percent, news magazines 7 percent, and radio 5 percent. In contrast to the television rating of 53 percent, for being most objective, newspapers got only 15 percent.)

It is likely that the question of image creation is concerned primarily with the medium of television. Even though factual information is highly condensed and limited, a sense of objectivity is conveyed by the "on-the-scene reports" that television can produce. Viewers have a sense of "being there" and come away with a feeling of participating somewhat directly in the situation.

Do the mass media produce exaggerated images of most disaster situations? The conventional wisdom of disaster watchers says that this is often so. Of the social scientists, Quarantelli (1980) has been the most persistent in accusing the mass media of keeping alive myths with regard to disaster reactions.

One example that has been documented is the Barseback "panic" in Sweden in 1973. A Swedish radio station broadcasted a fictitious account of a nuclear power station accident to highlight public interest in a discussion about nuclear energy risks and advantages. Although the broadcast took only 11 minutes, it was accepted by some people as an account of an actual situation. In studying media response to the situation, Rosengren et al. (1974) concluded that the media had exaggerated the extent to which the listening public had experienced strong reactions of fear and anger, and very much exaggerated or even invented the stories of panic flight that were supposed to have occurred. Thus, the image of panic regarding the incident was largely media-produced. (This incident is reminiscent of the "War of the Worlds" broadcast that received a similar kind of treatment from journalists and even social scientists in this country.)

The Barseback incident demonstrated several sources of false image creation. First, journalists, as well as social scientists, may overgeneralize from a few individuals to the general public. That is, they may project the actions, attitudes, and behavior of only a few individuals to a wider population. Journalists may be especially prone to overgeneralize if the atypical behavior observed is newsworthy. A second source of false images can occur when only a small number of people happen to converge on one point in the communication network. One thousand frightened people calling mass media switchboards or police stations represents a tremendous increase in the usual number of calls, even though one thousand people is only one tenth of 1 percent of a population of one million. To generalize to the population of one million would be a mistake. Of course, one thousand is still a significant number of frightened people if they all converge at one place in a short time span.

Dupont reviewed 13 hours of videotapes of nuclear energy broadcasts from the three major networks on their evening news programs between August 5, 1968 and April 20, 1979—a period encompassing the TMI accident. In DuPont's view, fear was the motif of the entire series of nuclear stories.

> Reporters do not play a reassuring role because there is interest in disaster, and because the reporters are worried that if the worst case should come up and they don't signal it in advance, they haven't given the facts to the people. They would be found guilty of minimizing a potential problem, a *what if*. They would be "in bed" with the "authorities," and they do not want to be found guilty of that. So they have got to talk about the risks and be cautious of reassurance. For example, at Three Mile Island the bottom line in the media coverage was not that no one was hurt. The bottom line was: we narrowly averted a nuclear holocaust, a nuclear catastrophe, the ultimate. As Walter Cronkite said, "The world has never known a day quite like

today. It faced . . . the worst nuclear power plant accident of
the atomic age." This is the bottom line of the public's awareness. The Three Mile Island experience is going to be a dominant image, probably for the next decade, because it has been
burned into the collective consciousness, largely through television news. (DuPont, 1980, pp. 13–14)

Many studies of emergency warnings *before* disasters occur have
been performed which document how information—including media information—contributes to public images and perceptions of a potential
disaster and its effects (Mileti et al., 1975). The conclusion is that the
media, along with other sources of information, are the key factor that
determines public response (Mileti et al., 1981).

How Do the Mass Media Actually Affect the Behavior of Individuals, Either Positively or Negatively, in Disaster Situations?

In terms of psychological effects, this is the bottom line question. One
must first define what is a positive or a negative reaction to disaster.
If an individual answers a questionnaire that he or she has "been much
more afraid since the disaster" or "become more demoralized since a
disaster" will the investigator be satisfied with this opinion, or search
further for the form of behavior that the fear or demoralization took?

It is necessary to look at behavior in terms of time sequences related to the disaster situation. There is more information available on
predisaster behavior and mass media than there is for either the immediate or long-run postdisaster phases. An overall conclusion is that the
media—which are the major "givers" of information to the public in
emergencies—have a profound effect on the predisaster behavior of individuals.

The process that research suggests as the best description of how
people come to respond to disaster warning information is relatively
straightforward (Mileti et al., 1981). First, people receive risk information. This information comes from a variety of sources including official warnings, neighbors and friends, and the like; however, most
comes from the media. Second, people evaluate the information that
is available to them. If information from multiple sources—or information from the same source over repeated communications—is consistent, that risk information is psychologically confirmed through
reinforcement with a resulting increase in trust and belief. If information
is inconsistent or confused it is less likely believed and people may
become confused or anxious. People typically seek confirmation and
reinforcement of risk information during times of receiving disaster

warning information from any source. Third, on the basis of available information, be it confirmed and reinforced or conflicting and unreinforced, people form situational perceptions of risk—be they accurate or not. Fourth, people respond to disaster warnings on the basis of the perception of risk that they hold.

This general process rarely operates in this straightforward a fashion in the real world. The process is typically altered by a number of real-world factors that reshape the general model. However, human response to emergency information or warnings is directly affected by the characteristics of the information received. Warning information is information to which people respond after that information is processed. Information differs in six important ways that affect human response. These are: (1) *warning content*—for example, information consistency, specificity, clarity, and message content; (2) *communication mode*—how the information is transmitted, for example, in person, or through the media; (3) *number received*—how many warning communications are actually received, for example, none, one, several, or dozens; (4) *perceived* certainty—how certain or sure the person giving the information seems to the person receiving the information; (5) *source*—who the information comes from, for example, a stranger, a friend, an official, or someone in a uniform; (6) *perceived trust*—how much the person receiving the information trusts the person giving the information.

More people will respond more appropriately to disaster warning information if those warnings—or risk information: (1) come from people they trust, respect or define as authority figures—the effect is enhanced if the givers of information are familiar persons, in uniforms, or high-ranking officials; (2) are delivered by the media with a good deal of certainty in reference to what information is being communicated; (3) are numerous, such that many communications are received rather than a few; (4) are delivered in some personal way or the information conveyed is personalized by the media rather than made general or vague; and (5) are consistent in content to enhance information reinforcement (rather than conflicting in content), clearly stated, and contain specific information rather than general information. These factors which affect human response are largely under the control of the media.

Put simply, people respond to disaster warning information differently because people respond to perceptions of risk or cognitive definitions of danger rather than to the danger that actually exists, and different people hold different perceptions of risk in disaster warning situations. Perhaps most significantly, risk perceptions are most strongly shaped by the varied dimensions and aspects of the disaster warnings—risk information—that are received from the media.

Immediately postdisaster, the mass media are concerned with providing information about the disaster situation. As the situation gradually becomes known by the general public, the media influence may have much more to do with conveying significance or meaning to the event rather than simply providing information.

MODEL OF MASS MEDIA-DISASTER RELATIONSHIPS

There has been a tendency in the communications field to use a straight linear model of effects of the mass media on a particular population or situation. A linear model implies a series of cause–effect relationships, somewhat analogous to a set of billiard balls in a straight line on a pool table. In the disaster area, a linear model would resemble the following chain of cause–effect: The disaster agent produces a situation that is assessed and reported by a disaster manager to representatives from the mass media, who then pass on the information to the general public, and individuals in the general public have certain psychological effects. In this model each stage or level is considered as a cause for the reaction that occurs in the next stage.

More recently, communications experts are using what was labeled by the National Academy of Sciences Workshop participants (Disasters and the Mass Media, 1980) as a flow model, which also might be labeled a cybernetic model. This is, a model that considers the interplay of forces on each other, as a total system of interdependent influences. An example is that disaster managers may give out selective information about the disaster agent in order to produce certain kinds of influences on the general public. In turn, the mass media reporters are influenced by impressions of what they feel the general public wants to know or should not know. The mass media have pressures on them for certain kinds of reporting and they impose these on the reporting situation. Newspapers and television stations are private enterprise companies, and may select to report or not report information which will effect their business. The disaster managers are strongly influenced, one might suppose, by their perceptions of how they think the public will react to whatever it is that they report. Thus, they are not simply reporting what they know about the disaster situation as unbiased observers, but they are anticipating how this information will be received by the general public. In turn, the general public is not a passive recipient of information but may directly or indirectly make certain demands on those who report the information to them.

A comprehensive analysis of the influence of the media on psychological effects of disaster should attempt to come to grips with at least the major dimensions of these interdependent forces. For example, it seems reasonable to believe that the reporting of TMI as an isolated incident could not be separated from the context of nuclear power as a controversial and generally emotional issue for many members of the general public. One might guess that media representatives were quite aware of the potential significance of TMI as related to this issue, and that this awareness may have influenced how they reported the event.

The bottom line, however, is that people respond and are affected by the information and the manner in which information is exchanged about an impending disaster. That information and its story line message is the basis for their perceived realities. During the TMI incident, for example, media-provided information may have been instrumental in determining public repsonse because the media largely controlled the factors that affect human response.

REFERENCES

Anderson, W.A. Disaster warning and communication processes in two communities. Journal of Communication, 1969, *19*, 92–104.

Anderson, W.A. Tsunami warning in Crescent City, California and Hilo, Hawaii. In The Great Alaska Earthquake of 1964: Human Ecology. Washington D.C.: National Research Council, National Academy of Sciences, 1970.

Bates, F.L., Fogelman, C.W., Parenton, V.I., et al. The Social and Psychological Consequences of a Natural Disaster. National Academy of Sciences National Research Council Disaster Study No. 18. Washington, D.C.: National Academy of Sciences, 1963.

Danzig, E.R., Thayer, P.W., Galanter, L.R. The Effects of a Threatening Rumor on a Disaster-Stricken Community. National Academy of Sciences, National Research Council Disaster Study No. 10. Washington, D.C.: National Academy of Sciences, 1958.

Disasters and the Mass Media, Washington, D.C.: National Academy of Sciences, 1980.

Drabek, T.E. Social processes in disaster: Family evacuation. Social Problems, 1969, *16*, 336–349.

DuPont, R.L. Nuclear Phobia—Phobic Thinking About Nuclear Power. Washington, D.C.: The Media Institute, 1980.

Frank, R.S. Message Dimensions of Television News. Toronto: Lexington Books, 1973.

Kreps, J.A. Research needs and policy issues on mass media disaster reporting. In Disasters and the Mass Media. Washington, D.C.: National Academy of Sciences, 1980.

Leik, R.K., et al. Community Response to Natural Hazard Warnings. University of Minnesota, Department of Sociology, 1981.

McLuckie, B.F. The Warning System: A Sociological Perspective. Department of Commerce, National Oceanic and Atmospheric Administration. Fort Worth, Texas: National Weather Service, Southern Region, 1973.

Mileti, D.S. A normative causal model analysis of disaster warning response. Doctoral thesis. Boulder: University of Colorado, Department of Sociology, 1974.

Mileti, D.S. Natural hazard warning systems in the United States: A research assessment. Boulder: University of Colorado Institute of Behavioral Science, 1975.

Mileti, D.S., Drabek, T., Haas, J. Human systems in extreme environments: A sociological perspective. Boulder: University of Colorado Institute of Behavioral Science, 1975.

Mileti, D.S., et al. Earthquake prediction response and options for public policy. Boulder: University of Colorado Institute of Behavioral Science, 1981.

Moore, H.E. And the Winds Blew. Austin, Texas: The Hogg Foundation for Mental Health, University of Texas, 1964.

Quarantelli, E.L. Some research emphases for studies on mass communication systems and disasters. In Disasters and the Mass Media. Washington, D.C.: National Academy of Sciences, 1980.

Quarantelli, E.L., Taylor, V. Some views on the warning problem in disasters as suggested by sociological research. Weather Service Disaster Preparedness Report, February 1978, Special Issue. Washington, D.C.: Department of Commerce, 1978.

Rosengren, K.E., Arvidson, P., Sturesson, D. The Barseback "panic": A radio programme as a negative summary event. Acta Sociologica, 1974, *18*, 303-321.

Turner, R.H., Nigg, J.M., Paz, et al., Community response to earthquake threat in Southern California, Part Ten, Summary and Recommendations. Los Angeles: Institute for Social Science Research, University of California, 1981.

14

Observations on the Media
and Disaster Recovery Period

Jacob D. Lindy
Joanne G. Lindy

Contemporary media have the capacity to exert powerful influence over the ways in which populations at risk prepare for, experience, and work through the material and psychological effects of disasters. This assertion is informed by the authors' experiences as consultants and primary service providers in several disaster situations and by our observations of the positive and negative impacts of the media in these situations.

To date, the subject of the psychological impact of media on the recovery process of disaster survivors has not been addressed in the mental health literature. A recent monograph on media and terrorists (Miller, 1982) approaches the subject but emphasizes political rather than emotional implications. The purpose of this contribution therefore is to report and discuss the phenomena we have observed in order to assist future disaster workers and sketch areas for additional reports and research. The specific disasters mentioned in this chapter include: the Buffalo Creek Dam collapse, the Xenia, Ohio, and Wichita Falls, Texas tornadoes, the Beverly Hills Supper Club fire, the mass suicide at Jonestown, Guyana, and the Crush at the "Who" Concert, Cincinnati, Ohio. A brief description of each of these events appears in the text as appropriate illustrations are made. See Chapter 3 for the role of the media in the volcanic eruption of Mount St. Helens.

For purposes of this report, the term "media" is defined as "the means of acquisition, processing, and dissemination of information to and from large numbers of people. These include but are not limited to radio, television, newspapers, and most importantly individual owners, reporters, technicians, and producers." (Lobue and Gressit, 1982). The media acquires, processes, and disseminates information at each of the major phases of disaster: warning, impact, rescue operations, inventory, short-term recovery, and long-term recovery. Throughout this chapter we shall be discussing the impact of media on survivors during each of these phases. As we do so we shall be viewing the phenomena from three points of reference: first, the internal experience of the survivors as they attempt to negotiate the external reality and internal psychological experiences of survival and recovery; second, the role(s) of media as it carries out society's tasks of becoming informed regarding the events of the time; third, the potential range of action of the mental health professional throughout the different phases, as these pertain to media.

WARNING PHASE

At each phase in the disaster situation media takes on functions in different relationship to the survivor. During the warning phase, media in our technological society has come to represent an extension of our perceptual apparatus. We have come to rely on radio and television in particular to warn us of natural hazards such as tornadoes, hurricanes, and flash floods. The reliability of this information represents part of our basic trust in authorities vested with responsibilities regarding protection of the populus at large. In this context during the warning phase of a disaster accurate information via media is processed into life-saving preparatory activities and the decreasing of life-endangering activities. At the same time there are powerful forces at work internally which act so as to deny the reality of the warnings transmitted. The audience at the Beverly Hills Supper Club fire, when first informed of the fire, thought it was part of the comedy act. Faulty perception of realistic danger may arise through denial of accurate warning or incorrect media communication. Deliberately faulty information is experienced with the most profound traumatic disillusionment and enduring distrust.

WICHITA FALLS TORNADO
The Wichita Falls, Texas tornado (1979) was one of the worst in this country's recent history in terms of extent of destruction, literally flattening a strip through the city one-half mile wide. It appeared remarkable that there were only five deaths.

Shortly after a tornado was sighted within potential striking distance of Wichita Falls, Texas radio and television broadcasts notified inhabitants of the precise positions they were to take with regard to shelter and protection in case the tornado moved into their city. Most houses did not have basements. People were instructed to climb into their tubs with their children on the ground floor and to place mattresses on top of the tubs to protect from overhead damage. People were cautioned not to be in their automobiles. Compliance with this public service announcement saved scores of lives in an otherwise devastating tornado. Successful warning was the first step in the community's effective banding together—a quality which sustained itself into the recovery phase.

THREE MILE ISLAND NUCLEAR ACCIDENT

A radio station near Harrisburg, Pennsylvania received contradictory material with regard to the potential hazards of the approaching nuclear meltdown at Three Mile Island. Radio officials chose to relay to nearby inhabitants the reassurances offered by company and state officials rather than to report the alarm expressed by scientists who were calling into the station and the indirect evidence that there was indeed a crisis at the reactor as measured by traffic flow to and from the plant. The misleading data with regard to degree of danger ultimately became a major psychological stressor when considered separately and have led to profound distrust of authority in that region. Later, the misleading data contributed to fragmentation in the recovery environment.

IMPACT PHASE

During the impact phase of disaster, the survivor is faced with unexpected devastation, threat to life, and loss of loved ones. Behavior is aimed at self-preservation and the safety of loved ones. Psychologically there is often the paradoxical presence of coping behaviors, psychic overload, and defenses against appreciating the reality of absurd events. From the vantage point of media the survivor now becomes the point of acquisition for information that will be broadly disseminated.

During the impact phase survivors' eyewitness accounts are now news. Their anguish, grief, and terror are the subjects of photographs, films, and videotapes. There is an asynchrony here between the needs of the survivor and the needs of media. For the survivor decreasing any unnecessary increment of traumatic input is central. The survivor needs time to recoil, to gather strength from loved ones, and only later is there a spontaneous need or "will to bear witness" (Deprès). Thus during this phase the needs of the media and the needs of the survivor are at odds with each other. Under these circumstances, there is the danger of potential damage that media interviewers and camera-operators may add to psychic overload in some survivors, contributing to long-remembered traumatic reactions.

During the impact phase of disaster, sensitive coverage of human catastrophe can bind survivors with a larger community of sympathetic neighbors while insensitive coverage of traumatic events exposes already vulnerable individuals to further traumatic intrusion, invading privacy, confidentiality, and provoking psychic overload.

Rarely is the mental health professional in a position to modify the dangers of traumatic overload at this point. However, an interesting intervention at a temporary morgue outside the Beverly Hills Supper Club is worth reporting.

BEVERLY HILLS SUPPER CLUB FIRE

The Beverly Hills Supper Club fire (1977) razed to the ground Greater Cincinnati's largest and most fashionable multipurpose supper club. More than 2500 people were inside the building when the fire started. There were 165 deaths.

Many of the deceased were transferred to a nearby temporary morgue where survivors and family anxiously gathered. Reporters quickly arrived on the scene. One family group had just identified a relative who had died. It was 10 minutes before the next regular newscast. A news team with reporter, without any introduction to this family, was about to televise a live impromptu interview. A mental health worker who had accompanied the family through the morgue could anticipate the added trauma this interview would likely cause. She intervened by speaking with the representative from the television crew and eliciting some of the television crew's own response to the disaster. Empathy worked. In the course of this several-minute contact, the reporter changed his strategy with the family and decided to sit down with them and spend some time getting to know them. Later an interview was broadcast which appeared effective and respectful.

RESCUE PHASE

During the rescue phase of a catastrophe, media provide the neurons which connect the emergency relief operation. Mass media announcements contribute in keeping roads cleared and calling in needed expertise. More limited media, such as citizen band (CB) radio, addresses specific needs of survivors. If mental health emergency "relief" is to be included, it must tap into that media network at this phase. It was the use of CB radio which provided the communication network for clergy of the Greater Cincinnati Area to set up a family reception center for families of the deceased (in conjunction with Red Cross, coroner's office, and other agencies) after the Beverly Hills Supper Club fire.

A negative side effect of media's role during the rescue phase is that occasionally unscreened or poorly processed media messages expose volunteers to hardships they are ill-prepared to master.

In the hours following the Beverly Hills Supper Club fire it became clear to those working with the coroner at the temporary morgue that many bodies (the total at that time was unknown) would be unrecognizable because of being charred in the blaze. A needed resource would be dental technicians to take teeth imprints from such remains in order to establish positive identification of the dead. Dental technicians responded to radio broadcast requests that there was need for their services. Poorly prepared for the grotesque sights and smells which were to come, these dental technicians intending to help in the rescue operation became traumatized by their overexposure to the grotesque. In several instances clear posttraumatic stress disorder followed.

Finally, large-scale disruption may wipe out usual centers of communication. In one instance, media and mental health simply switched roles; during the Xenia tornado, it happened that the mental health center, the only building not hit, voluntarily took on the position of being the major switchboard for relief services.

INVENTORY

During the inventory phase media reports on the extent of damage and loss. It provides urgent news to pockets of evacuated survivors regarding the fate of others. Media also begins to focus on the set of conditions that precipitated the disaster. There is an urgent, and often incomplete search for responsibility. In natural disasters this tends to focus on faulty reporting of early warning signs of disaster or faulty communication of accurate reports. In man-made disasters there is a search for inadequate inspections or inadequate equipment. Out of these early assessments come the first wave of more generalized vantage points from which society as a whole is beginning to see the nature of the particular catastrophe. These generalized media viewpoints have a major impact on the recovery process psychologically with survivors.

The survivors, beginning to come to grips with the extent of their losses, are keenly interested in the cause of the disaster as well. Intrapsychically this is a period of intense survivor guilt (why is it that I survived and others died) as well as its projection—excessive blame. In one instance, media coverage during the inventory phase blamed the survivors themselves and contributed to both an increase in survivor guilt and defensive rage against the accusation.

CRUSH AT "THE WHO" CONCERT
Thousands of teenagers and young adults stood in near-freezing temperatures in an open square for hours awaiting the opening of the doors of Riverfront Coliseum for the "Who" rock concert. One door was opened, and music from inside the building drifted to the crowd. A rumor quickly spread that the concert had begun, and the large mass pressed against the single doorway like toothpaste being squeezed through an opening that is too small. Many people fainted or fell in the congestion; 11 were crushed to death.

On the day following the disaster an article appearing in the Chicago paper explained the event as being the result of "young barbarians."

The article served as an added noxious stimulus. It tapped into a latent anti-"rock," anti-adolescent bias; and was in danger of dividing the community's support ("they got what they deserve") at a point when it was most needed ("these are the children of all of us"). Clinicians manning a disaster "hotline" became aware of the additional pain teenagers and young adults, already stressed and grieving, were experiencing as a result of this media "assault on the survivors." Many youngsters in fact had made even heroic efforts to engage the police (who were standing nearby) in an effort to organize the waiting crowd; others had literally risked their lives in saving others.

In this instance mental health professionals through media activity made a concerted effort at a local level (and national) to offer a countertone (more empathic to the survivors and their parents) which portrayed more compassionately the experience of those who had gone through the disaster, with good results.

SHORT-TERM RECOVERY PHASE

Two aspects of media activity during the first year following disaster are of special importance: (1) public education and outreach, and (2) a consolidating viewpoint with regard to the nature of the disaster.

Public Education
Previously healthy individuals exposed to trauma and loss in disaster need not feel alarmed if they experience transient episodes of some sleep disturbance, nightmares, difficulty concentrating, and irritability. Families and naturally occurring support groups should be encouraged to talk about the events and to offer support. More severe instances of stress reaction should be referred to specially trained clinicians. A wide variety of means exists in the recovery phase to communicate these and other messages to survivors, including public service announcements, local news "spots," newspaper columns and feature articles, television specials, talk shows, and so forth.

The Mental Health Professional Relies Heavily on Media Collaboration in Outreach Programs in the Aftermath of Disaster
Following the Beverly Hills Supper Club fire, media actively assisted mental health professionals in contacting nearly 500 survivors. One hundred and fifty agreed to participate in extensive research. In the course of that work (Lindy et al., 1981) we learned several points: (1) media can be an effective arm for mental health outreach, and (2) survivors drawn to outreach by different types of media constitute differing groups in terms of stress and impairment. For example, those respond-

ing to newspaper, radio, and television were more significantly impaired than those responding to letter or telephone. Further, written media (magazines and newspaper columns) were more effective means for bringing severely impaired survivors to treatment than were television or radio. We speculated that such differences might be the result of a survivor's tendency to wish to "turn off" unwanted stimuli which tend to recreate intrusive imagery: thus media that are available at the time that the survivor wishes to make use of them (as in an article) tend to be more useful than visual stimuli which unexpectedly activate traumatic memory.

LONG-TERM RECOVERY PHASE

Later in the recovery phase, the media through editorials or more thoughtful pieces, attempts to put the disaster in some context or perspective. The precise wording used, for example, "flood" or "dam collapse," or "stampede" or "crush," become important in fixing this particular event and the nature of the experience of those who went through it. For example, inaccurate early assessments by the Governor of West Virginia at the Buffalo Creek Dam collapse termed the disaster an "act of God," a flood. Later, reference to the defective slag dam which caused the flood became explicit in media coverage, and the event was termed the Buffalo Creek Disaster.

At times the dominant media perspective has been sharply at odds with the dominant perception of the survivors themselves. This, for example, was the case of American media coverage of the returning Vietnam veteran during most of the first decade following that war. Preoccupations with the Cally Trial and with the national sense of shame at both the conduct and outcome of the war cast a tarnished light on those who risked their lives for their country, depriving them of the patriotic return home. Here the contrast in media presentation from the veteran as causative agent in a shameful war to patriotic combatant survivor of a political and military error has been crucial in the recovery process.

Similarly recent Israeli coverage of the evacuation of cities in the Sinai such as Yamit and Ophira tended to view the returning settlers as enraged radicals rather than as involuntary refugees who were giving up their dreams with dignity. Mental health workers on the scene in this instance were unable to influence the media perspective (J. Rosenfeld, personal communication, 1983).

Anniversary coverage of a major disaster appears to be a standard practice both locally and nationally. Media, here, seem to be responding to a societal need to mark major events by observing the anniversary. Survivors, anticipating such attention, and fleeing from the impact of internally driven "anniversary reactions," fear and avoid exposure to such media activity.

Interestingly, this dilemma may offer some creative opportunities for mental health workers in collaboration with the media. One year after the Beverly Hills fire there was an effort on the part of national media to utilize the network built through mental health efforts at outreach as a means to gather access to a relevant group of survivors for anniversary broadcasts. Concurrently there was an effort by mental health professionals to offer a public format for meaningful working through within this context. In one instance a black newscaster from a national network was so moved that he spontaneously joined the singing of the gospel choir severely traumatized by the Beverly Hills fire. His presence in the brief newsclip over national television provided an instance of linking the group tragedy with a compassionate response from the nation as a whole.

Anniversary coverage of major disasters places local journalists sometimes in an unique relationship with certain traumatized families. It is common that in order to meet the need for anniversary news coverage they will return to families whom they have interviewed one year earlier. Where relationships are good between media and mental health professionals, such supportive contact over time had led to successful referral in otherwise highly traumatized and isolated family units.

In any discussion of the media and disaster from a mental health perspective we would be remiss if we did not include some discussion of the mental health risk to those whose role it is to cover major disasters for the media. Camera operators, announcers, and technicians are exposed for long hours to traumatic conditions and to overexposure to the grotesque. Those working in such roles often do so for long hours without regard to the effects of their own mental health. Media personnel are at high risk for the development of posttraumatic stress disorder. Like other rescue workers in the line of duty they stand the risk of being overexposed to the traumatic events. In our research group's public presentation at the Ohio Hospital Association Meeting, Spring of 1978 we were struck by the number of people in the press who had and continued to have symptoms of posttraumatic stress disorder as a result of their exposure to the Beverly Hills fire.

Another more severe illustration of this was the media coverage of the mass suicide at Jonestown, Guyana. For days there was little to do but to photograph hundreds of decaying and bloated bodies. Stress reactions in the camera crews were severe (H. Sukdheo, personal

communication, 1980). Members of the media may become survivor—chronicles of disaster.

SUMMARY

Our experience has shown that each phase of disaster aftermath offers
opportunities for the media to assist or to impede survivors' recovery.
During the warning phase, accurate communication of potential danger with specific steps to minimize damage helps maintain a trusting
attitude between victims and survivors and the authority structure of
the community, and facilitates recovery. Inaccurate information during the warning phase which unnecessarily places at risk exposed
population (as in Three Mile Island) results in long-lasting suspiciousness and hostility toward authority and impairs recovery. During the
impact phase, perceived exploitation by media in efforts to cover the
human interest aspects of disaster constitutes added psychic trauma
and therefore impairs recovery. During inventory and recovery phases,
assessment of responsibility on to the disaster victims themselves,
stimulates rage and survivor guilt and impairs recovery. Accurate, compassionate overviews of the responsibility for a disaster promote a recovery environment conducive toward resolution of trauma and loss.

To the degree that mental health activities are viewed within the
context of overall community disaster emergency services and to the
degree that alliances with media have been built during earlier stages
of planning and work, media can become a cooperative and effective
partner in carrying out specific mental health activities such as public
service announcements and outreach. With this increased awareness
of the power of the media it behooves mental health professionals to
study in more systematic ways some of the themes outlined in this
chapter. Furthermore, a broadly based preventive psychiatry stance
calls on the mental health professional to develop alliances with our
colleagues in the media that permit consultation and collaboration
throughout the recovery process.

REFERENCES

Lindy, J., Grace, M., Green, B. Survivors: Outreach to a reluctant population,
    American Journal of Orthopsychiatry, 1981, *51* 3, 468.
Lobue, A., Gressit, S. Editorial, Psychiatry and the Media, 1982, *1*, 1.
Miller, A. Terrorism, the Media and the Law. New York: Transnational Publica-
    tions, 1982.

Epilogue: The Blizzard

[This is a personal account by Dr. Laube of her experience in the "Blizzard of '78" in Indianapolis.]

I had spent 7 years in the study of disaster, but had never experienced a disaster myself. Suddenly I was "on the other side." For myself, it was little more than inconvenience. However, for many around me it was much more.

It was Wednesday. I had to stay late at work to keep some appointments. About 4:30 P.M. someone came into my area and said there was a news bulletin—that a heavy snow storm was coming and that driving would be impossible. At that time it was too late to cancel my 5:00 P.M. appointment, but I did call my 7:00 P.M. appointment. I told her the news and asked if she would like to change her appointment. Her response was that an Indiana blizzard doesn't mean anything—after all she was from Minnesota and she was used to driving in much worse than anything that could occur in Indiana! I must have been in agreement as I stayed and kept the appointment. I put the storm warnings out of my mind, which was not difficult to do, as I was in a windowless room.

At 8:15 P.M., I left the building and went out into the STORM. Snow was coming down hard, and the wind was blowing at 35 to 40 miles per hour. I had difficulty in walking to my car parked less than a block away because of the strong wind and snow obscuring my vision.

Driving home was difficult. Snow was blowing into the windshield, and the window wipers iced up considerably, decreasing visibility. I was very cold as the car was slow to heat. I came to a red light and slid crosswise through the intersection. Thankfully, no car was coming through. Very few cars were on the road. I was wishing that I wasn't on the road with my car!

I could not get home through my usual route. I tried different approaches to avoid steep hills that could not be traversed. I, as well as my few fellow travelers, had to make dangerous U-turns in the dark, icy streets that proved to be impassable. My travel time that evening was 1 hour and 30 minutes; the usual travel time is 20 minutes. I did reach home safely, though, and found my family all home, safe. I listened to the news reports informing the listeners that we were in a blizzard, that travel warnings were in effect, and that conditions would not change for several hours. My husband decided to check in at the hotel where he worked. He made it in safely. That was the last time I saw him until the roads were sufficiently clear for him to make it back Saturday afternoon, 3 days later!

Now, what did I do in this crisis? How did I cope? Well, in the first place, I was home and knew the whereabouts of my family—that they were safe. Following the steps I have outlined previously in this book, my next step was to report to my previously assigned duty post, if I had one. This was not so in my case. Next step was to be available by telephone for a call from the Red Cross or authorities of the Medical Center where I taught and to listen to the radio or television for requests for additional disaster workers. With no calls, and because I could not travel (I could not get out of my driveway because of the 6-foot snowdrifts), I stayed at home with my son but experienced some feelings of guilt because I was not involved in rescue efforts or disaster work.

What were the effects of the blizzard? The winds and snow began on Wednesday, January 25. On Thursday morning the following announcement was given through one radio station: "All schools are closed, all offices are closed, all businesses are closed, Indianapolis is closed." The Friday morning headlines of the Indianapolis Star read: "Worst Blizzard in Its History Makes a Ghost Town of Indy." Passengers were stranded. Airline travelers were either shuttled to hotels which soon were bursting at their seams or they were marooned at the airport along with the terminal workers. Bus, train, and car passengers were housed in Red Cross shelters, churches, and even private homes.

Both adventure and horror stories have come out of the blizzard about Indiana travelers. To illustrate: a southbound Floridian train was snowbound in Bainbridge, a small town just west of Indianapolis. The following excerpt from a newspaper account tells the rest of the story for that group.

> The Bainbridge fire department, in conjunction with two Lousville and Nashville locomotives brought to the other side of the drift, did the job (rescue). Passengers and crew were ferried to the fire station and then to Bainbridge United Methodist Church. All were safe and starting to get warm by 6:00 A.M. Friday. "We ate like kings," Cummings recalled later

about the homecooked cuisine. Sleeping on the church pews covered with foam pads brought no complaints. Bainbridge residents opened their homes to the stranded visitors for showers and phone calls. Local residents brought toys, games and even their own small children to entertain the 14 youngest passengers. A songfest was held Saturday morning which roused any late sleepers in the church.

By 3:00 P.M. Saturday, Gonzalez had arranged the beginning of the end of the adventure. Local officials had volunteered North Putnam school buses to make the trip to Indianapolis, and Amtrak had lined up rooms in the Holiday Inn.

The Floridian passengers and crew left Bainbridge to the accompaniment of an emotional scene with many vowing to return. Plans already have been started for a reunion next fall to coincide with a fall festival at Bainbridge. (Rubenton, 1978)

During this same time period, a northbound Floridian also became snowbound. From the same newspaper account comes the fate of that group of passengers and crew.

Passengers on the northbound Floridian, which was stuck in Lafayette, were not so lucky. The 27 travelers, plus crew members, stayed on the train for almost three days before checking into a motel early Sunday morning. By Sunday evening, 15 passengers remained stranded . . . the Amtrak crew kept the train well heated, and three meals a day were catered on board. Passengers complained, however, that some were threatened with arrest if they tried to disembark. (Rubenton, 1978)

"Where'd Everybody Go?" This was one Indianapolis Star headline that captured the scene of Indianapolis and most of Indiana during this period. The only people able to travel were those with snowmobiles, skis, four-wheel-drive vehicles, snow plows, or helicopters. These people, aided considerably by citizens' band radio operators, took the sick and injured to hospitals and delivered food, emergency supplies, and medicine to the stranded people. With supplies somewhat low but sufficient, hospitals and hotels were filled to capacity.

On Monday, January 30, Indianapolis was slowly returning to "business." Businesses reopened, and people were beginning to make their way on the slick, but generally passable, major roads to their places of work. Snow emergency and curfew orders were lifted, limited metro bus service resumed, stranded travelers moved on to their planned destinations, and law enforcement agencies returned to full capacity for the first time since the blizzard struck the area late Wednesday, January 25.

How were people handling their emotions during the storm? Reports from local crisis units and emergency rooms vary as to psychological reactions. "Cabin fever" was the greatest complaint with accompanying restlessness, agitation, and/or active aggression. One "C.B.er" said that while he was monitoring Channel 9 (the emergency channel), a call came from a man to be taken to a psychiatric unit because he kept beating his wife and children. When dispatching this message for assistance, the "C.B.er" said he received resistance in that it was not perceived as a medical emergency. However, he persevered in his request and was successful in securing transportation for the man. As the "C.B.er" said, "One or more lives may have been saved in that action."

Losses due to the storm were high. Over 14 deaths were attributed to the blizzard. In addition, there were a number of personal injuries, frostbite cases, and illnesses directly attributed to the weather and related conditions. Economic losses, although hard to measure, were estimated to be high. With the closing of a highly industrialized and commercialized area, the total loss ran into the millions.

How do you end a story on the Blizzard of '78? The Mayor of Indianapolis organized a 1-year anniversary party. T-shirts were distributed with the following imprinted on the front: "I survived the blizzard of '78." However, the impact of that blizzard will long be felt.

How do I feel now that I have experienced, albeit in a somewhat small way, a disaster? There is a feeling of inadequacy, of having witnessed a scene that cannot be totally expressed, but there is a feeling of warmth toward my neighbors as I recall how we had checked on each other's welfare during the storm. We exchanged needed food and supplies and cooperated in securing someone with a heavy snowplow to shovel our driveways and street. My lingering feelings are sorrow for those who suffered losses and thankfulness for my own and my family's safety and well-being.

REFERENCES

Rubenton, N. Some travelers won't forget Indiana. The Indianapolis Star, January 30, 1978.

Appendix: Summary Table of Behavior Symptoms and Treatment Options

The Institute for the Studies of Destructive Behaviors and the Los Angeles Suicide Prevention Center

SUMMARY TABLE OF BEHAVIOR SYMPTOMS AND TREATMENT OPTIONS: AGE GROUP — 1 THROUGH 18*

Ages	Behavior Symptoms			Possible Treatment Options
	Regressive	Body	Emotions	
1–5	Resumption of bed-wetting, thumbsucking, fear of darkness	Loss of appetite Indigestion Vomiting Bowel or bladder problems, e.g., diarrhea, constipation, loss of sphincter control Sleep disorders	Nervousness Irritability Disobedience Intractability Tics (muscle spasms) Speech difficulties, e.g., appearance of stammering or stuttering Refusal to leave proximity of parents	Give additional verbal assurance and ample physical comfort, e.g., holding and caressing. Warm milk and comforting bedtime routines Permit child to sleep in parents' room temporarily if necessary; if symptoms persist, refer to professional. Provide opportunity and encouragement for expression of emotions through play activities, e.g., finger painting, clay modeling, physical reenactment of disaster.
5–11	Increased competition with younger siblings for parents' attention	Headaches Complaints of visual or hearing problems Persistent itching and scratching	School phobia Withdrawal from play group and friends Withdrawal from family contacts	Give additional attention and consideration. Gentle but firm insistence on relatively more responsibility than would be expected from younger child

Age	Behavior	Approach
	Sleep disorders	Temporarily lessen requirements for optimum performance in school and home activities.
	Unusual social behavior, e.g., fighting with close friends or siblings	Encourage verbal expression of thoughts and feelings about the disaster.
	Loss of interest in previously preferred activities	Provide opportunity for structured but not demanding chores and responsibilities at home.
	Inability to concentrate and drop in level of school achievement	Rehearse safety measures to be taken in future disasters
11–14	Competing with younger siblings for parental attention	Give additional attention and consideration.
	Failure to carry-out chores previously completed without complaint	Temporarily lower expectations of performance at school and home.
	School phobia	Encourage verbal expression of feelings.
	Reappearance of earlier speech and behavior habits	Provide structured but undemanding responsibilities and rehabilitation activities.
	Headaches	Encourage and assist child to become involved with same-age group activities.
	Complaints of vague aches and pains	Future disaster rehearsal
	Loss of appetite	
	Bowel problems	
	Sudden appearance of skin disorders	
	Sleep disorders	
	Loss of interest in peer social activities	
	Loss of interest in hobbies and recreations	
	Increased difficulty in relating with siblings and parents	
	Sharp increase in resisting parental or school authority	

(continued)

311

SUMMARY TABLE OF BEHAVIOR SYMPTOMS AND TREATMENT OPTIONS: AGE GROUP — 1 THROUGH 18 *(continued)*

Ages	Behavior Symptoms			Possible Treatment Options
	Regressive	*Body*	*Emotions*	
14–18	Resumption of earlier behaviors and attitudes	Bowel and bladder complaints	Marked increase or decline in physical activity level	Encourage discussion of disaster experiences with peers and extrafamily significant others.
	Decline in previous responsible behavior	Headaches	Frequent expression of feelings of inadequacy and helplessness	If adolescent chooses to discuss disaster fears within family setting, such expression is to be encouraged but not insisted upon.
	Decline in emancipatory struggles over parental control	Skin rash	Increased difficulties in concentration on planned activities	Reduce expectations for level of school and general performance temporarily.
	Decline in heterosexual interests and activities	Sleep disorders		Provide opportunity for involvement in rehab planning and participation to fullest extent possible.
		Disorders of digestion		Encourage and assist in becoming fully involved in peer social activities.
				Future disaster rehearsal.

*This research was supported by Contract No. 278-75-0018 (SM), Mental Health Disaster Assistance Section, Division of Special Mental Health Programs, National Institutes of Mental Health, August 1, 1976.

Index

Tables are indicated by *t;* figures are indicated by *f.*